TAEKWONDO
Defense Against Weapons

TAEKWONDO
Defense Against Weapons

Weapons, Sparring, and Patterns from Taekwondo's Technical Founder

KIM, BOK MAN

YMAA Publication Center
Wolfeboro, N.H., USA

YMAA Publication Center, Inc.
Main Office
PO Box 480
Wolfeboro, NH, 03894
1-800-669-8892 • www.ymaa.com • info@ymaa.com

Cover Design: Axie Breen
Edited by Dolores Sparrow
Photographs provided by the author.
Additional material for the second edition provided by Brad Shipp.

ISBN-13: 978-1-59439-227-6
ISBN-10: 1-59439-227-7

Second edition, originally published 1979 by Sun Light Publishing.

10   9   8   7   6   5   4   3   2   1

Publisher's Cataloging in Publication
Kim, Bok Man.
    Taekwondo : defense against weapons / Kim, Bok Man. -- 2nd ed. --
Wolfeboro, NH : YMAA Publication Center, c2012.

        p. ; cm.
        ISBN: 978-1-59439-227-6
        "Originally published 1979 by Sun Light Publishing."--T.p. verso.

        1. Tae kwon do--Defense. 2. Tae kwon do--Handbooks,
    manuals, etc. 3. Self-defense. 4. Martial arts. I. Title. II. Title:
    Tae kwon do : defense against weapons.

    GV1114.9 .K56 2012   2012932168
    796.815/7--dc23   1210

Editor's Note: The spelling of 'tae kyon' and other Korean words has been retained for this edition. However, spelling of some words will vary at certain times (e.g., 'Taekwondo') depending on the usage of the word. Where rules of the World Taekwondo Federation are quoted, those spellings have been left unchanged.

Warning: While self-defense is legal, fighting is illegal. If you don't know the difference you'll go to jail because you aren't defending yourself, you are fighting—or worse. Readers are encouraged to be aware of all appropriate local and national laws relating to self-defense, reasonable force, and the use of weaponry, and to act in accordance with all applicable laws at all times. Understand that while legal definitions and interpretations are generally uniform, there are small—but very important—differences from state to state and even city to city. To stay out of jail, you need to know these differences. Neither the authors nor the publisher assumes any responsibility for the use or misuse of information contained in this book.
Nothing in this document constitutes a legal opinion nor should any of its contents be treated as such. While the authors believe that everything herein is accurate, any questions regarding specific self-defense situations, legal liability, and/or interpretation of federal, state, or local laws should always be addressed by an attorney at law. When it comes to martial arts, self-defense, and related topics, no text, no matter how well written, can substitute for professional, hands-on instruction. These materials should be used for academic study only.

Printed in USA.

Contents

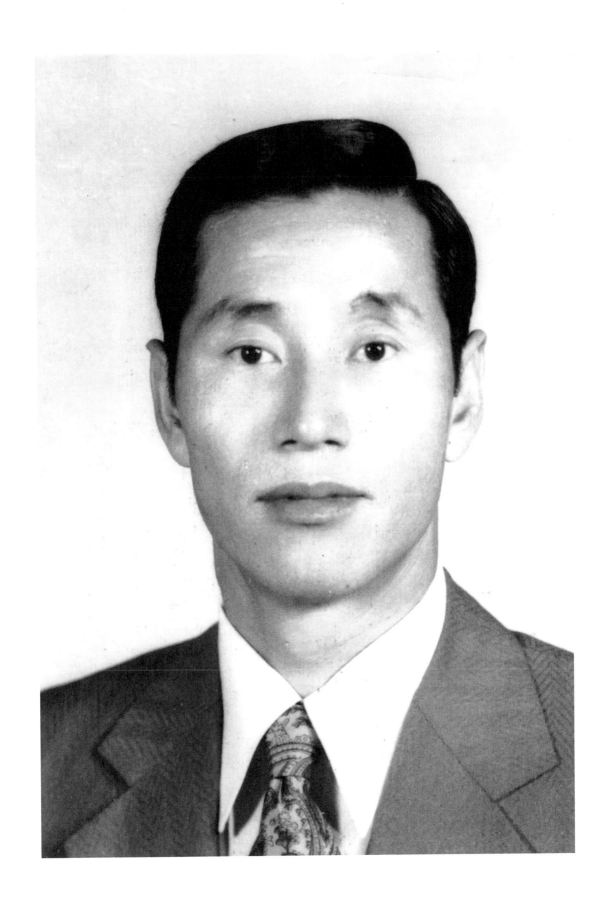

金福萬師傅八段黑帶雅正

勤習跆拳

健身之道

震霈周淬敬題

Foreword by Dr. Peter C. Y. Wong

A short time after being introduced outside Korea, taekwondo became one of the most popular martial arts in the world. The success in the spreading of taekwondo depends on two basic facts. Firstly, it is a most scientific, easy to learn and extremely effective means of self-defense and for building up physical stamina. Secondly, at all times, promotion of the art is most active and untiring. It is a pity, however, that textbooks on the instruction of the art are comparatively and incredibly few.

Mr. Kim, Bok Man was the pioneer in promoting and instructing taekwondo in many countries particularly in Southeast Asia. Throughout his sixty years of experience as a leading instructor, he has become painstakingly clear about what the students need and how to communicate with them so that they can learn and comprehend to the best extent possible. At the same time, he has also invented many new techniques and patterns of training especially for life-threatening situations. These techniques and patterns are very effective against the attacks of weapons like the knife, baton, or bayonet.

Thirty years ago, Mr. Kim determined to write a textbook to contribute to the teaching methods of taekwondo using his own experience gained with his continuous teaching. He has constantly reviewed and studied the different movements and techniques and practiced them in actual sparring with the students and other instructors in order to make them perfect. Later on, he started to take thousands of photographs, as he believed that illustrations would make the students better understand and absorb more. Finally, he personally took a lot of time compiling the whole textbook.

I am sure this book will benefit all the taekwondo practitioners who are longing for more refined and advanced movements in the techniques of taekwondo. I wish to congratulate Mr. Kim and his associates on being able to produce such a masterpiece, and I hope they will continue with their untiring effort in the promotion of taekwondo in the future.

Dr. Peter C. Y. Wong
Honorary President
Hong Kong Taekwondo Association

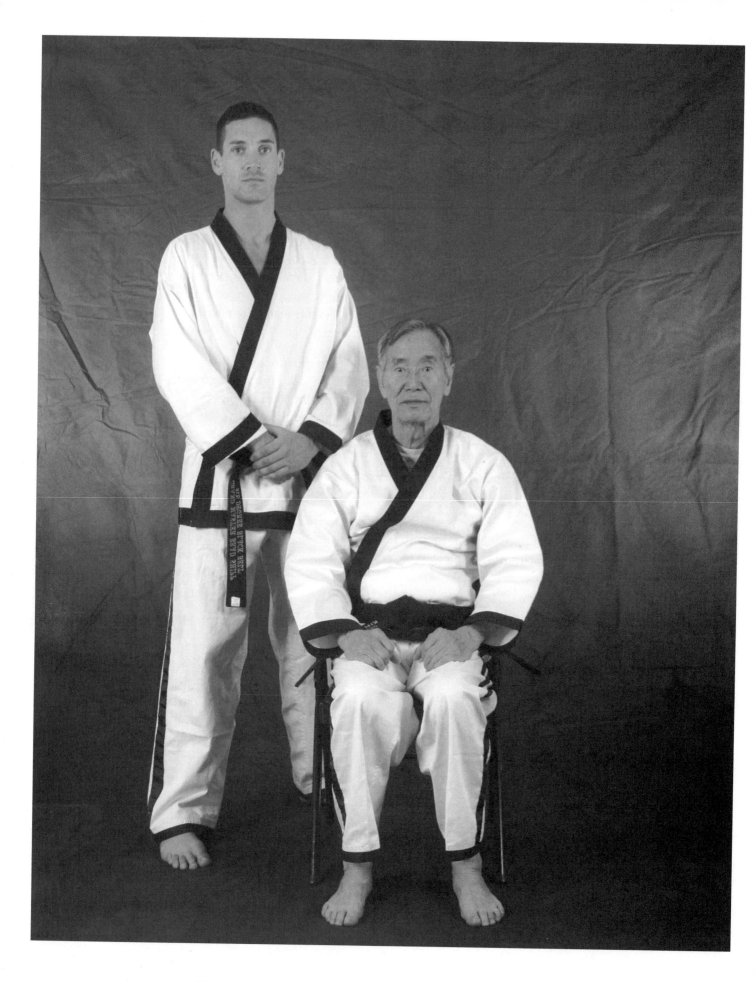

Foreword by Brad Shipp

I am proud that Supreme Master Kim, Bok Man has agreed to republish his first book *Practical Taekwon Do,* which is now this new book, *Taekwondo—Defense Against Weapons.* Supreme Master Kim has devoted his entire life to teaching and perfecting the traditional Korean martial arts. Supreme Master Kim spent many hours with General Choi in Malayasia in 1963 developing his first book. He felt very strongly that all techniques should have a proper title and all patterns should be balanced in terms of left and right. Supreme Master Kim is considered the technical founder of taekwondo because of his input in cataloging by name all of the techniques of the art. When he parted ways with General Choi in 1966, he was unhappy with the political and technical status of taekwondo, which is why in 1967 he began to work on his own book, *Practical Taekwondo,* published in 1979.

This new book, *Taekwondo—Defense Against Weapons,* highlights many of the techniques that are lost in today's sport version of taekwondo. These techniques were taught to soldiers preparing for war and were tested on the battlefield. Supreme Master Kim is proud that the art he helped to create has reached the highest level of competition possible, an official Olympic Sport. Still we must not forget that taekwondo is first and foremost a martial "killing" art developed for self-defense by the Korean military, not to score a point or win a gold medal. The techniques demonstrated in this book will not only teach you how to defend yourself against weapons, but will also promote overall health and well being. Martial arts is one of the best exercises you can do to develop your mind, body, and spirit throughout your lifetime. The cardiovascular workout from training will keep your heart strong and ensure healthy circulation throughout the entire body. The muscles, tendons, and ligaments will remain strong yet flexible. The mental discipline required promotes focus and concentration while accumulating skill and knowledge. A healthy mind and body promotes a positive attitude, a sense of well being.

Now at age 78, Supreme Master Kim continues to independently teach the true practical Korean art of self-defense. I am truly grateful to be able to spend each day training and teaching with such a great Master. Currently, Supreme Master Kim and I are in the final stages of completing his six-volume *Korean Martial Art Encyclopedia.* We continue to work together to develop new advanced techniques based on his experience and skill. If you are interested in organizing a seminar for your martial art group, he keep in mind that Dr. Kim still enjoys traveling the world teaching seminars and promoting his martial art.

Brad Shipp
Technical Director
World Chun Do Federation

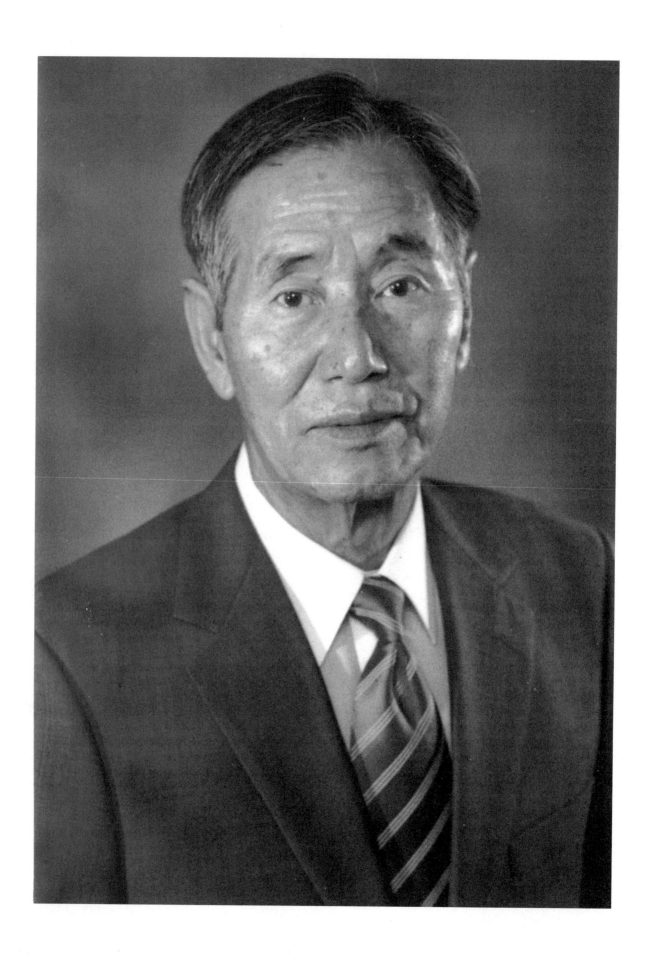

Preface

Although taekwondo has traversed a long passage through time and techniques have been improved and refined, a lot of work remains in bringing the martial art of self-defense to yet unexplored heights.

A phenomenon, which evidently is very widespread and which jeopardizes the practitioner's attainment and development of skills and techniques in taekwondo, should necessarily be explained and its problems cast aside.

Specifically, in practicing the sport, there is absolutely no shortcut in the route to achieve advanced technical skill. As in all sports, intensive, dedicated, and harsh training, coupled with diligence, patience, confidence, and sacrifice are prerequisites for ultimate victory and success.

Every fundamental movement is a stepping-stone toward increased mastery of skill and technique. What cannot be over-emphasized is that an individual's physical and mental capacities determine what he himself needs to follow in a certain program. In other words, strict standardization inhibits rather than enhances a person's progress. This, however, does not imply overall irregularity. Taekwondo should allow each person to practice according to his individual and unique capabilities.

I hope that the contents of this book will strengthen the above points. The techniques defined can be indiscriminately selected, studied, and practiced to the full advantage of the participant.

I must give special thanks to my black-belt students for posing for the pictures; to my daughter Angela, who sacrificed many hours to prepare the entire manuscript; and to Dr. Peter C. Y. Wong, who helped me with much of the editorial work and with seeking out new techniques; and finally to Grandmaster Brad Shipp for his help in republishing this book.

Kim, Bok Man
Founder and President
World Chun Kuhn Do Federation

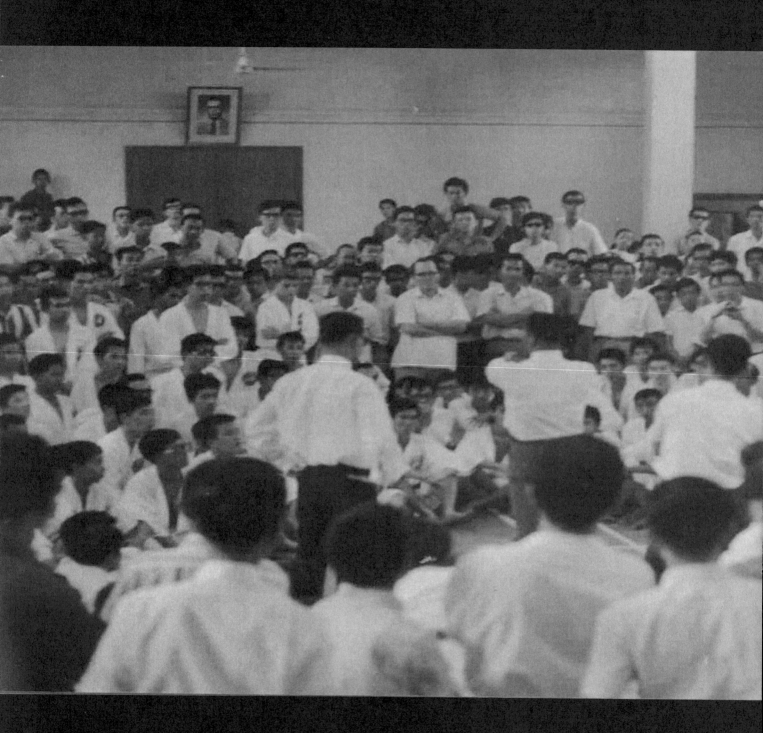

CHAPTER 1
INTRODUCTION

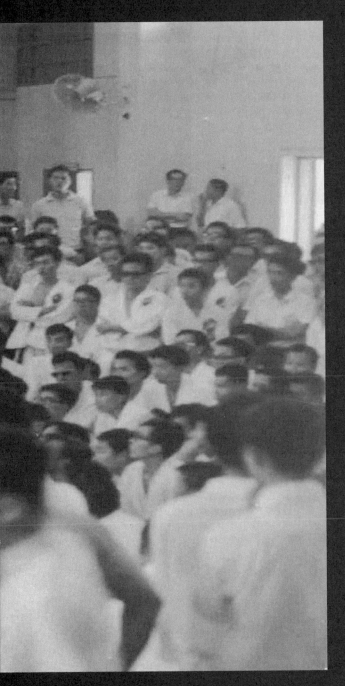

The martial art of taekwondo, literally meaning "art of hand and foot fighting," is more than two thousand years old. Yet its physical and spiritual content has never been so vigorously sought after and practiced as it is now.

Taekwondo is considered the oldest self-defense martial art in the world and uniquely developed in Korea. It was first recorded in the Koguryo dynasty founded in 37 B.C. of whose vast territory included the Korean Peninsula north of the Han River and the Manchurian territory of China. Taekwondo is a sport that responds to survival needs in a powerful and rational manner and maintains, as well, an orderly system uniformly related to the inner and outer spheres of the human being. The immense power of taekwondo stems directly from the scientific use of the body systems. The power is so formidable that several bricks, roof tiles, or wooden boards can be broken merely with the bare hands or fists. Taekwondo employs almost every part of the body in defensive and offensive moves. Its techniques comprise units combined together for maximum efficiency in free fighting. These practice units are body drill in postures, punching, kicking, striking, blocking, combinations of these moves in formal patterns, pre-arranged attacks and counterattacks, and more. Conscientious training in these areas not only results in the ultimate self-defense techniques, but also in a mental discipline, which creates the strength of character necessary for success in many fields of endeavor.

History of Taekwondo

Taekwondo may be considered as old as history itself. Since man first learned to protect himself, it could be said that the primitive features of taekwondo had spontaneously arisen. This form of self-defense became an essential part of daily life that was gradually streamlined and organized into a unique and powerfully efficient weapon for survival.

In the process of the development of taekwondo, a new sense of awareness of both physical and mental potential in the human body was discovered. Through a myriad of thought, stimuli, experimentation, and experience, this skill of unarmed combat became what is today, a martial art technically moralized and scientifically formalized.

Before the birth of Christ, the three kingdoms of Koguryo, Baek-je, and Silla had been established on the peninsula now known as Korea. In each of these kingdoms, the skills and techniques su bak or kwon bupsu, later on called tae kyon, the predecessors of taekwondo, were already highly sophisticated. They were a basic component of the military training of soldiers as a weapon based solely on fists, hands, and feet.

Some of the earliest known features of taekwondo can be found in the murals of the royal tombs of Kakjeochong and Mooyongchong of the Koguryo period. These murals clearly show physical combat movements, fighting stances, and skills closely resembling the present movements of taekwondo.

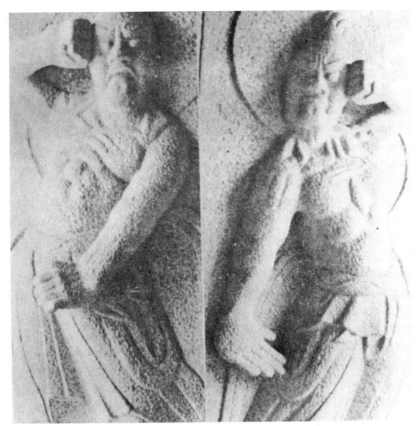

Some of the earliest known features of Taekwondo can be found in the murals
of the royal tombs of Kakjeochong and Mooyongchong of the Koguryo period.

From the murals, we can visualize that taekwondo was then already familiar to the
people of Koguryo. And because it was such a highly respected sport among the people, it
was thus depicted in murals and paintings in tombs.

Substantial documentary evidence of the martial arts spirit in Baek-je also exist. In
that era, the sport was officially encouraged, and not only the military had their soldiers
trained in taekwondo, archery, and horse riding, the general populace too were warriors
who excelled in the arts.

The temples and shrines during the Silla dynasty produced a great many stone engrav-
ings depicting a variety of taekwondo forms. During the reign of Chin Heung, twenty-
fourth king of Silla, Korean culture and martial arts rose to flourishing heights. Silla, at the
time, was a mere weak and tiny kingdom, constantly harassed and threatened by its more
powerful neighbor kingdoms of Koguryo and Baek-je. But Silla did not stir and proving
itself with national character of strength and integrity, existed for 992 years.

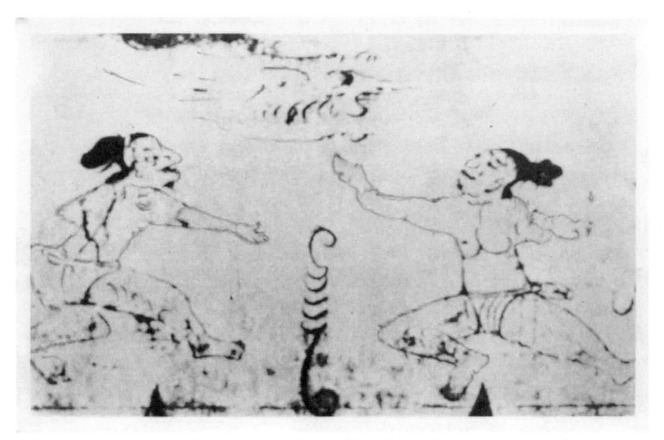

The mural painting at Kak-je tomb, painted at the time of the tenth king of Koguryo, shows sparring of joo bak.

At the time the most outstanding contribution to the development of the martial arts emanated from an elite officer corps called Hwa Rang Do—a military and social organization for noble youths formed by King Chin Heung. The Hwa Rang Do were well trained not only in the usual sports of archery, target practice, and horsemanship, but also practice of mental and physical discipline, as well as many forms of hand and foot fighting. Through their unrelenting efforts to conquer turbulent rivers and rugged terrain, the group of young knights grew strong and fearless. Their merciless strife to defend their country and their refinement of their souls became well known throughout the peninsula. Their victories helped to advance the movement for the unification of the three separated kingdoms for the first time in the history of the Korean Peninsula.

The Koguryo dynasty (A.D. 935–1392) further popularized the study of unarmed combat. It was during this period that the martial arts were scientifically analyzed and systematized. They were later adopted into the Yi era (A.D.1392–1910). However, strong anti-military sentiment soon pervaded among the ruling classes and tae kyon was generally and openly debased. By the end of the Yi dynasty, the martial arts appeared to have lost all traces of their original vigorousness and liveliness in the midst of the period of civil enlightenment.

For several decades after the turn of the twentieth century, the Japanese occupation of Korea forbid the practice of any of the martial arts. Only in secrecy were the arts passed on to a small number of students and kept alive by ardent proponents, such as Song, Duk Ki and Han, Il Dong.

After Korea was liberated in 1945, many dojang (martial arts institutes) sprang forth, each announcing its presence with its own particular standard of style and method. It was nevertheless the dawning of a new day for the ancient art of tae kyon. Its revival in various forms can explain that it has successfully remained deeply implanted in the fabric of Korean society to be able to flower and blossom once again to its full colors.

A decade later, taekwondo was selected as the new name of the national martial art. The name resembles the old name of tae kyon and it perfectly describes the art (do) of hand (tae) and foot (kwon).

Theory of Power

The effective application of power in taekwondo demands that a person be qualified in appreciating and understanding the fundamentals of physical balance, concentration, speed and respiration. The intelligent use of them literally means that untapped power of immense proportions could be successfully attained. In our present discussion on the theory of power, we shall focus on the truncal twist which is more difficult to learn but which has been considered the supreme contributor in the whole process of power generation.

In any action, there is one form of reaction, as for example, a side kick where one leg is thrust out in one direction while at the same time, the upper portion of the body, i.e. head, shoulder and trunk, moves in the opposite direction. In this manner, the reactionary force of the latter movement adds to the former, thus effecting much more power.

But, whatever the power that is generated, its maximum is not achieved without truncal movements. The central trunk twist plays the principle role in physical movement. Indeed, the very first bodily movement should begin from the trunk, twisting on a vertical axis of the body, rotating the pelvis in turn to carry the leg, torso, and shoulders into their finals paths.

Sufficient practice of the twisting of the trunk will in time lead to spontaneous truncal twist in each and every action. A good test on whether a person is developing mastery of the truncal twist is the elbow breaking of boards. A truncal countertwist on a vertical axis, and delivery of an elbow strike onto a pile a thick boards requires proper practice and employment of the countertwist.

This brings us to the interesting aspect regarding the distribution of the variety of strikes. A strike, whether by kicking, punching, or other use of body parts for attacking, produces a direct effect on the known target. And it is the effect, such as the extent of target damage, tissue injury, contact time, area of displacement, etc., which ultimately determines the characteristic of the strike itself.

In striking a target, if contact time and displacement are zero or minimal, the strike would be of the First degree, as it is in free sparring. A Second-degree strike renders the target maximal extent of damage for the gravity of the force used. The total energy is dispersed instantaneously. For a Third-degree strike, contact time is relatively longer than the First- and Second-degree strikes because this time the attacking force pushes a target for a variable distance whereby all of the power is administered throughout the total displacement.

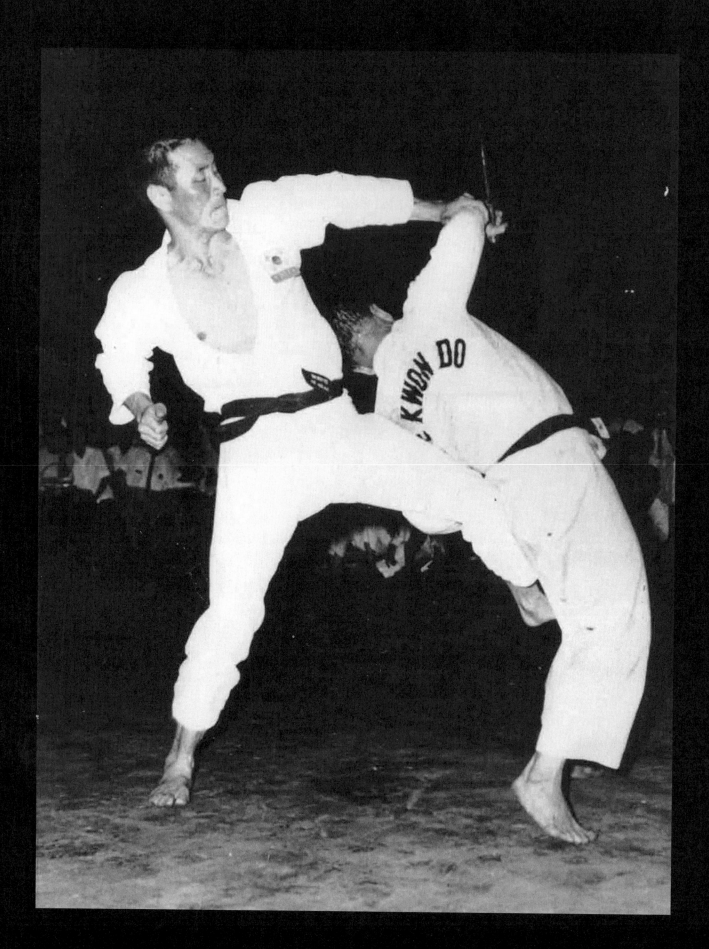

CHAPTER 2
DEFENSE AGAINST WEAPONS

In self-defense, situations involving armed attackers, either single or multiple, each situation is extremely dangerous and more complex than any type of unarmed attack. Accordingly, defense techniques must be learned thoroughly and executed as automatic responses to any series of happenings, if serious injury is to be avoided.

In facing an armed attacker, it is of foremost importance to observe his facial tone and his entire state of body preparedness, such as the sort of weapon being used, how he is going to use it, etc. Having these mentally assimilated, you should next gauge your distance accurately in order to fully control and exploit your defense techniques. By this time, two choices are open to you—one is to get outside of the swing zone, the other to get inside of the swing zone. Dodging too far from your attacker may make it virtually impossible to counterattack in time, while being too close could well hamper your motions. Two steps away from your attacker does not offer the advantage of a better striking range than one step does. Clearly, it is undesirable to attack with more than two steps distance.

In other situations, you are sometimes caught off-guard as the attacker moves in on you, and then it is even more necessary to exercise keen reflexes of eyes and limbs under such circumstances. Immediately determine what area of target he is aiming at, then gauge your distance precisely thereby enabling you to apply those blocking and/or attacking techniques most suited to you.

The following defense technique described may be practiced to develop self-control, balance, speed, concentration, and to gain experience as if under actual encounters with armed attackers. The various techniques can be explored and studied and then compared for the purpose of finding the most effective ones to meet the student's physical capabilities.

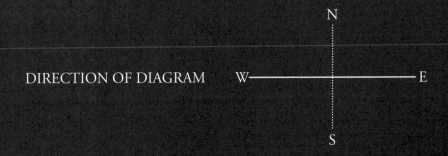

The exercise is performed under the assumption that the attacker (A) and the defender (D) stand on line EW facing each other.

For the reader's convenience, each exercise sequence in this chapter begins with a bolded caption.

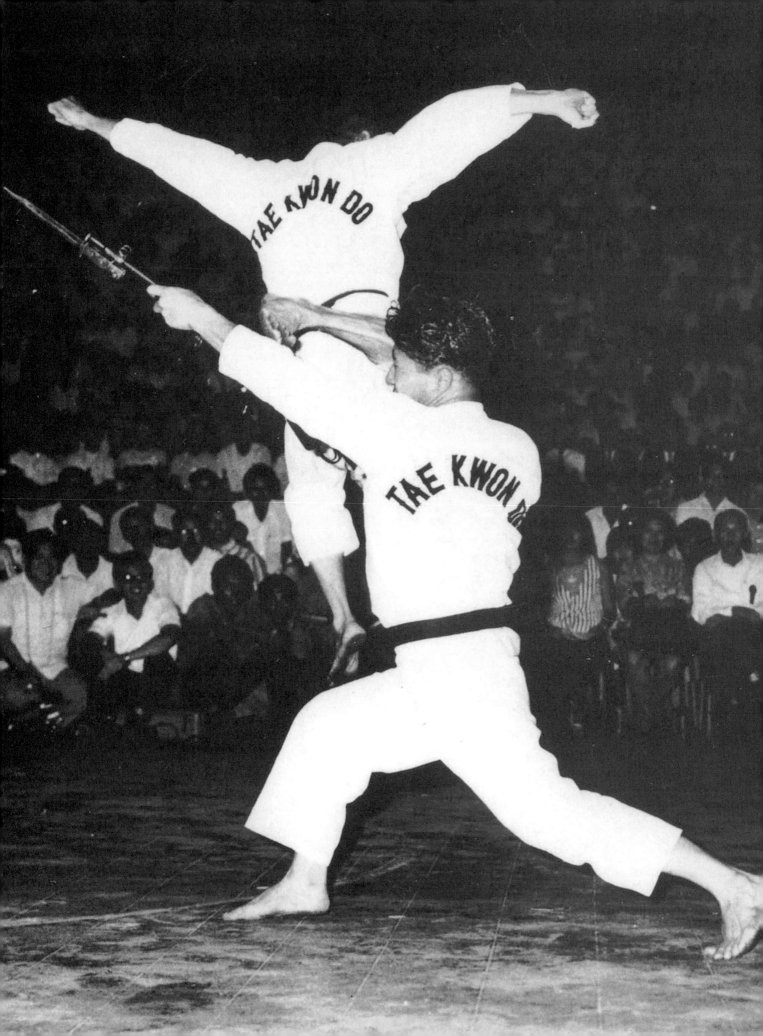

How to Release from a Knife Attack

The defender should not become excited, but carefully study his attacker to discern what direction the attacker is going to move his knife. The defender must always keep his body away from the knife and stay in a counterattacking position ready to counter any thrusts by the attacker. The defender's movements should always be brisk and accurate, and include the truncal twist. With skill in the execution of the twist, improvement in the art of self-defense would surely be hindered if the truncal twist technique is not all together acquired. To release from a knife attack, you should also select the attacker's weakest parts as the first targets for the counterattack to be truly effective.

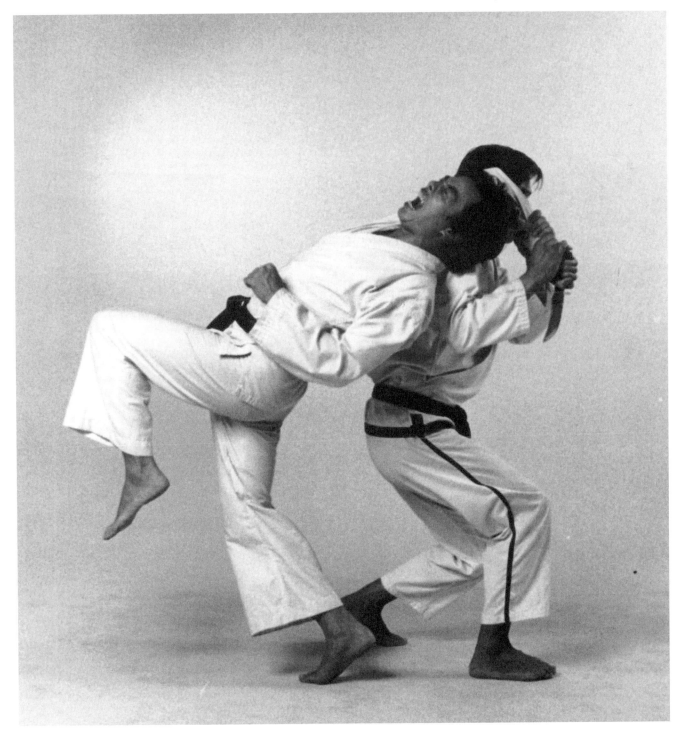

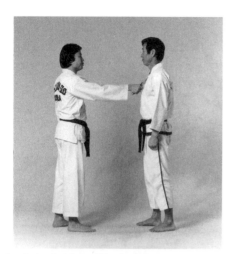

A: Point knife at D's windpipe.

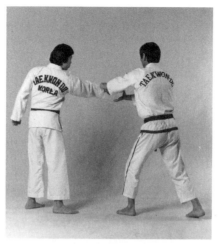

D: Grab A's arm with left hand while turning body clockwise pivoting on the left foot.

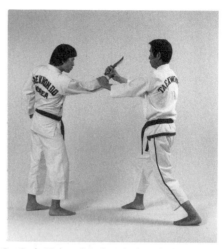

D: Grab A's hand with right hand while moving left foot backward.

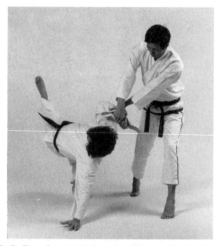

D: Pull and twist A's hand while turning body counterclockwise, pivoting on both feet.

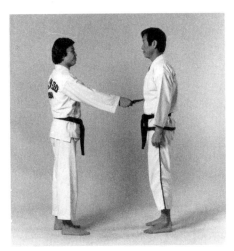

A: Point knife at D's solar plexus.

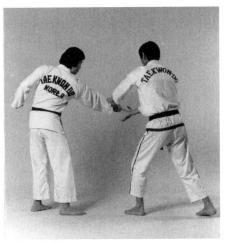

D: Grab A's arm with left hand while turning body clockwise pivoting on left foot.

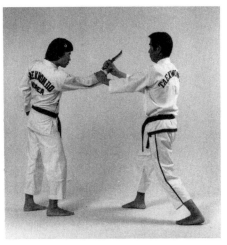

D: Grab A's hand with right hand while moving left foot backward.

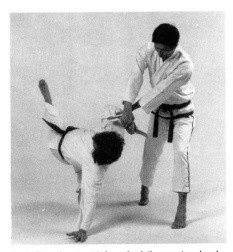

D: Pull and twist A's hand while turning body counterclockwise, pivoting on both feet.

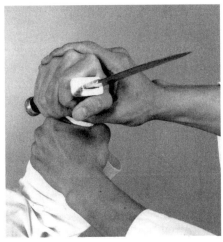

Close-up of grab, pull, and twist.

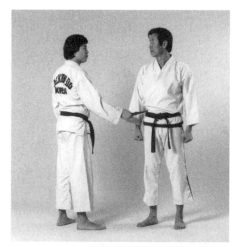

A: Point knife at D's side floating ribs.

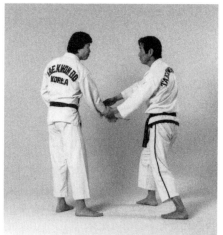

D: Grab A's arm with left hand while moving right foot to the right, and turn body clockwise pivoting on left foot.

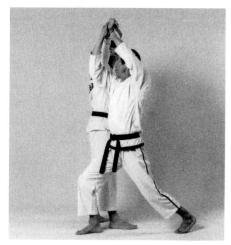

D: Grab A's arm with right hand and raise it over head while moving right foot forward.

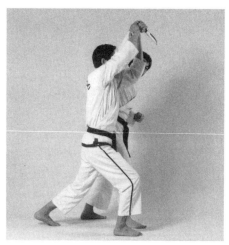

D: Twist A's arm while moving left foot backward and turn body counterclockwise, pivoting on right foot.

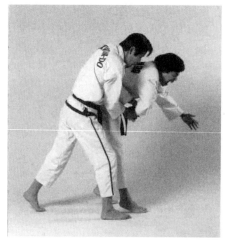

D: Pull A's arm and force the knife backward toward A's body.

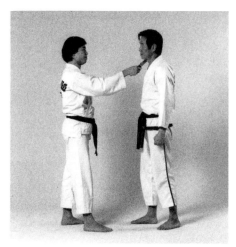

A. Hold knife against right side of D's neck.

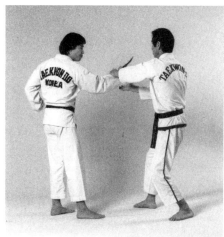

D: Grab A's arm with left hand while moving left foot to the left.

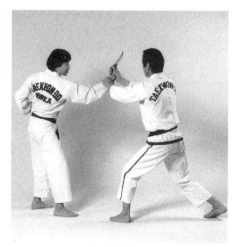

D: Grab A's hand with right hand while moving right foot backward.

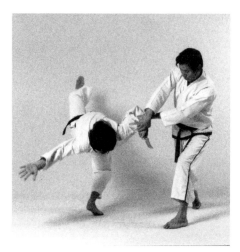

D: Twist A's wrist counterclockwise.

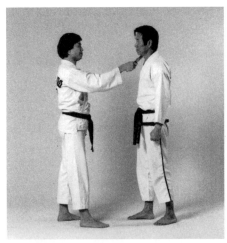

A. Hold knife against right side of D's neck.

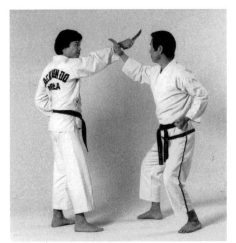

D: Execute pushing-block at A's arm with right knife-hand while moving left foot to the left.

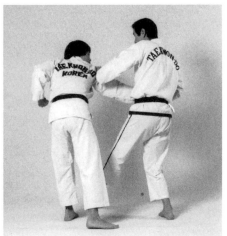

D: Grab A's arm with right hand while moving left foot forward, and place left palm on A's left shoulder joint.

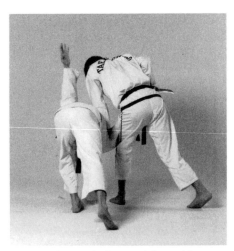

D: Twist A's arm clockwise while pushing down on A's shoulder joint.

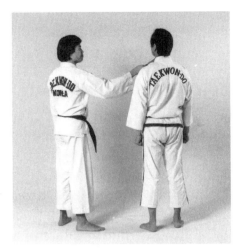

A: Hold knife against D's throat.

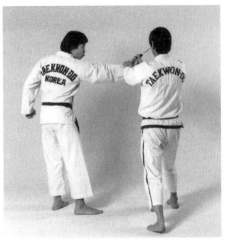

D: Grab A's arm with left hand while moving left foot backward.

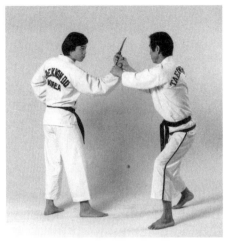

D: Grab A's hand with right hand while turning body counterclockwise, pivoting on left foot.

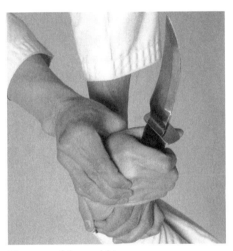

Close-up of the grabbing.

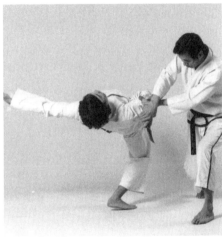

D: Twist A's hand counterclockwise and push it downward.

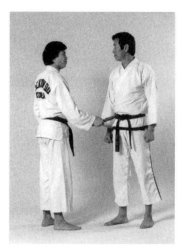

A: Point knife at D's left ribs.

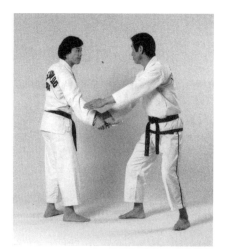

D: Grab A's arm with right hand while turning body counterclockwise, pivoting on right foot.

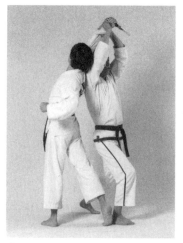

D: Grab A's arm with left hand and raise it over head while moving left foot forward, and turn body clockwise pivoting on right foot.

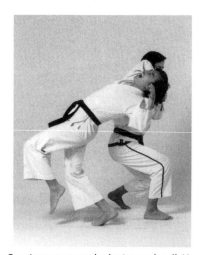

D: Continue to turn clockwise and pull A's arm downward.

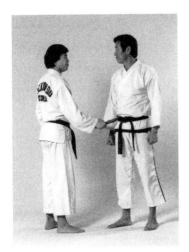

A: Point knife at D's left ribs.

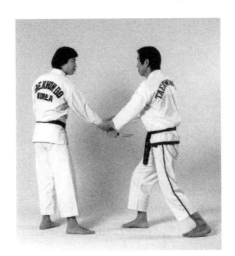

D: Grab A's arm with left hand while moving left foot backward.

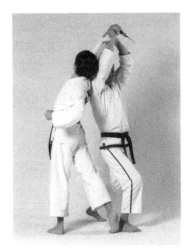

D: Grab A's arm with right hand and raise it over head while moving left foot forward, and turn body clockwise pivoting on right foot.

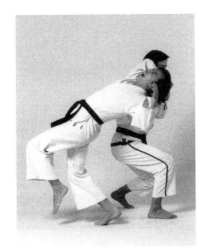

D: Continue to turn clockwise and pull A's arm downward.

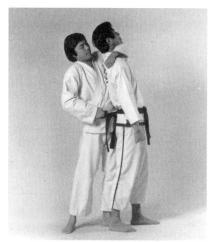

A: Lock D's neck with left arm from behind and point knife at D's kidney.

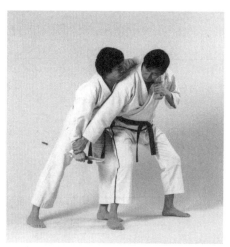

D: Grab and pull down A's left arm with left hand, and grab and push A's right arm with right hand while moving left foot forward.

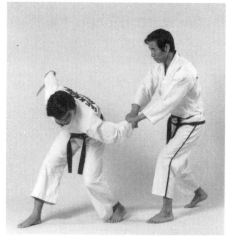

D: Move right foot backward and turn body clockwise, pivoting on left foot while grabbing and twisting A's left hand with both hands.

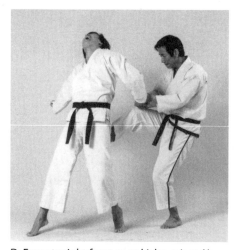

D: Execute right front snap kick against A's coccyx.

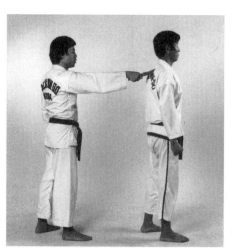

A: Point knife at D's upper back.

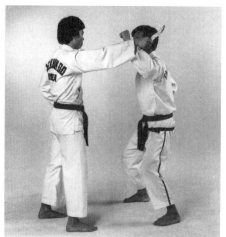

D: Execute strike-block at A's arm with left outer forearm while turning body counterclockwise, pivoting on left foot.

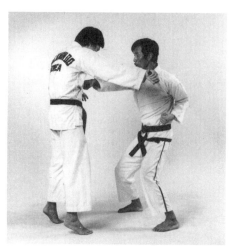

D: Execute right punch against A's solar plexus.

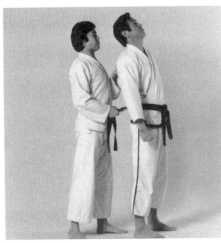

A: Grab D's left hand from behind and twist it backward while pointing knife at D's back.

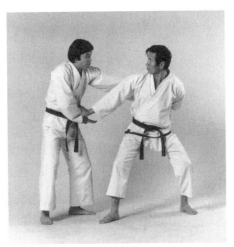

D: Execute pushing-block at A's arm with right arc-hand, while moving left foot forward and turning body clockwise.

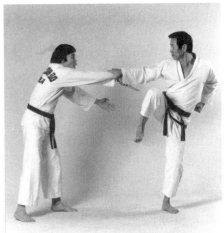

D: Grab A's arm with right hand and raise right leg.

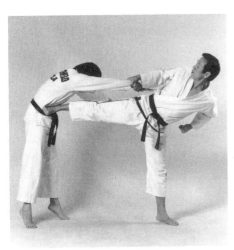

D: Execute snap and pushing kick against A's stomach.

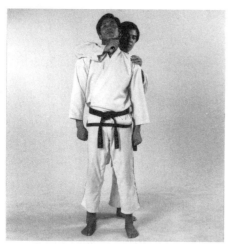

A: Lock D's neck from behind with right knife and grab D's clothes on left shoulder.

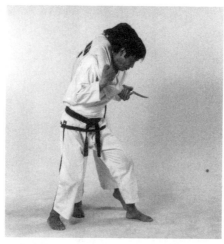

D: Grab A's arm with right hand and grab A's hand with left hand while pulling A's arm downward and lowering body by sliding right foot sideways.

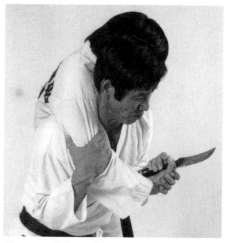

Close-up of the grabbing.

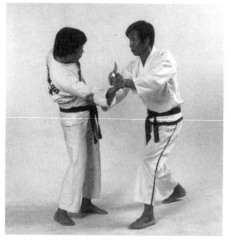

D: Pull A's arm with right hand while moving right foot backward and turn body clockwise, pivoting on left foot.

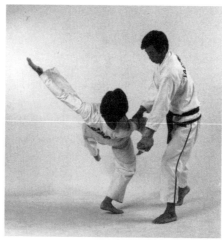

D: Pull and twist A's arm with right hand and push A's hand with left hand.

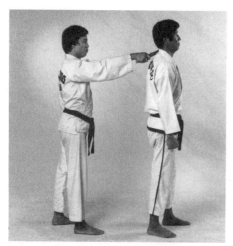

A: Hold knife against D's left side neck.

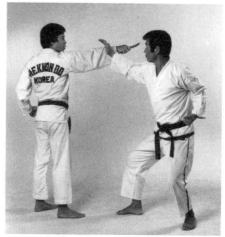

D: Execute strike-block at A's arm with right knife-hand while turning body clockwise, pivoting on right foot.

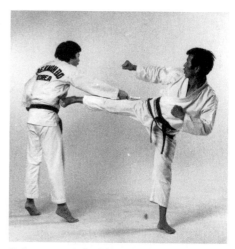

D: Execute a right side-snapping kick against A's floating ribs.

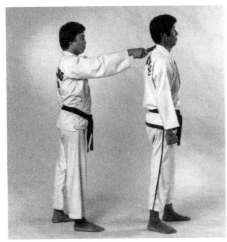

A: Hold knife against D's left side neck.

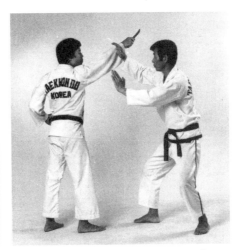

D: Execute pushing-block at A's arm with right palm while turning body clockwise, pivoting on right foot.

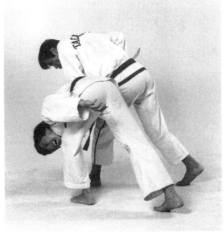

D: Grab and twist A's arm with right hand and press A's shoulder joint downward with left palm.

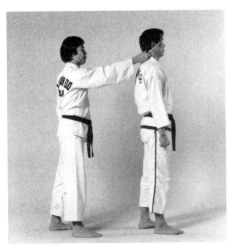

A: Hold knife against D's right side-neck.

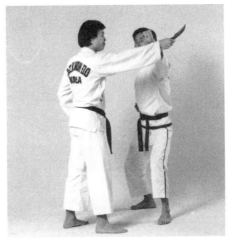

D: Execute pushing-block at A's arm with left forearm while turning body counterclockwise, pivoting on left foot.

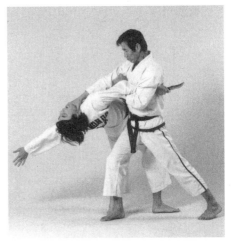

D: Move right foot forward and lock A's arm with left forearm while grabbing and pushing at A's Adam's apple with right arc-hand.

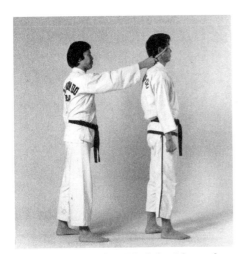

A: Hold knife against D's right side-neck.

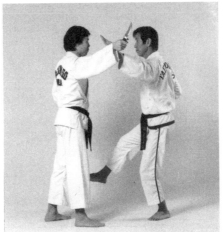

D: Execute strike block at A's arm with left knife-hand while turning body counter-clockwise, pivoting on left foot.

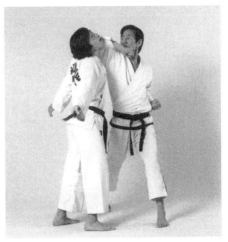

D: Execute right side-elbow strike against A's jaw.

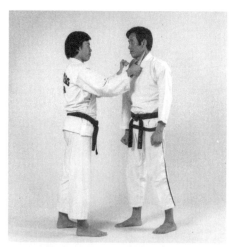

A: Grab D's clothes on right shoulder from front with left hand and hold knife against D's left side-neck.

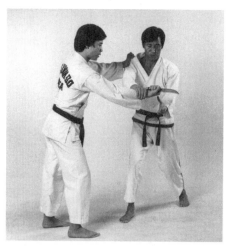

D: Grab A's arm with right hand while turning body counterclockwise, pivoting on right foot.

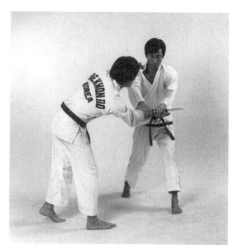

D: Grab A's hand with left hand and twist it counterclockwise while moving right foot backward.

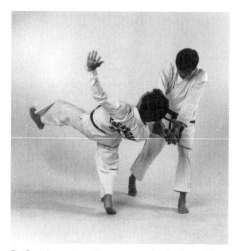

D: Continue to twist counterclockwise while pushing A's hand downward.

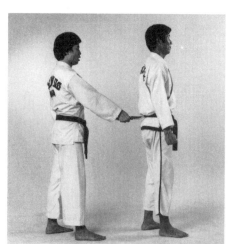

A: Point knife at D's lower back.

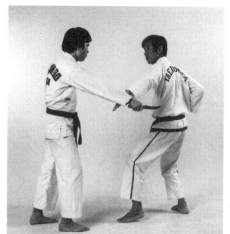

D: Execute strike-block at A's arm with left knife-hand while turning body counter-clockwise, pivoting on left foot.

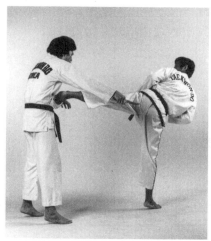

D: Execute left side-snapping kick against A's stomach.

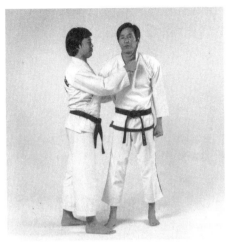

A: Grab D's right arm from the side, twist it upward and hold knife against D's neck.

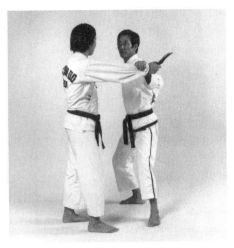

D: Grab and push A's arm with left hand while moving right foot backward.

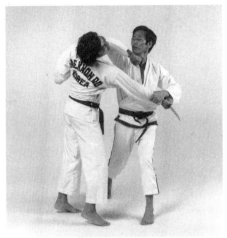

D: Execute right elbow strike against A's jaw.

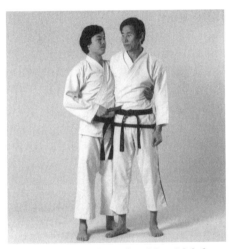

A: Hold D's waist from the side with left arm and point knife at D's floating ribs.

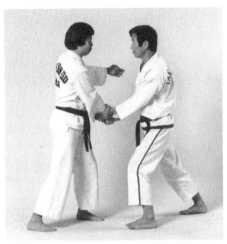

D: Grab A's arm with left hand while turning body clockwise, pivoting on left foot.

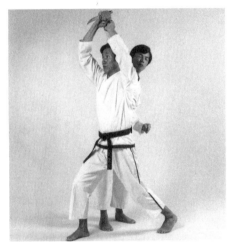

D: Grab A's arm with right hand and raise it over head while moving right foot forward.

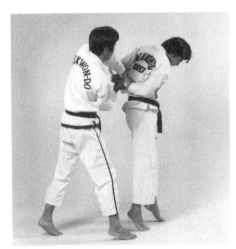

D: Twist A's arm while moving left foot backward and turn body counterclockwise, pivoting on right foot.

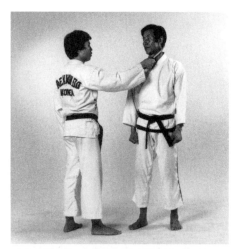

A: Hold knife against D's left side-neck.

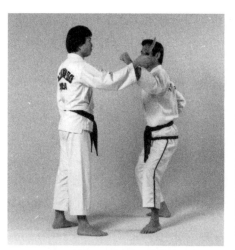

D: Execute pushing-block at A's arm with left outer forearm while moving right foot to the right.

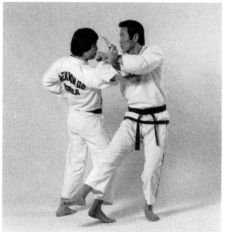

D: Lock A's elbow with right forearm and pull it forward while pushing left arm and moving right foot forward.

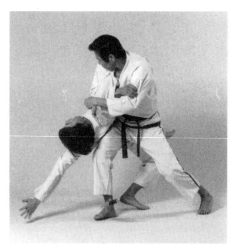

D: Continue pulling and pushing A's arm downward.

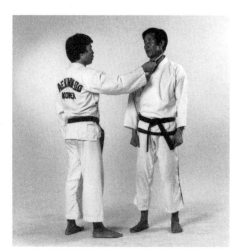

A: Hold knife against D's left side-neck

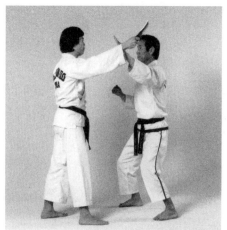

D: Execute strike-block at A's arm with left knife-hand while moving right foot to the right.

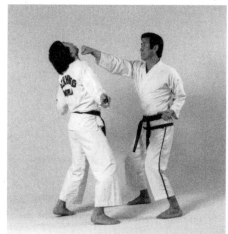

D: Execute right punch against A's philtrum.

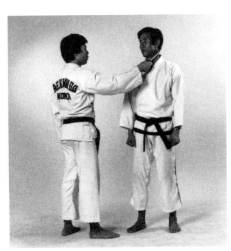

A: Hold knife against D's left side-neck

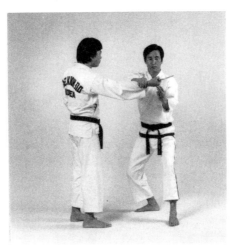

D: Grab A's arm with right hand while moving right foot to the right.

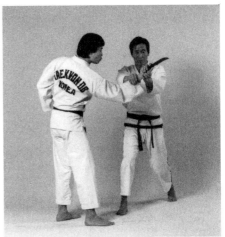

D: Grab A's hand with left hand while moving left foot backward.

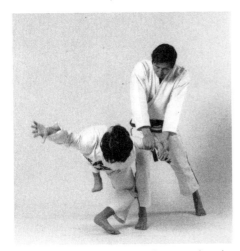

D: Twist A's wrist counterclockwise and push it downward.

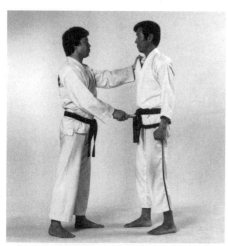

A: Hold knife at D's stomach and grab D's shirt on the right shoulder.

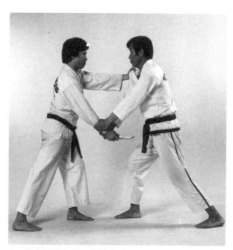

D: Grab A's arm with both hands while moving left foot backward.

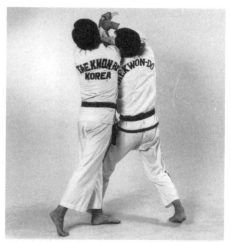

D: Twist A's arm over head while moving left foot forward and turn body clockwise, pivoting on right foot.

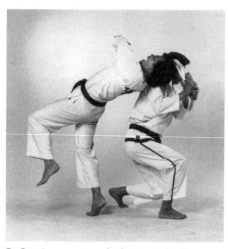

D: Continue to turn clockwise and pull A's arm downward.

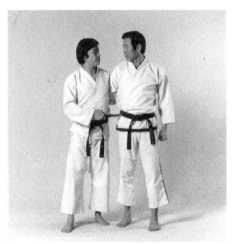

A: Grab D's right hand from the side, twist it upward and point knife at D's floating ribs.

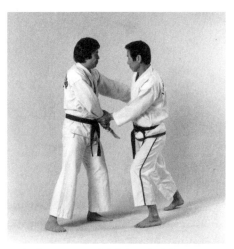

D: Grab A's arm with left hand while turning body clockwise, pivoting on left foot.

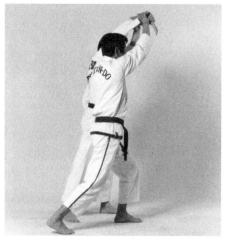

D: Grab A's arm with right hand and raise it over head while moving right foot forward.

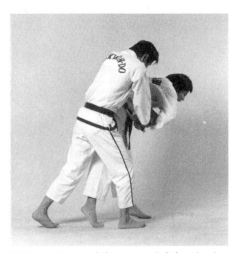

D: Twist A's arm while moving left foot backward and turn body counterclockwise, pivoting on right foot.

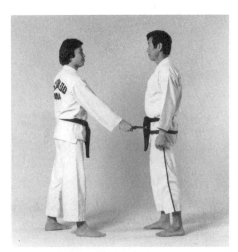

A: Point knife at D's stomach.

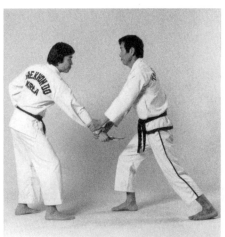

D: Grab A's arm with both hands while moving left foot backward.

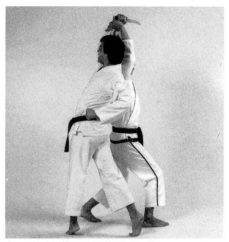

D: Twist A's arm over head while moving left foot forward and turn body clockwise, pivoting on right foot.

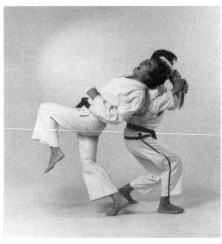

D: Pull A's arm downward.

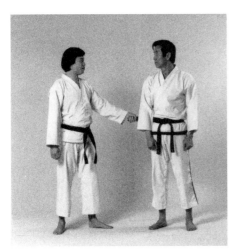

A: Point knife at D's left ribs.

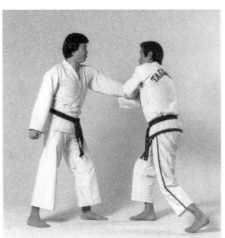

D: Turn body counterclockwise, pivoting on right foot and block A's arm with left forearm while moving right foot.

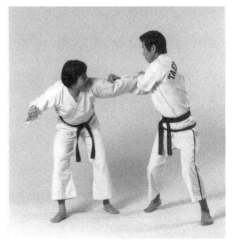

D: Grab A's hand with left hand and push it forward while pressing A's elbow with right forearm and turning body counter-clockwise, pivoting on both feet.

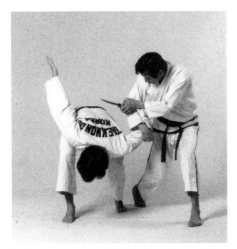

D: Continue to push A's hand and press A's elbow down.

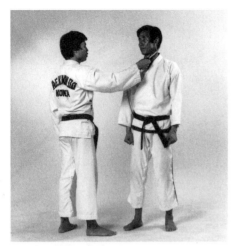

A: Hold knife against D's neck.

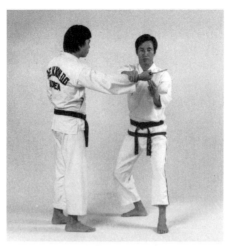

D: Grab A's arm with right hand while moving right foot backward.

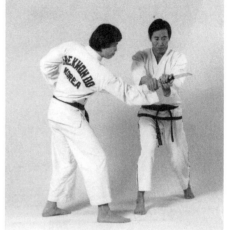

D: Grab A's hand with left hand and twist it counterclockwise while moving left foot backward.

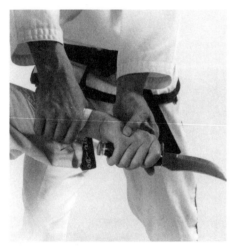

Close-up of the grabbing.

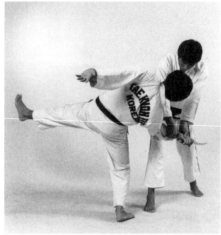

D: Continue to twist counterclockwise and push A's hand downward.

Defense Against a Sudden Attack with Knife

Attacks may arise at the most unpredictable circumstances. The defender should, in all situations, be totally aware even when no direct offensive motive is visible, such as when a relaxed conversation is taking place between himself and his attacker. The attacker has the advantage of surprise assaults; however, a well-trained taekwondo student will be able to defeat or counter any surprise attack. The attainment of good skills in sparring and experience in the realism of good skills in counterattacking will further accelerate him toward achieving acuity and keenness of reflexes.

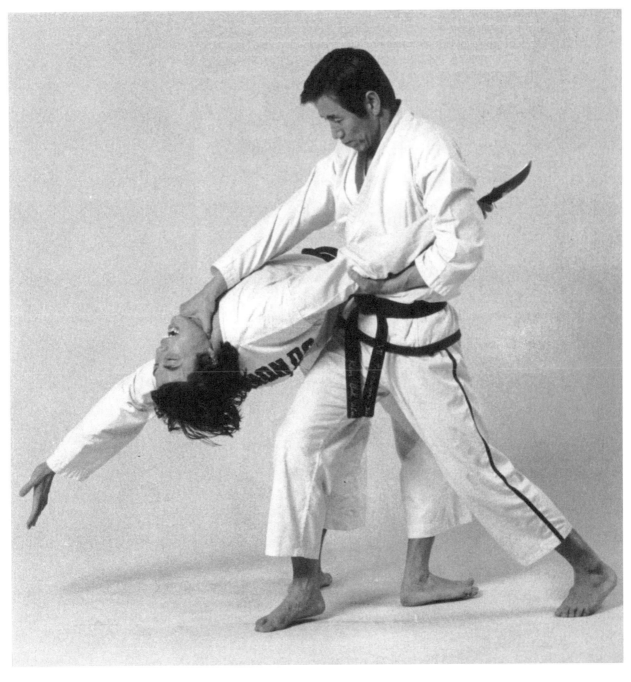

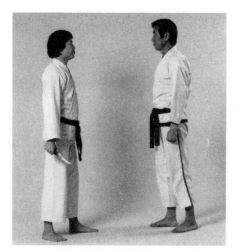

A. Hold knife in right hand facing D.

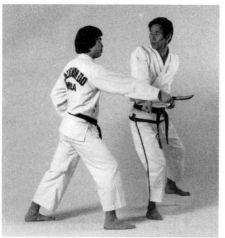

A: Stab toward D's epigastrium while moving right foot forward.

D: Exert block at A's arm with right inner forearm while turning body counterclockwise, pivoting on right foot.

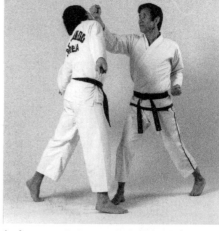

D: Execute a right back fist strike against A's jaw.

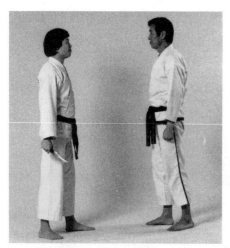

A. Hold knife in right hand facing D.

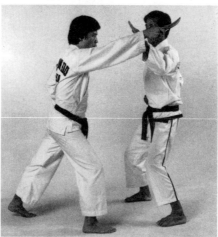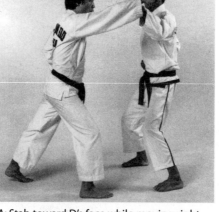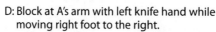

A: Stab toward D's face while moving right foot forward.

D: Block at A's arm with left knife hand while moving right foot to the right.

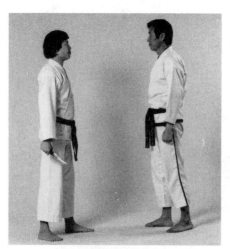

D: Execute a right punch against A's jaw.

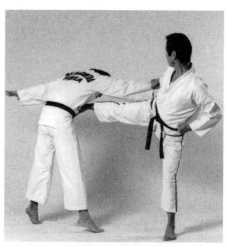

A. Hold knife in right hand facing D.

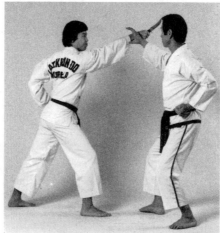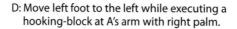

A: Stab toward D's face while moving right foot forward.

D: Move left foot to the left while executing a hooking-block at A's arm with right palm.

D: Grab A's arm with right hand and pull while executing a right turning kick against A's solar plexus.

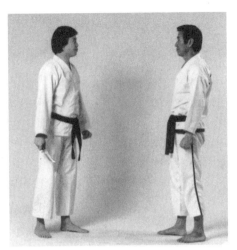

A. Hold knife in right hand facing D.

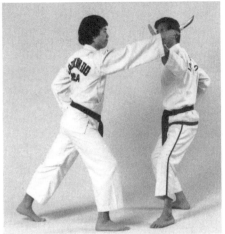

A: Slash diagonally downward toward D's body while moving right foot forward.

D: Move right foot to the right while blocking A's arm with left knife-hand.

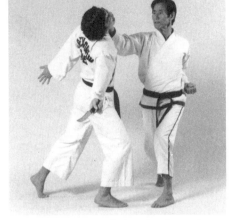

D: Execute a right knife-hand strike against A's neck.

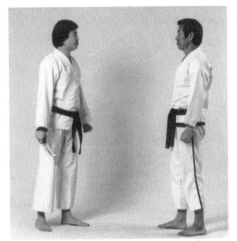

A. Hold knife in right hand facing D.

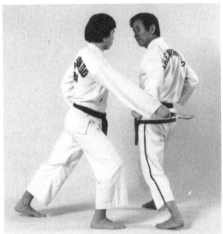

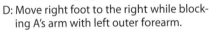

A: Slash diagonally upward toward D's body while moving right foot forward.

D: Move right foot to the right while blocking A's arm with left outer forearm.

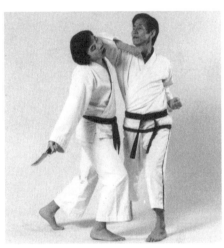

D: Execute a right elbow strike against A's jaw.

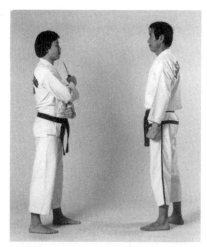

A. Hold knife in right hand facing D.

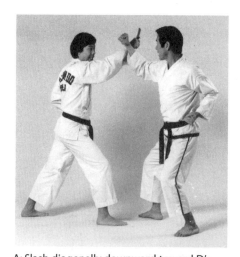

A: Slash diagonally downward toward D's body while moving right foot forward.

D: Move left foot to the left while blocking A's arm with right outer forearm.

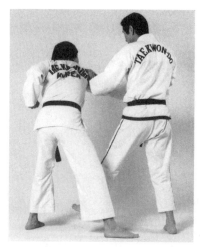

D: Grab A's arm with right hand while moving left foot forward, and place left palm at A's shoulder joint.

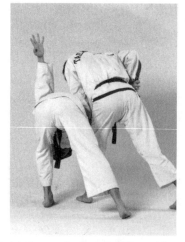

D: Twist A's arm clockwise while pushing downward at A's shoulder joint.

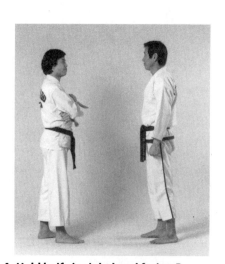

A. Hold knife in right hand facing D.

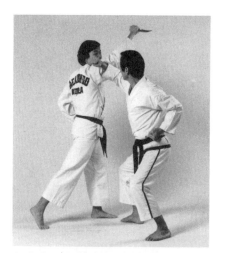

A: Stab diagonally downward toward D's front chest while moving left foot forward.

D: Move left foot to the left while blocking A's arm with right forearm.

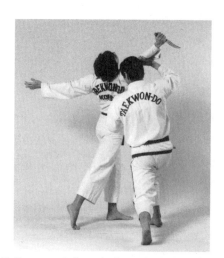

D: Execute a left vertical punch against A's kidney.

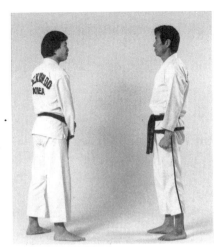

A. Hold knife in right hand facing D.

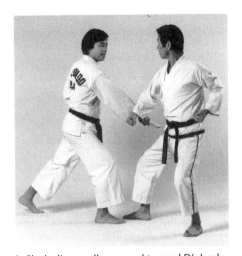

A: Slash diagonally upward toward D's body while moving right foot forward.

D: Move left foot to the left while blocking A's arm with the right outer forearm.

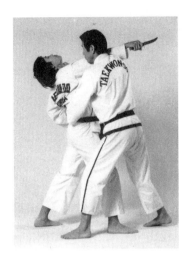

D: Grab A's neck with right arc-hand and hold A's back ribs with left hand while moving left foot forward.

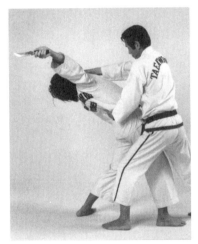

D: Push A's neck with right hand and pull A's back waist with left hand.

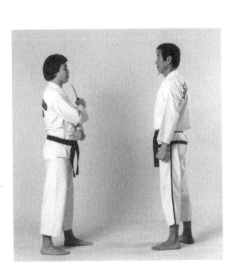

A. Hold knife in right hand facing D.

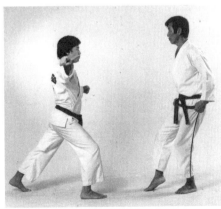

A: Slash horizontally toward D's neck while moving right foot forward.

D: Move left foot backward while dodging the knife, and raise right foot.

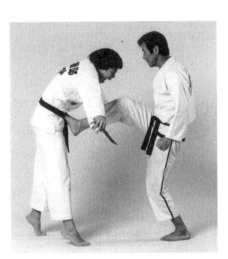

D: Execute a right front snap kick against A's epigastrium.

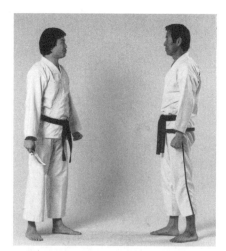

A. Hold knife in right hand facing D.

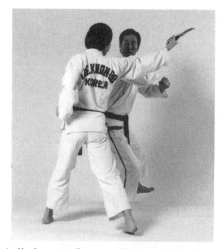

A: Slash vertically upward toward D's middle chest while moving left foot forward.

D: Turn body counterclockwise, pivoting on right foot while dodging the knife.

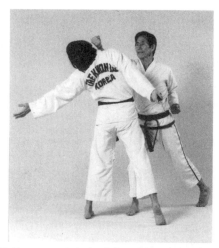

D: Execute a right back fist strike against A's jaw.

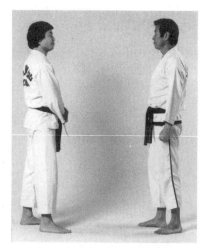

A. Hold knife in right hand facing D.

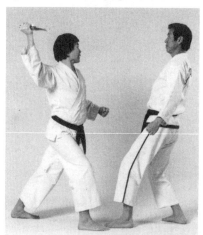

A: Slash diagonally upward toward D's body while moving right foot forward.

D: Move right foot backward while dodging the knife.

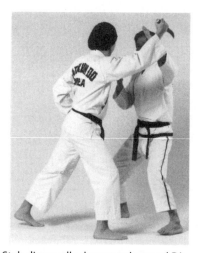

A: Stab diagonally downward toward D's front chest.

D: Execute a left outer forearm block at A's arm.

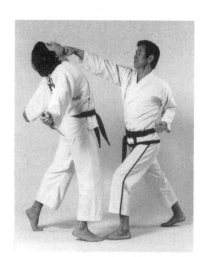

D: Execute a right punch against A's philtrum.

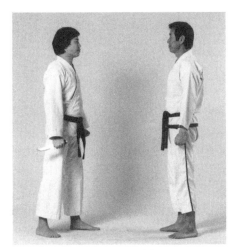

A. Hold knife in right hand facing D.

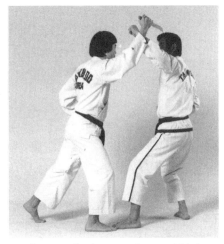

A: Stab vertically downward toward D's face while moving right foot forward.

D: Move right foot to the right while striking block at A's arm with left knife-hand.

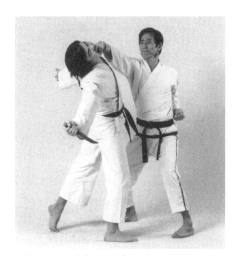

D: Execute a right punch against A's jaw.

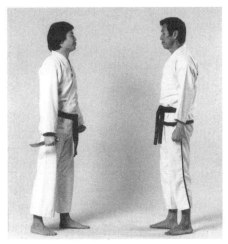

A. Hold knife in right hand facing D.

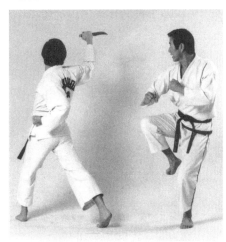

A: Slash diagonally upward toward D's body while moving left foot forward.

D: Move left foot backward while dodging the knife, and raise right leg.

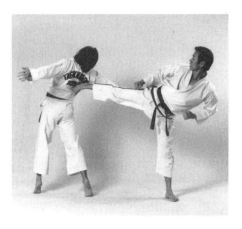

D: Execute a right side-snapping kick against A's kidney.

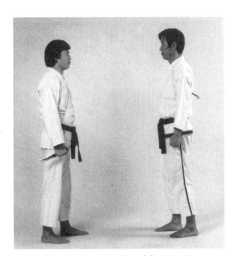

A. Hold knife in right hand facing D.

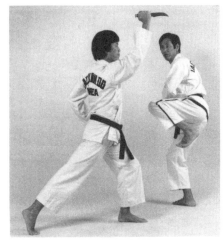

A: Slash vertically upward toward D's middle chest while moving left foot forward.

D: Step to the right with right foot and raise left leg.

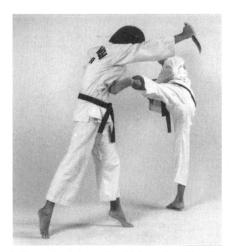

A: Execute a left turning kick against A's solar plexus.

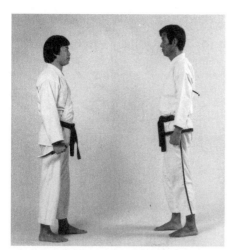 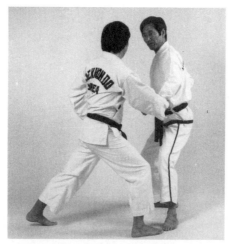 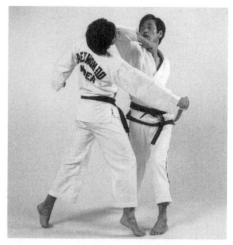

A. Hold knife in right hand facing D.

A: Slash diagonally upward toward D's body while moving right foot forward.

D: Move right foot to the right while blocking A's arm with left outer forearm.

D: Execute a right elbow strike against A's jaw.

Defense Against a Knife Attack

The defender should remain as calm as possible and adjust his position according to the attacker's position. The defender's body must keep away from the attacker's knife. The defender should carefully gauge the distance between himself and the attacker and be ready to counterattack immediately. When the attacker thrusts the knife from a specific direction, the defender counterattacks by intercepting the knife and throwing or pushing the attacker away in the same direction that he is moving.

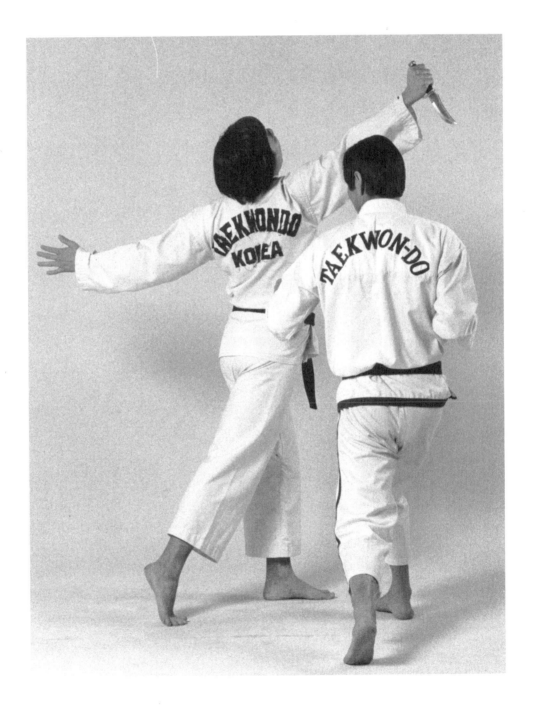

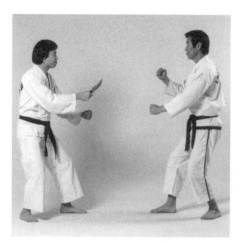

A. Face D and hold knife in right hand.

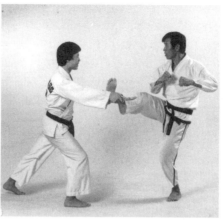

A: Stab toward D's solar plexus while moving right foot forward.

D: Execute right crescent kick at A's arm.

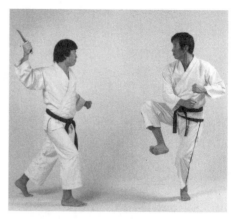

D: Be ready to kick again.

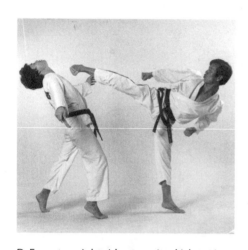

D: Execute a right side-snapping kick against A's upper neck.

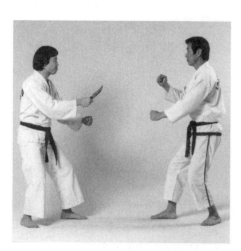

A. Face D and hold knife in right hand.

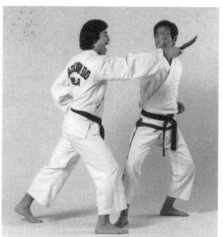

A: Stab toward D's face while moving right foot forward.

D: Execute block at A's arm with right outer forearm while turning body counterclockwise, pivoting on right foot.

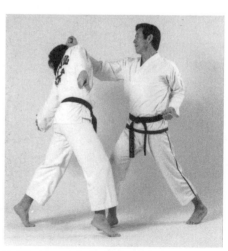

D: Execute a right back-fist strike against A's jaw.

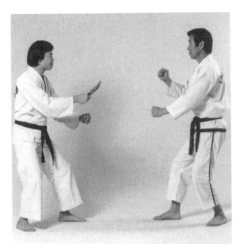

A: Face D and hold knife in right hand.

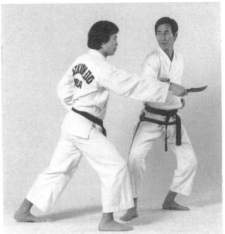

A: Stab toward D's stomach while moving right foot forward.

D: Exert pushing-block at A's arm with the right palm while turning body counterclockwise, pivoting on right foot.

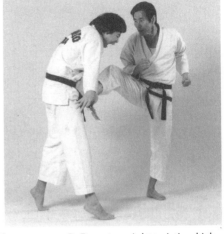

D: Execute a right twisting kick against A's stomach.

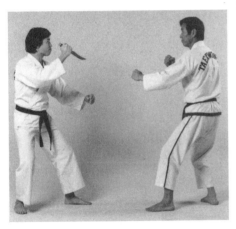

A: Face D and hold knife in right hand.

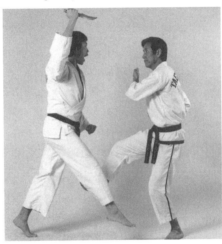

A: Stab toward D's face from above while moving right foot forward.

D: Move right foot to the right while dodging the knife.

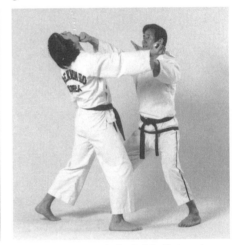

A: Block A's arm with the left knife-hand while executing right punch against A's jaw.

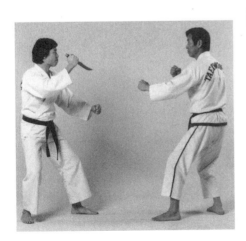

A: Face D and hold knife in right hand.

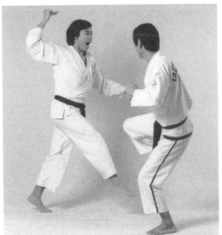

A: Stab toward D's face from above while moving right foot forward.

D: Step to the left with left foot and raise right leg.

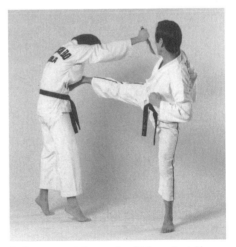

D: Execute a right turning kick against A's solar plexus.

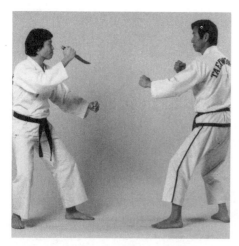

A: Face D and hold knife in right hand.

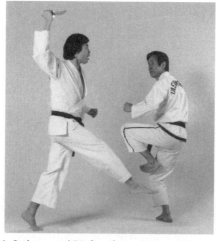

A: Stab toward D's face from above while moving right foot forward.

D: Step to the right with right foot and raise left leg.

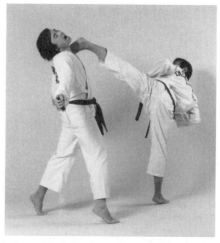

D: Execute a left side-snapping kick against A's upper neck.

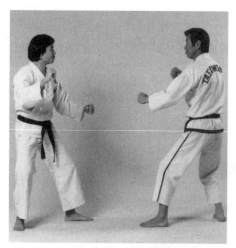
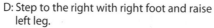

A: Face D and hold knife in right hand.

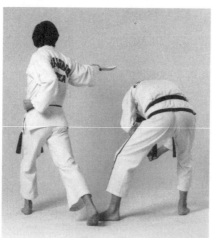

A: Slash horizontally toward D's neck while moving right foot forward.

D: Bend over to dodge the knife.

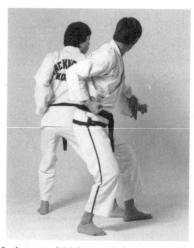

A: Stab toward D's lower abdomen while turning body clockwise.

D: Exert left knife-hand block at A's arm while turning body clockwise, pivoting on left foot.

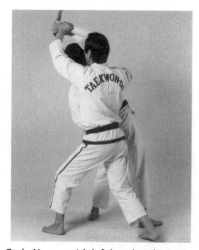

D: Grab A's arm with left hand and raise it up while moving left foot backward.

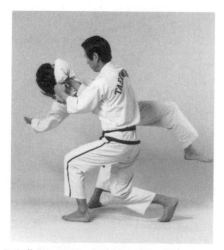

D: Pull A's arm downward and push against A's shoulder joint with right palm.

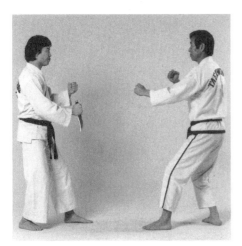

A: Face D and hold knife in right hand.

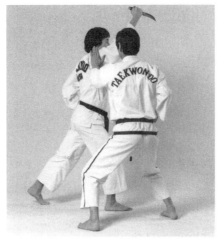

A: Slash upward at D's middle chest while moving right foot forward.

D: Block A's side-shoulder with left palm while turning body clockwise, pivoting on left foot.

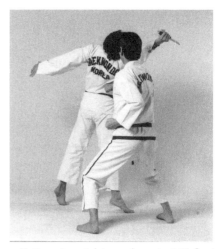

D: Execute a right punch against A's floating ribs.

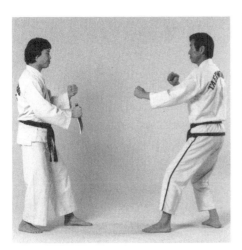

A: Face D and hold knife in right hand.

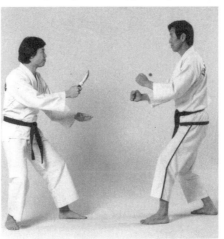

A: Stab toward D's solar plexus while moving right foot forward.

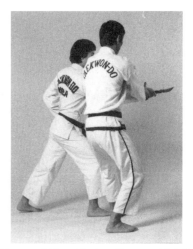

D: Exert grabbing block at A's arm with left hand while turning body clockwise, pivoting on left foot.

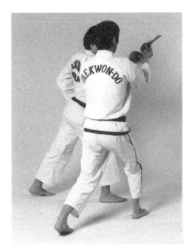

D: Grab A's hand with right hand while moving left foot backward.

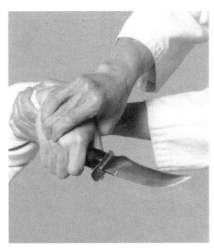

Close-up of the grabbing.

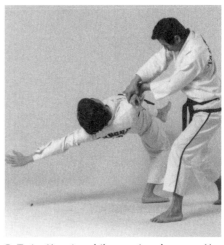

D: Twist A's wrist while pressing down on A's hand.

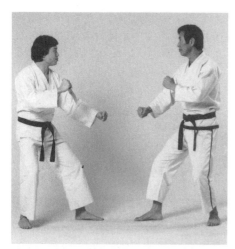

A: Face D and hold knife in right hand.

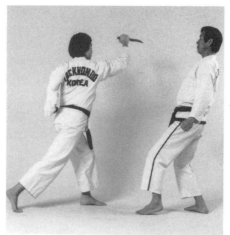

A: Slash diagonally upward toward D's body while moving left foot forward.

D: Move right foot backward while dodging the knife.

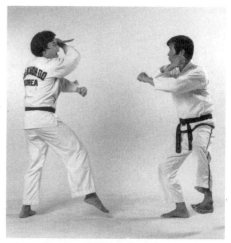

A: Move right foot forward.

D: Move left foot to the left.

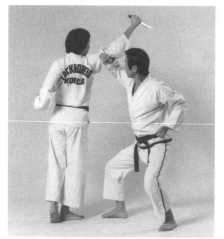

A: Stab toward D's face from above while jumping forward.

D: Block A's upper arm with right outer forearm.

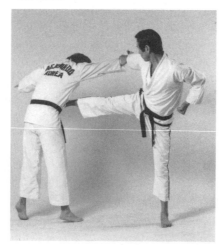

D: Grab A's arm with right hand while executing right turning kick against A's solar plexus.

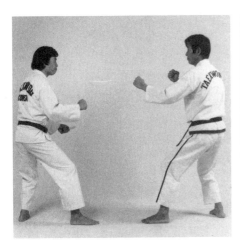

A: Face D and hold knife in left hand.

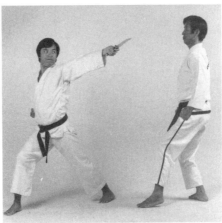

A: Slash diagonally upward toward D's body while moving left foot forward.

D: Slide backward while dodging the knife.

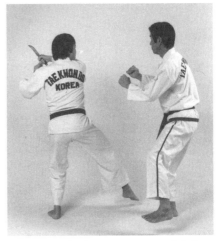

A: Turn body clockwise pivoting on left foot while passing the knife to right hand.

D: Move left foot to the left while preparing to block.

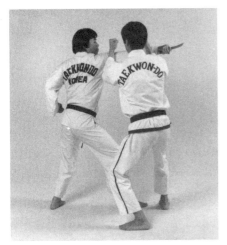

A: Slash horizontally outward toward D's neck.

D: Block A's arm with both outer forearms.

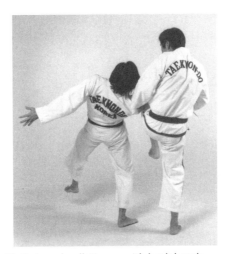

D: Grab and pull A's arm with both hands while executing left knee kick against A's elbow.

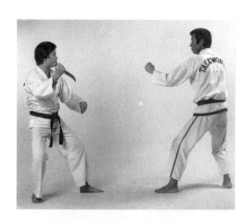

A: Face D and hold knife in right hand.

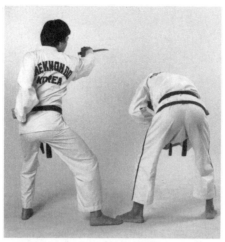

A: Slash horizontally inward toward D's neck while moving right foot forward.

D: Bend over to dodge the knife.

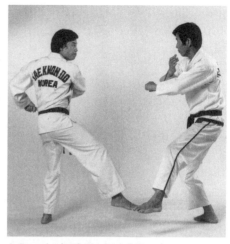

A: Pass the knife to the left hand.

D: Move left foot to the left and prepare to block.

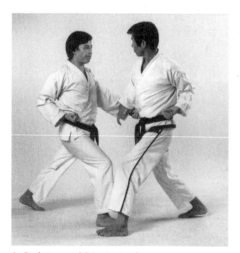

A: Stab toward D's stomach.

D: Exert right knife-hand block at A's arm.

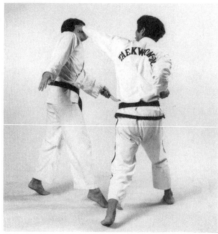

D: Execute a left punch against A's jaw.

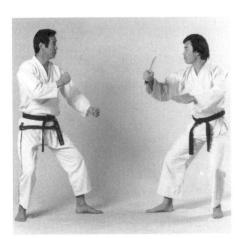

A: Face D and hold knife in right hand.

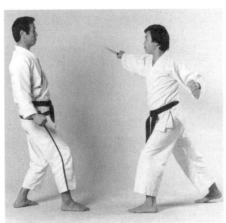

A: Slash horizontally outward toward D's ribs while moving left foot forward.

D: Move left foot backward while dodging the knife.

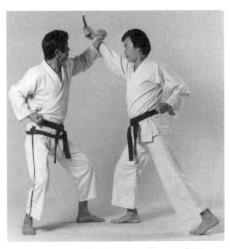

A: Slash diagonally downward toward D's neck while moving right foot forward.

D: Move right foot backward while blocking A's arm with left outer forearm.

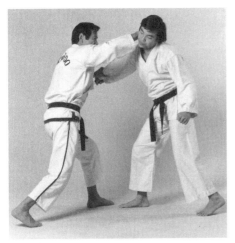

D: Grab A's arm with left hand while pushing A's neck with right hand.

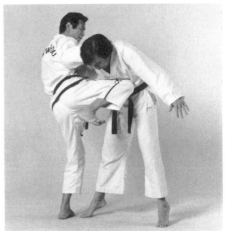

D: Pull A's neck with right hand while executing right knee kick against A's ribs.

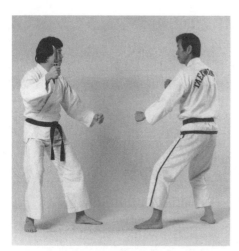

A: Face D and hold knife in right hand.

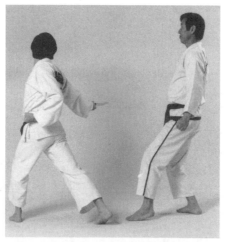

A: Slash diagonally downward toward D's body while moving right foot forward.

D: Move right foot backward while dodging the knife.

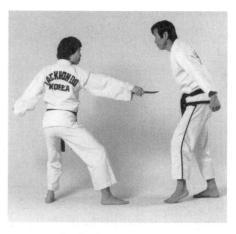

A: Slash horizontally outward toward D's ribs while sliding forward.

D: Slide backward while dodging the knife.

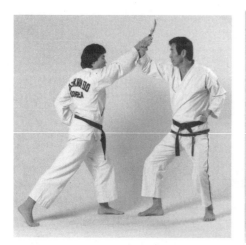

A: Slash diagonally downward toward D's body while moving left foot forward.

D: Move left foot backward while blocking A's arm with right outer forearm.

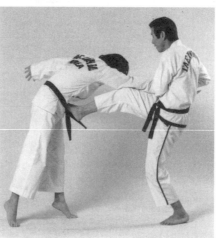

D: Grab and pull A's arm with both hands while executing right front snap kick against A's floating ribs.

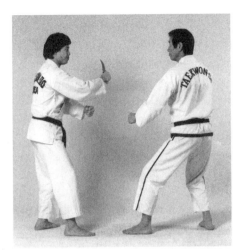

A: Face D and hold knife in right hand.

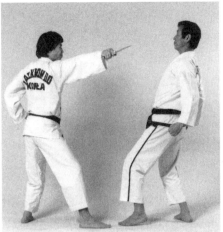

A: Slash horizontally toward D's face while sliding forward.

D: Slide backward while dodging the knife.

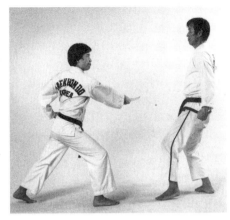

A: Slash diagonally downward toward D's face while sliding forward.

D: Slide backward while dodging the knife.

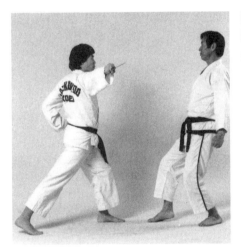

A: Slash horizontally toward D's neck while moving left foot forward.

D: Move left foot backward while dodging the knife.

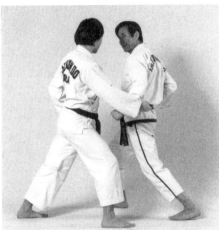

A: Slash diagonally downward toward D's ribs while moving right foot forward.

D: Move right foot to the right while blocking A's arm with left forearm.

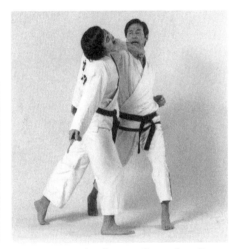

D: Execute a right elbow strike against A's jaw.

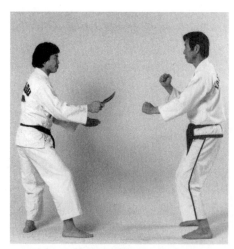

A: Face D and hold knife in right hand.

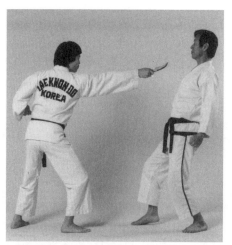

A: Stab toward D's face while sliding forward.

D: Move left foot backward while dodging the knife.

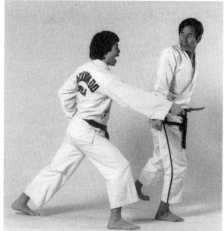

A: Stab toward D's lower abdomen while sliding forward.

D: Execute a strike-block at A's arm with right inner forearm while turning body counter-clockwise, pivoting on right foot.

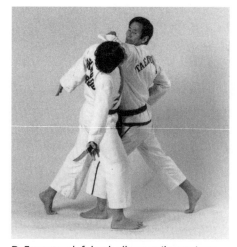

D: Execute a left back elbow strike against A's jaw.

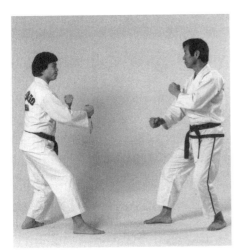

A: Face D and hold knife in right hand.

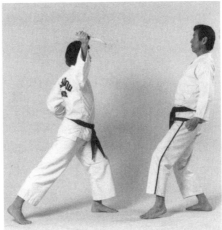

A: Slash diagonally upward toward D's body while moving left foot forward.

D: Move right foot backward while dodging the knife.

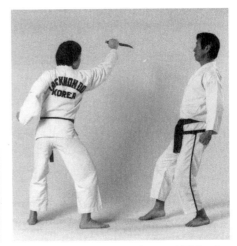

A: Slash diagonally upward toward D's body while moving right foot forward.

D: Move left foot backward while dodging the knife.

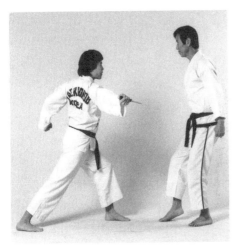

A: Slash horizontally toward D's ribs while moving left foot forward.

D: Slide backward while dodging the knife.

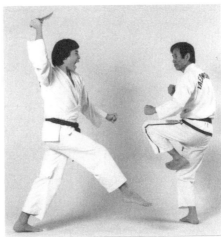

A: Stab toward D's face from above while moving right foot forward.

D: Step to the right with right foot and raise left leg.

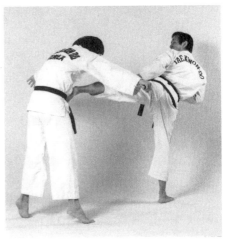

D: Execute a left side-snapping kick against A's floating ribs.

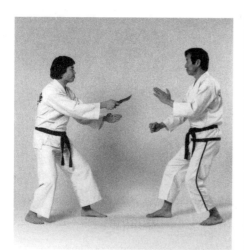

A: Face D and hold knife in right hand.

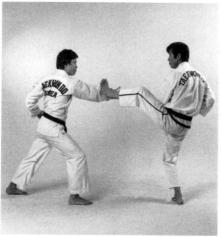

A: Stab toward D's umbilicus while moving right foot forward.

D: Execute a left crescent kick at A's arm.

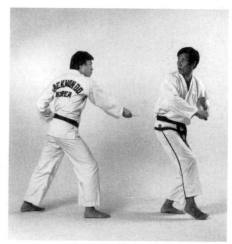

D: Lower the left foot in front of the right foot while turning body clockwise pivoting on left foot.

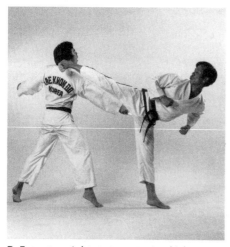

D: Execute a right reverse turning kick against A's neck.

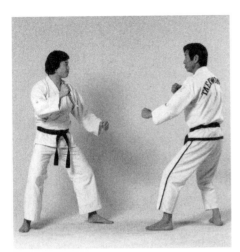

A. Face D and hold knife in right hand.

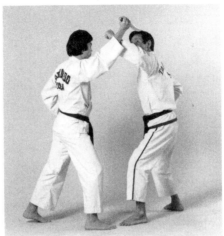

A: Stab toward D's face from above while moving right foot forward.

D: Move right foot to the right while blocking A's arm with left outer forearm.

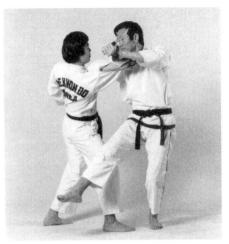

D: Lock A's elbow with right forearm and pull it forward while pushing with left arm and moving right foot forward.

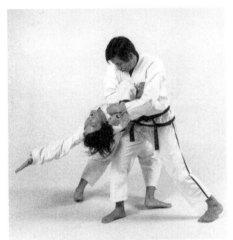

D: Continue pulling and pushing A's arm downward.

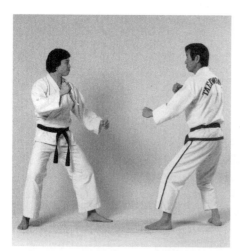

A: Face D and hold knife in right hand.

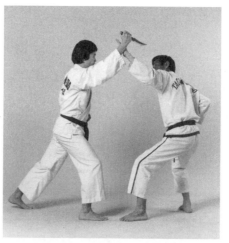

A: Stab toward D's face from above while moving right foot forward.

D: Move right foot to the right while blocking A's arm with left knife-hand.

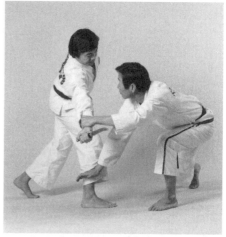

D: Grab A's arm with left hand and pull it down while striking A's right ankle with right knife hand.

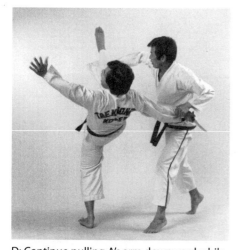

D: Continue pulling A's arm downward while grabbing A's ankle and raising it up.

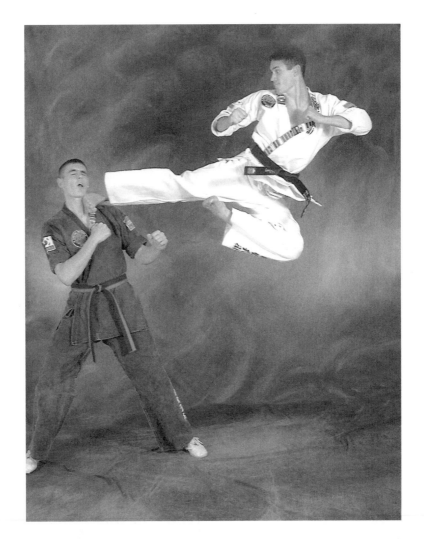

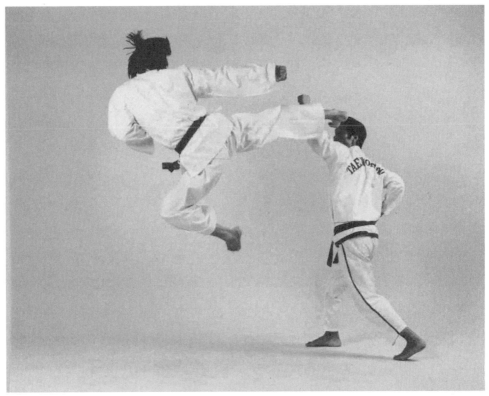

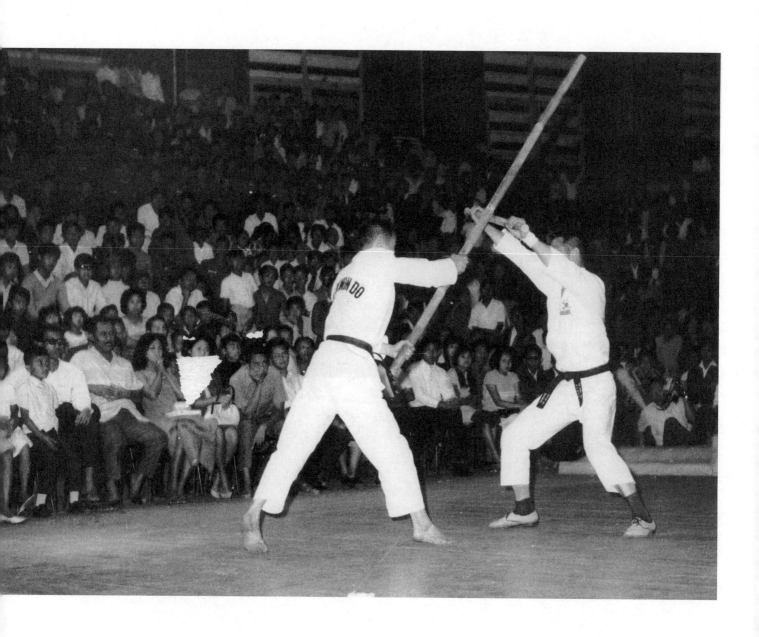

Defense Against a Sudden Attack with Baton

You should gauge the distance between yourself and the attacker precisely. Do not attempt to block a strike from a baton. It is dangerous. Only when the attacker swings the baton, may you then try to block his arm when opportunity allows. Or you may dodge from a thrusting baton. Dodging too far from your attacker, however, may make it impossible to counterattack in time. In a similar way as in a knife attack, the defender must always be on guard in every situation, despite unobservable motives on the part of the attacker.

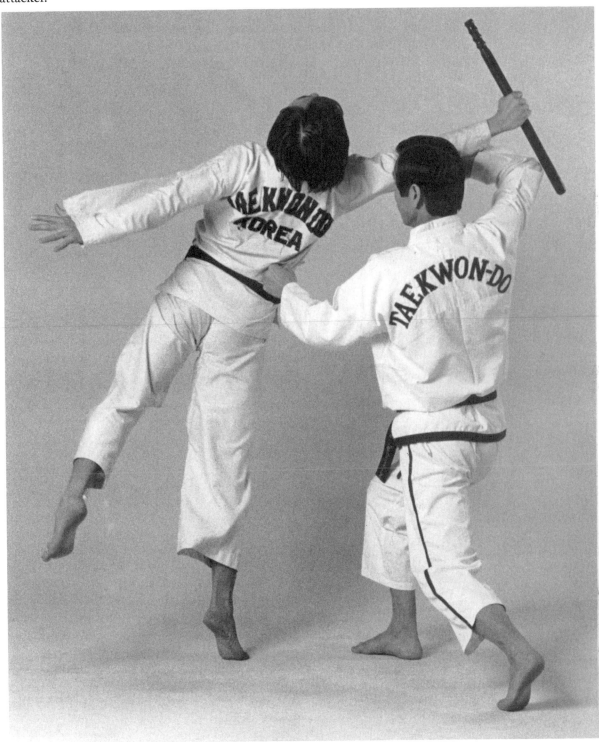

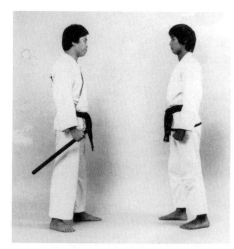

A: Face D and hold baton in right hand.

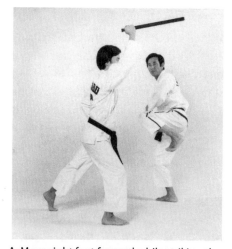
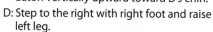

A: Move right foot forward while striking the baton vertically upward toward D's chin.

D: Step to the right with right foot and raise left leg.

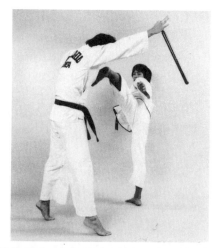

D: Execute a left turning kick against A's solar plexus.

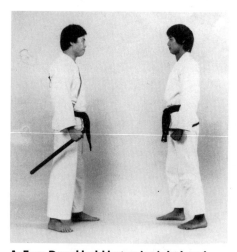

A: Face D and hold baton in right hand.

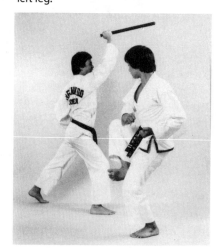

A: Move right foot forward while striking the baton vertically upward toward D's scrotum.

D: Step to the left with left foot and raise right leg.

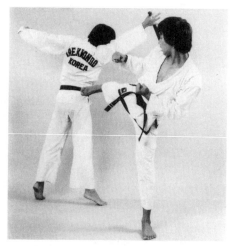

D: Execute a right side-snapping kick against A's kidney.

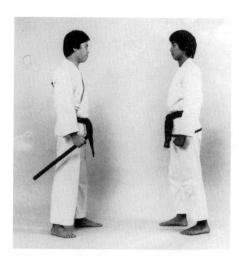

A: Face D and hold baton in right hand.

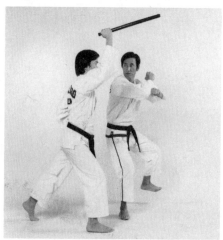

A: Move right foot forward while striking the baton vertically upward toward D's chin.

D: Turn body counterclockwise while pivoting on right foot, and prepare for a back-fist strike.

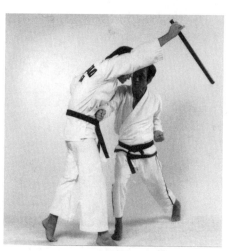

D: Execute a right back-fist strike against A's epigastrium.

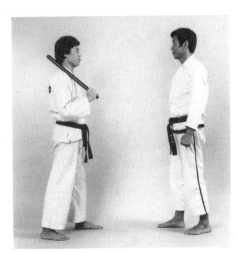

A: Face D and hold baton resting on shoulder.

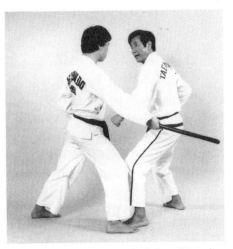

A: Move right foot forward while striking the baton diagonally downward toward D's knee.

D: Move right foot to the right while blocking A's arm with left outer forearm.

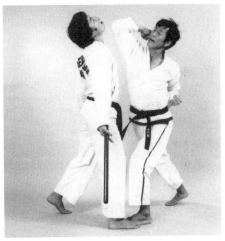

D: Execute a right upward elbow strike against A's chin.

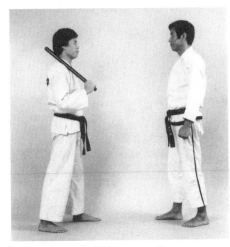

A: Face D and hold baton resting on shoulder.

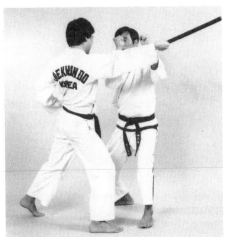
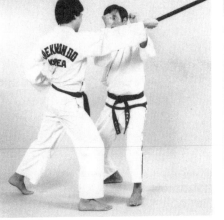
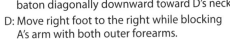

A: Move right foot forward while striking the baton diagonally downward toward D's neck.

D: Move right foot to the right while blocking A's arm with both outer forearms.

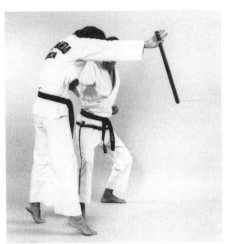

D: Execute a right back-elbow thrust against A's stomach while turning body counterclockwise, pivoting on right foot.

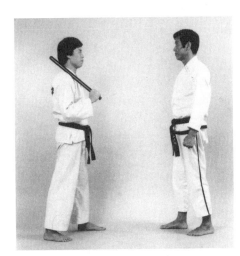

A: Face D and hold baton resting on shoulder.

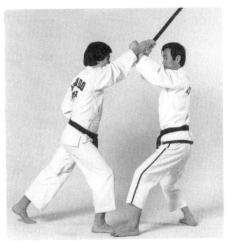
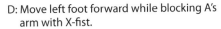

A: Move right foot forward while striking the baton vertically downward toward D's head.

D: Move left foot forward while blocking A's arm with X-fist.

D: Execute a back-fist strike against A's solar plexus while turning body counterclockwise, pivoting on right foot.

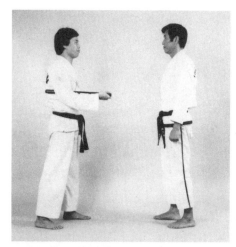

A: Face D and hold baton under the arm-pit.

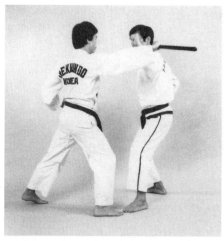

A: Move right foot forward while striking the baton horizontally inward toward D's neck.

D: Move right foot to the right while blocking A's arm with left outer forearm.

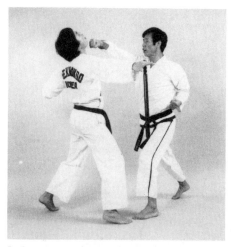

D: Execute a right punch against A's chin.

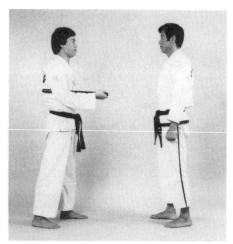

A: Face D and hold baton under the arm-pit.

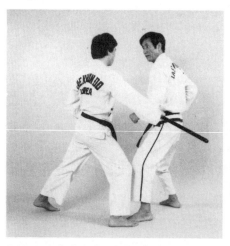

A: Move right foot forward while striking the baton diagonally upward toward D's knee.

D: Move right foot to the right while blocking A's arm with left outer forearm.

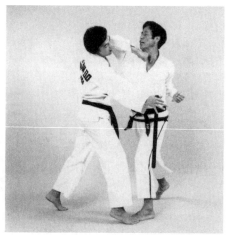

D: Execute a right side-elbow strike against A's jaw.

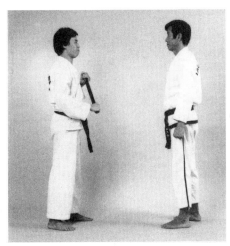

A: Face D and hold baton in both hands.

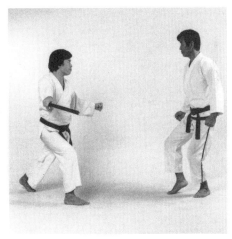

A: Move right foot forward while striking the baton horizontally outward toward D's neck.

D: Move left foot backward while dodging the baton.

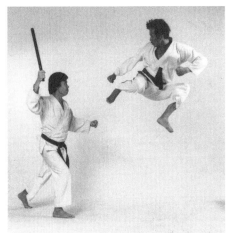

A: Prepare for a vertically downward strike at D's knee.

D: Jump to dodge the baton.

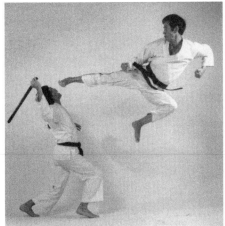

D: Execute a right flying side-snapping kick against A's face.

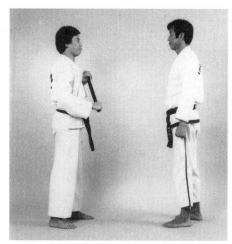

A: Face D and hold baton in both hands.

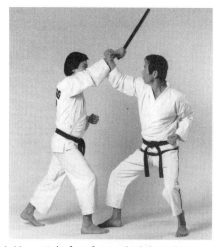

A: Move right foot forward while striking diagonally downward toward D's shoulder.

D: Move left foot to the left while blocking A's arm with right outer forearm.

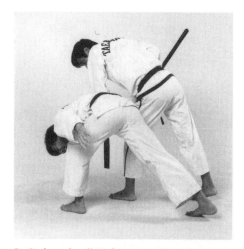

D: Grab and pull A's forearm with right hand and move left foot forward while pushing A's shoulder with left palm.

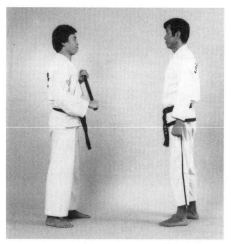

A: Face D and hold baton in both hands.

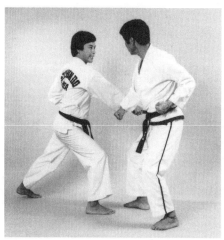

A: Move right foot forward while striking the baton diagonally downward toward D's knee.

D: Move left foot to the left while blocking A's forearm with right outer forearm.

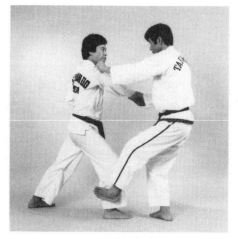

D: Grab A's arm with right hand and grab A's shoulder with left hand while raising left leg.

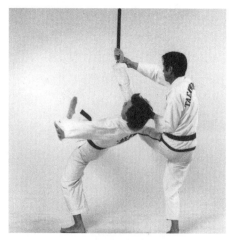

D: Execute a sweeping-kick against A's right ankle while pulling A's shoulder.

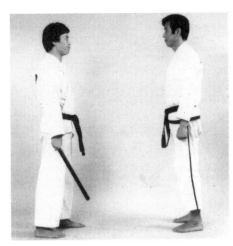

A: Face D and hold baton in right hand.

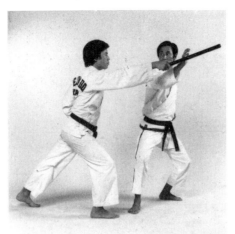

A: Move right foot forward while thrusting the baton toward D's face.

D: Block A's baton with right palm while turning body counterclockwise, pivoting on right foot.

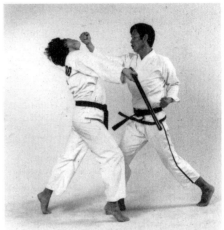

D: Execute a right back-fist strike against A's jaw.

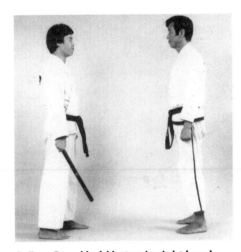

A: Face D and hold baton in right hand.

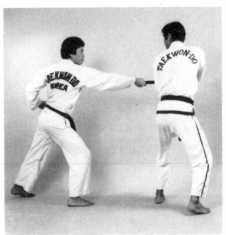

A: Move right foot forward while thrusting the baton toward D's solar plexus.

D: Move right foot backward and turn body clockwise, pivoting on left foot while grabbing A's baton with both hands.

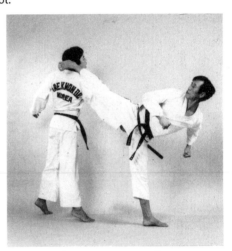

D: Execute a right reverse turning kick against A's upper neck.

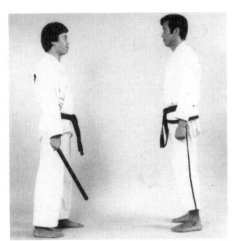

A: Face D and hold baton in right hand.

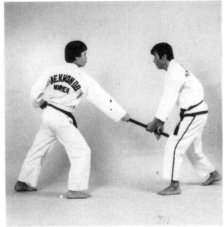

A: Move right foot forward while thrusting the baton toward D's stomach.

D: Move right foot backward while grabbing block at A's baton with both hands.

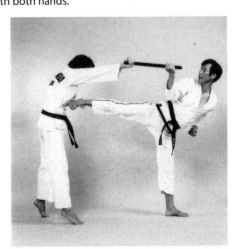

D: Raise up A's baton while executing right snap and pushing kick against A's stomach.

Defense Against a Baton Attack

When defending against a baton attack, the defender should check the distance between the attacker, the baton, and himself. Although the striking power of a baton is greater than a knife, the movement is comparatively slower because of the baton's length and weight.

Warning: To prevent serious injury, the defender should always move his body sideways in the direction the baton is swung as an extra precaution in case he fails to defend against the attack properly. When counterattacking, the defender should concentrate on the end of the baton nearest the attacker's hand because this is the part that is moving more slowly, and is less powerful.

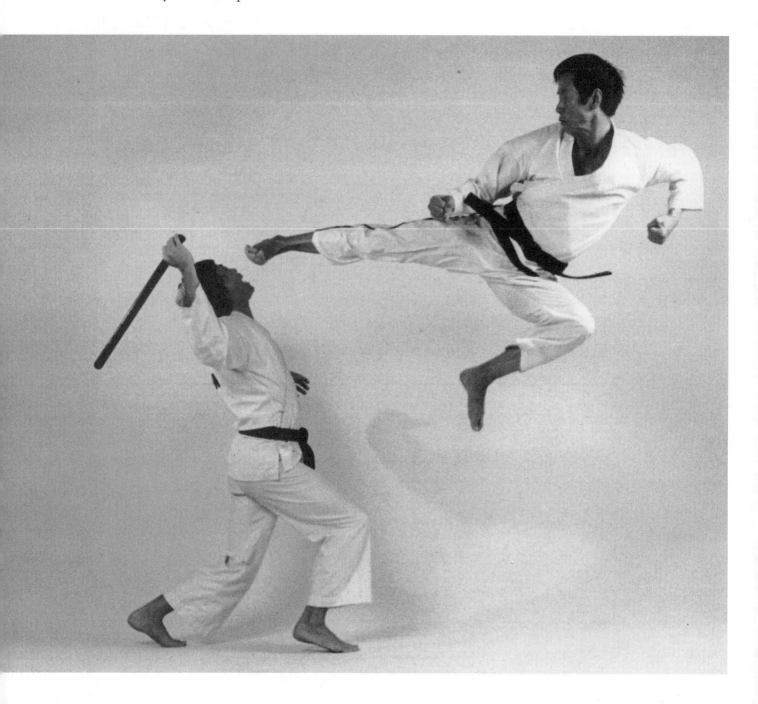

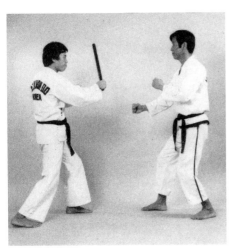

A: Face D and hold baton in right hand.

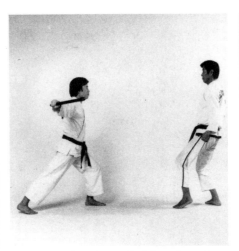

A: Move left foot forward while striking the baton horizontally toward D's neck.

D: Move right foot backward while dodging the baton.

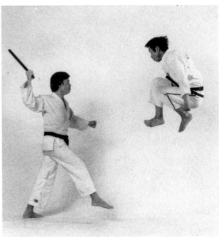

A: Move right foot forward while striking the baton diagonally downward toward D's knee.

D: Jump up to the right while dodging the baton.

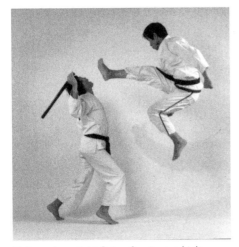

D: Execute a right flying front snap kick against A's chin.

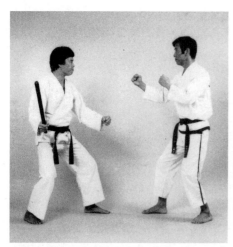

A: Face D and hold baton in right hand.

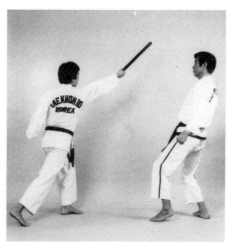

A: Move left foot forward while striking the baton diagonally upward toward D's ribs.

D: Move right foot backward while dodging the baton.

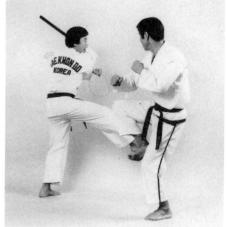

A: Move right foot forward while striking the baton vertically downward toward D's shoulder.

D: Step to the left with left foot and raise right leg.

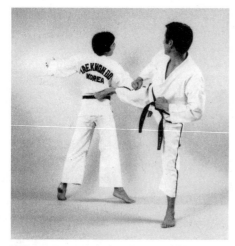

D: Execute a right side-snapping kick against A's kidney.

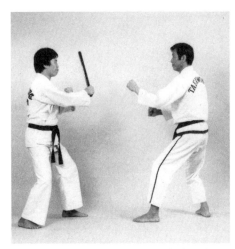

A: Face D and hold baton in right hand.

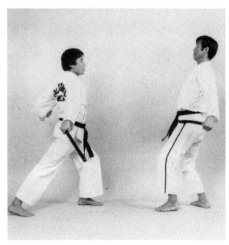

A: Move left foot forward while striking the baton diagonally downward toward D's shoulder.

D: Slide backward while dodging the baton.

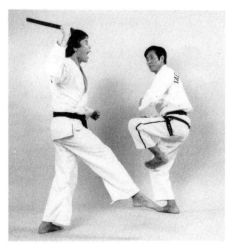

A: Move the right foot forward while striking the baton vertically downward toward D's head.

D: Step to the right with right foot and raise left leg.

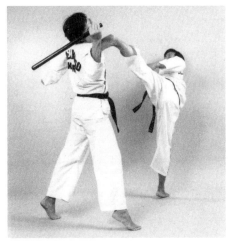

D: Execute a left side-snapping against A's upper neck.

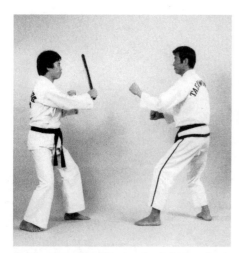

A: Face D and hold baton in right hand.

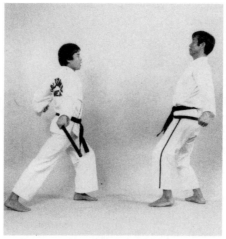
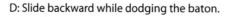

A: Move left foot forward while striking the baton diagonally downward toward D's shoulder.

D: Slide backward while dodging the baton.

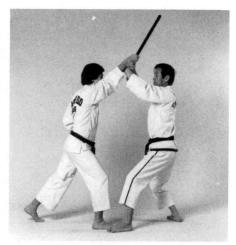

A: Move right foot forward while striking the baton diagonally downward toward D's shoulder.

D: Move right foot to the right while blocking A's arm with X-fist.

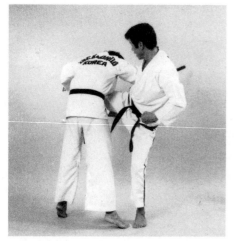

D: Grab A's arm with right hand and pull downward while executing right knee kick against A's stomach.

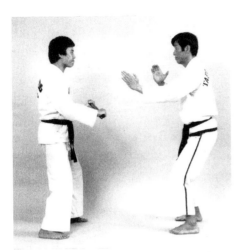

A: Face D and hold baton in both hands.

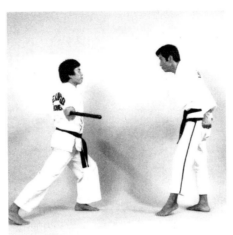

A: Move left foot forward while striking the baton horizontally toward D's ribs.

D: Move right foot backward while dodging the baton.

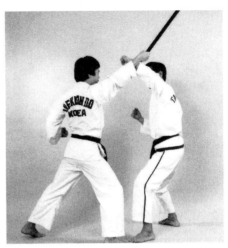

A: Move right foot forward while striking the baton diagonally downward toward D's neck.

D: Move right foot to the right while blocking A's arm with left outer forearm.

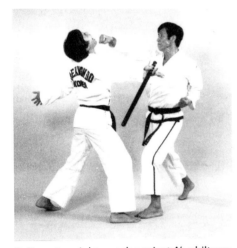

D: Execute a right punch against A's philtrum.

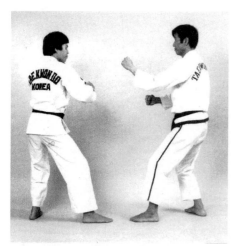

A: Face D and hold baton in both hands.

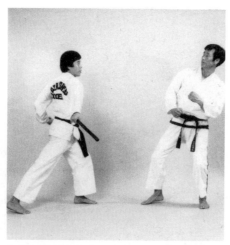

A: Move left foot forward while striking the baton diagonally downward toward D's shoulder.

D: Move left foot backward while dodging the baton.

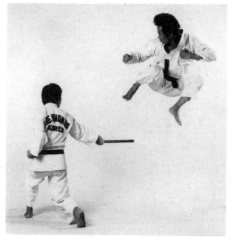

A: Move right foot forward while striking the baton horizontally inward toward D's knee.

D: Jump up to dodge the baton.

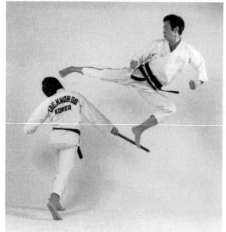

D: Execute a right flying side-snapping kick against A's face.

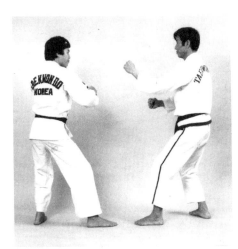

A: Face D and hold baton in both hands.

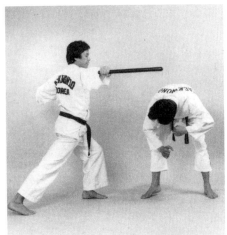

A: Move left foot forward while striking the baton horizontally outward toward D's neck.

D: Move left foot backward while bending over to dodge the baton.

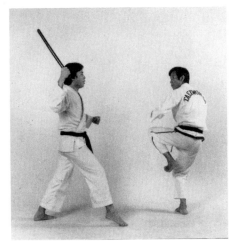

A: Move right foot forward while striking the baton vertically downward toward D's upper neck.

D: Step to the right with right foot and raise the left leg.

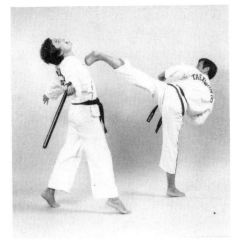

D: Execute a left side-snapping kick against A's upper neck.

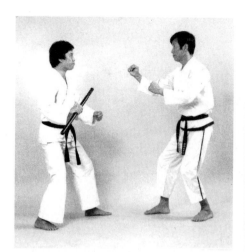

A: Face D and hold baton in right hand.

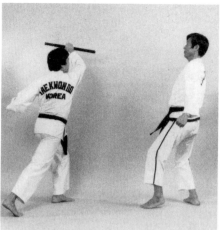

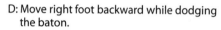

A: Move left foot forward while striking baton diagonally upward toward D's upper neck.

D: Move right foot backward while dodging the baton.

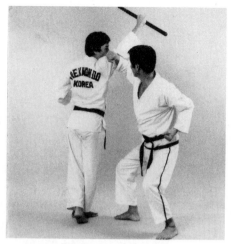

A: Thrust the baton downward toward D's windpipe while jumping the right foot forward.

D: Move left foot to the left while blocking A's upper arm with right outer forearm.

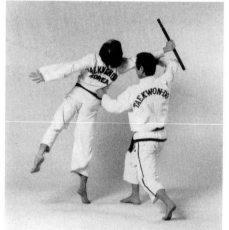

D: Grab and pull A's upper arm with right hand while executing left vertical punch against A's kidney.

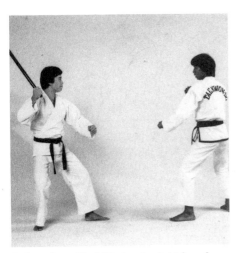

A: Face D and hold baton in right hand.

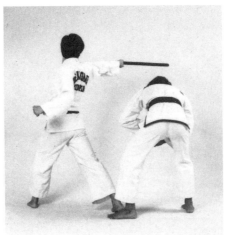

A: Move right foot forward while striking the baton horizontally inward toward D's neck.

D: Bend body to dodge the baton.

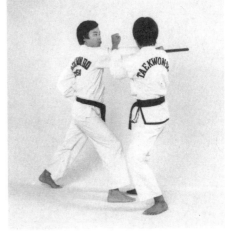

A: Strike the baton diagonally outward toward D's face.

D: Move left foot backward while blocking A's arm with both outer forearms.

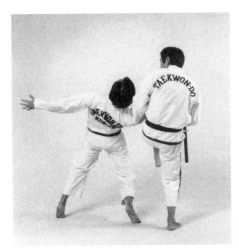

D: Grab A's arm with both hands and pull it down while executing left knee kick against A's elbow.

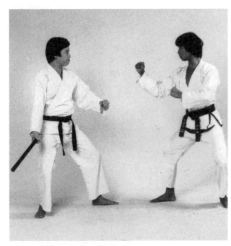

A: Face D and hold baton in right hand.

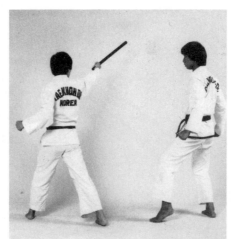

A: Move right foot forward while striking the baton diagonally upward toward D's ribs.

D: Move right foot backward while dodging the baton.

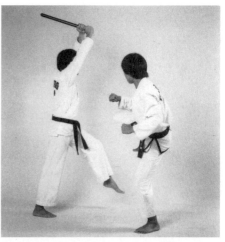

A: Move left foot forward while striking the baton vertically downward toward D's head with both hands.

D: Step to the left with left foot and raise the right leg.

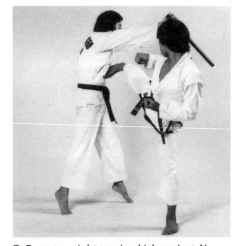

D: Execute a right turning kick against A's solar plexus.

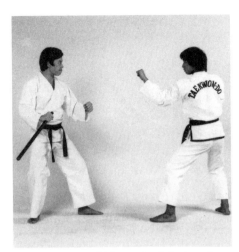

A: Face D and hold baton in right hand.

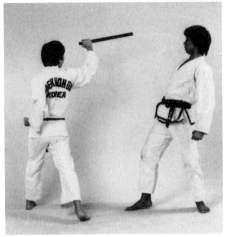

A: Move right foot forward while striking the baton diagonally upward toward D's knee.

D: Move left foot backward while dodging the baton.

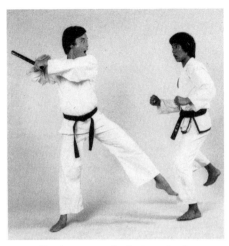

A: Turn body counterclockwise, pivoting on right foot while passing the baton to the left hand.

D: Move right foot backward and raise both arms preparing to block.

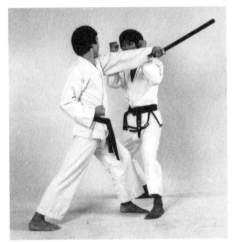

A: Strike the baton horizontally outward toward D's neck.

D: Block A's forearm with both outer forearms.

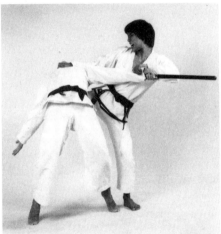

D: Grab A's arm with left hand and pull A's neck backward with right hand while executing right knee kick against A's kidney.

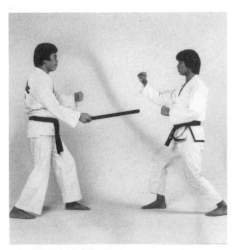

A: Face D and hold baton in right hand.

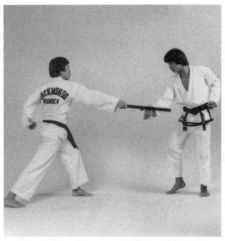

A: Move left foot forward while thrusting the baton toward D's epigastrium.

D: Slide backward while blocking A's baton with right palm.

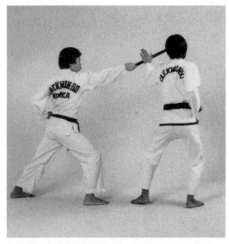

A: Move right foot forward while thrusting the baton toward D's face.

D: Move right foot backward while blocking A's baton with left palm.

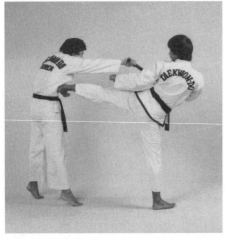

D: Execute a left side-snapping kick against A's ribs.

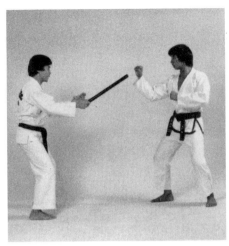

A: Face D and hold baton in right hand.

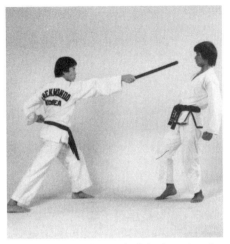

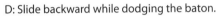

A: Move left foot forward while thrusting the baton toward D's face.

D: Slide backward while dodging the baton.

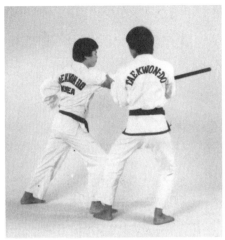

A: Move right foot forward while thrusting the baton toward D's solar plexus.

D: Move right foot backward and turn clockwise, pivoting on left foot while executing grasping block at A's arm with both hands.

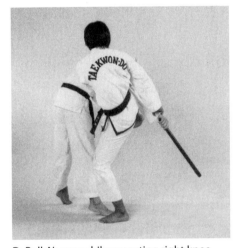

D: Pull A's arm while executing right knee kick against A's stomach.

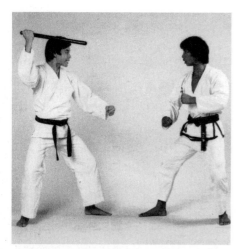

A: Face D and hold baton in right hand.

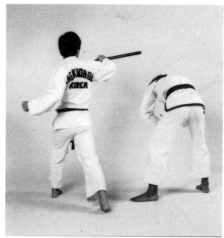
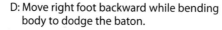

A: Move right foot forward while striking horizontally toward D's neck.

D: Move right foot backward while bending body to dodge the baton.

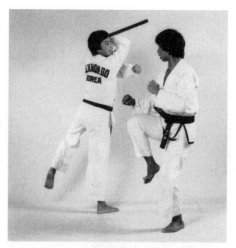

A: Thrust the baton downward toward D's lower back.

D: Step to the left with left foot and raise right leg.

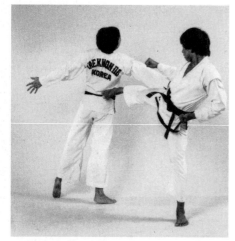

D: Execute a right side-snapping kick against A's kidney.

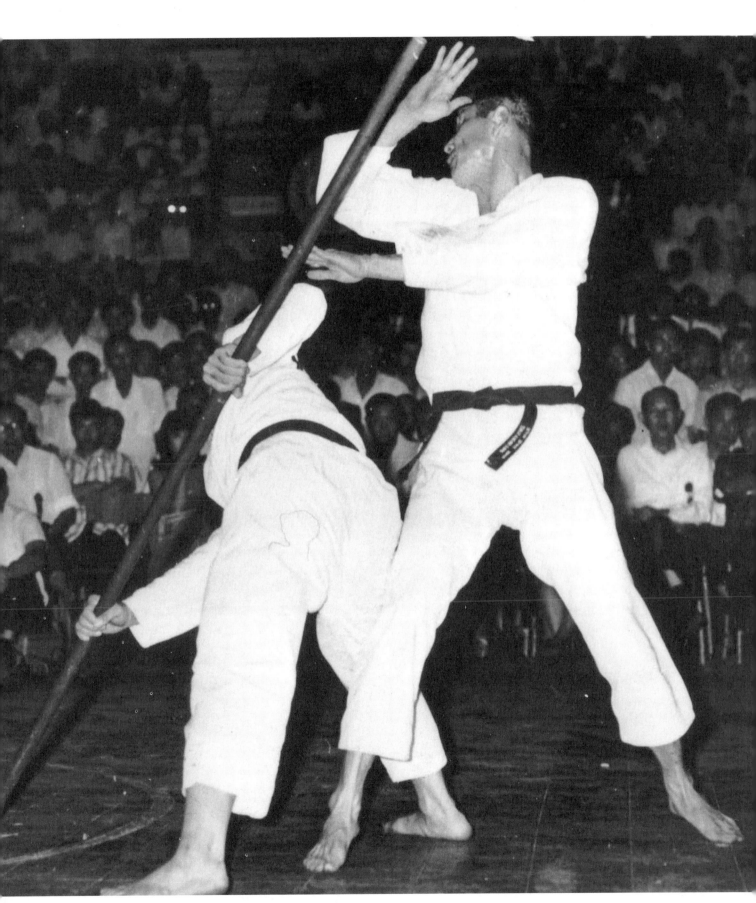

81 / Defense Against a Baton Attack

Defense with Baton Against a Pole Attack

The defender does not have to get too close to the attacker with the pole because the defender actually has the advantage. A pole is much longer than a baton, but it is also more unwieldy and much slower than a baton, and this allows the defender more time for thought and correct positioning to counter the attack. Since the major concentration of force is at the outer end of the pole, this part should not be blocked. Instead, it is best to block the middle-lower portion of the pole where its striking force is comparatively much weaker.

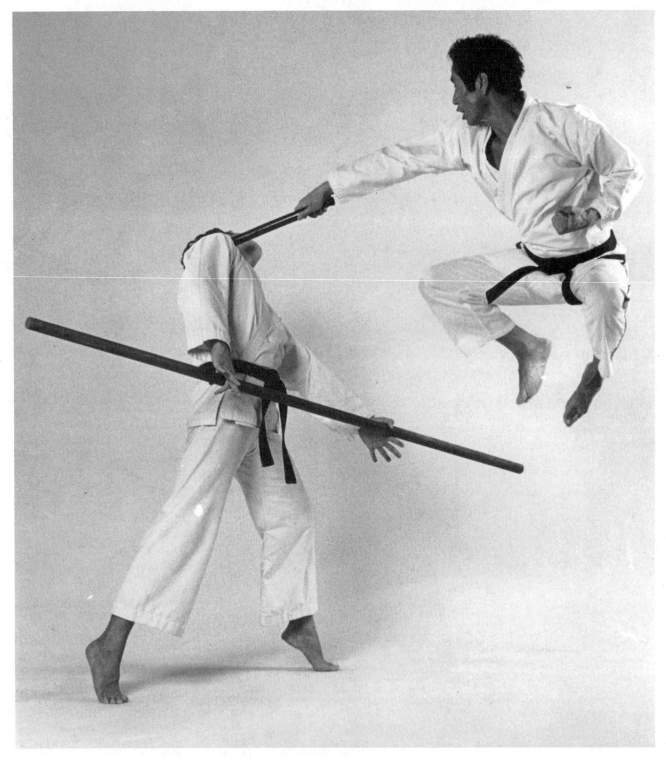

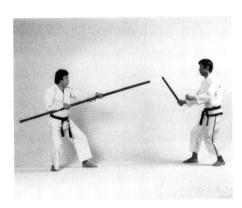

A: Point pole at D.
D: Hold baton in right hand facing A.

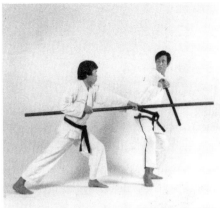

A: Move left foot forward while thrusting the pole toward D's epigastrium.

D: Block the pole with baton while turning body counterclockwise, pivoting on right foot.

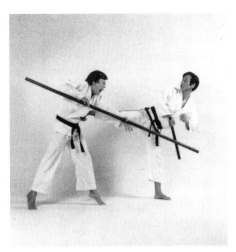

D: Execute a right side-snapping kick against A's floating ribs.

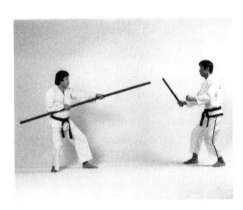

A: Point pole at D.
D: Hold baton in right hand facing A.

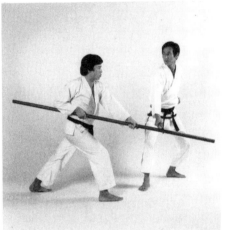
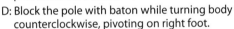

A: Move right foot forward while thrusting the pole toward D's sternum.

D: Block the pole with baton while turning body counterclockwise, pivoting on right foot.

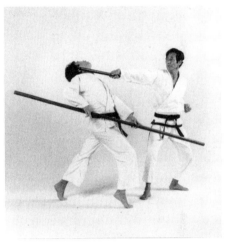

D: Execute a baton strike against A's Adam's Apple.

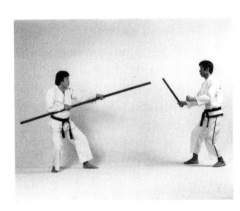

A: Point pole at D.
D: Hold baton in right hand facing A.

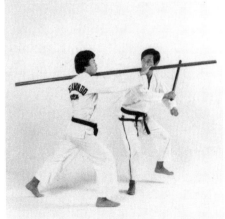

A: Move right foot forward while striking the pole vertically upward toward D's scrotum.

D: Turn body counterclockwise, pivoting on right foot.

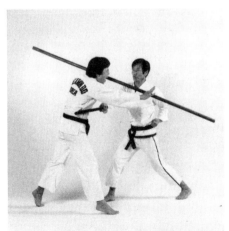

D: Move right foot to the right while executing baton strike against A's ribs.

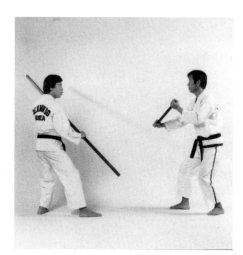

A: Hold pole facing D.
D: Hold baton facing A.

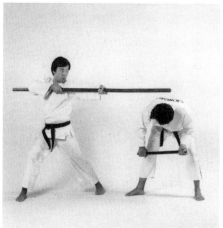
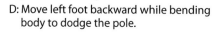

A: Move left foot forward while striking the pole horizontally toward D's neck.
D: Move left foot backward while bending body to dodge the pole.

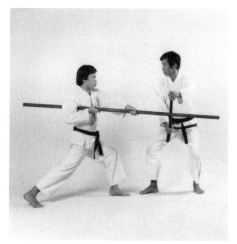

A: Strike the pole diagonally upward at D's body.
D: Block the pole with baton.

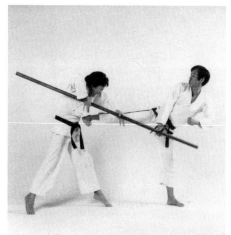

D: Execute a right side-snapping kick against A's floating ribs.

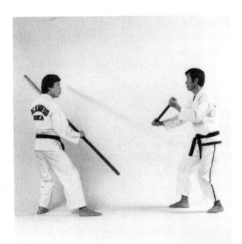

A: Hold pole facing D.
D: Hold baton facing A.

A: Move left foot forward while striking the pole vertically downward at D's head.
D: Turn body counterclockwise, pivoting on right foot and prepare to strike.

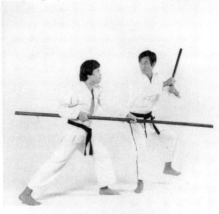

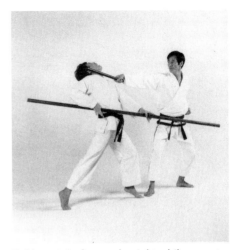

D: Move right foot to the right while executing baton strike against A's neck.

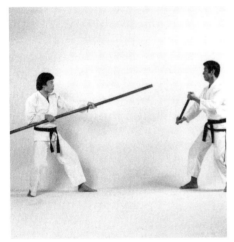

A: Point pole at D.
D: Hold baton in right hand facing A.

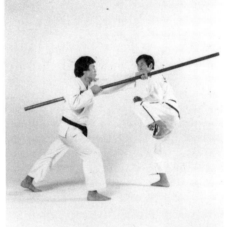

A: Move right foot forward while thrusting the pole toward D's face.
D: Step to the right with right foot and raise left foot.

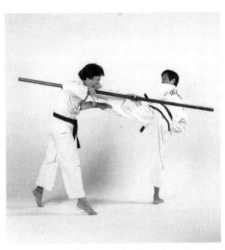

D: Execute a left turning kick against A's solar plexus.

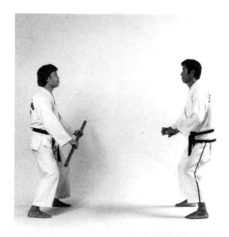

A: Hold pole facing D.
D: Hold baton facing A.

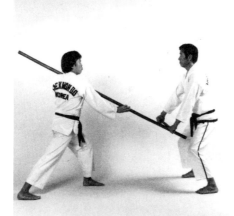

A: Move left foot forward while striking the pole vertically upward toward D's scrotum.
D: Block the pole with the baton while sliding backward.

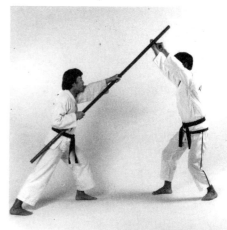

A: Strike the pole vertically toward D's head.
D: Move left foot backward while blocking the pole with baton.

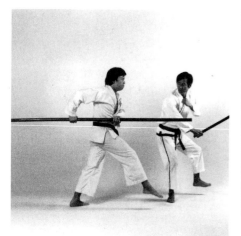

A: Step forward with right foot.
D: Hold baton in right hand while preparing to block.

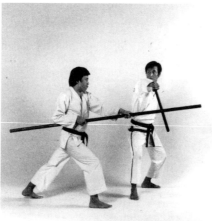

A: Thrust the pole toward D's umbilicus.
D: Block the pole with baton while turning body counterclockwise, pivoting on right foot.

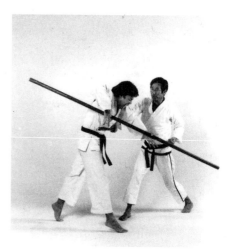

D: Execute a baton strike against A's stomach.

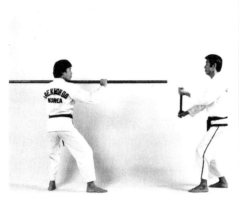

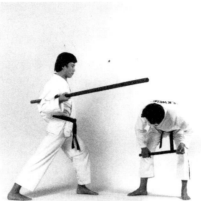

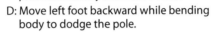

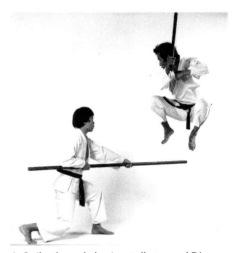

A: Hold pole facing D.
D: Hold baton facing A.

A: Move left foot forward while striking the pole horizontally toward D's neck.

D: Move left foot backward while bending body to dodge the pole.

A: Strike the pole horizontally toward D's knee.

D: Jump up to dodge the pole.

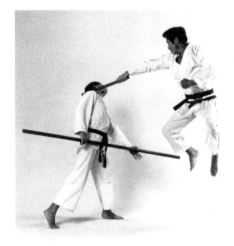

D: Hold baton in right hand while executing baton strike against A's neck.

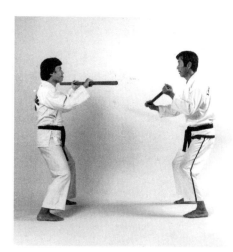

A: Hold pole facing D.
D: Hold baton facing A.

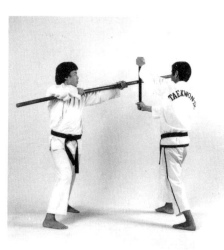

A: Strike the pole horizontally inward toward D's neck while turning body clockwise pivoting on both feet.

D: Block the pole with the baton while turning body clockwise pivoting on both feet.

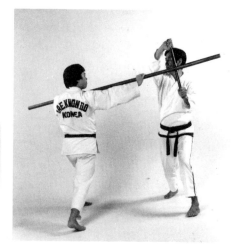

A: Strike the pole horizontally toward D's upper body while turning the body counterclockwise.

D: Block the pole with baton while turning body counterclockwise, pivoting on both feet.

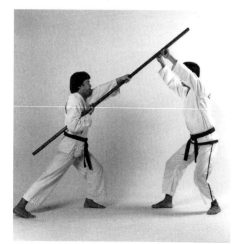

A: Move left foot forward while striking the pole vertically downward on D's head.

D: Move left foot backward while blocking the pole with baton.

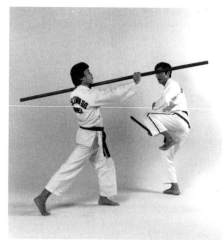

A: Strike the pole vertically upward toward D's scrotum.

D: Step to the right with right foot and raise left leg.

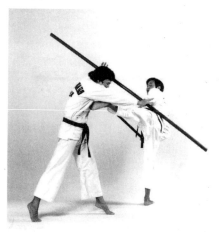

D: Execute a left turning kick against A's floating ribs.

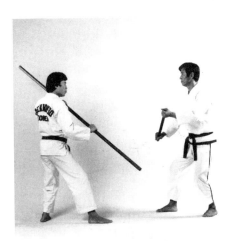

A: Hold pole facing D.
D: Hold baton facing A.

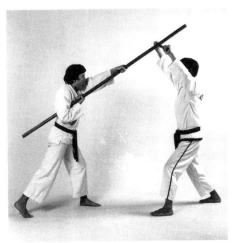

A: Move left foot forward while striking the pole vertically downward toward D's head.

D: Move right foot backward while blocking the pole with baton.

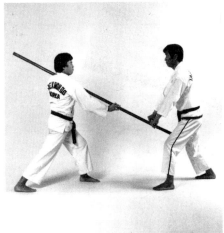

A: Strike the pole vertically upward toward D's scrotum.

D: Block the pole with baton.

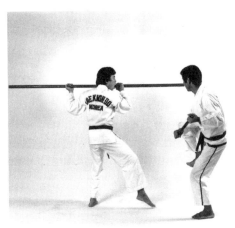

A: Move right foot forward while thrusting the pole toward D's face.

D: Step to the left and raise right leg.

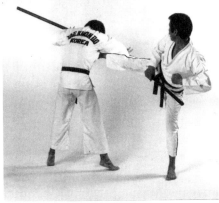

D: Execute a right turning kick against A's solar plexus.

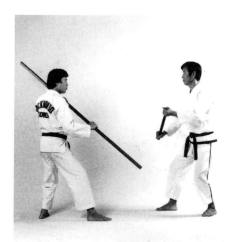

A: Hold pole facing D.
D: Hold baton facing A.

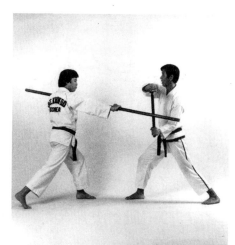
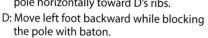

A: Move left foot forward while striking the pole horizontally toward D's ribs.

D: Move left foot backward while blocking the pole with baton.

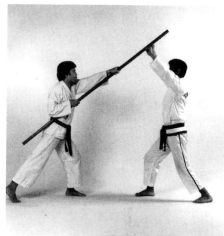

A: Strike the pole vertically downward toward D's head.

D: Block the pole with baton.

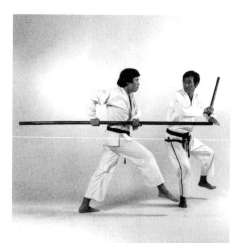
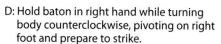

A: Prepare to thrust while moving right foot forward.

D: Hold baton in right hand while turning body counterclockwise, pivoting on right foot and prepare to strike.

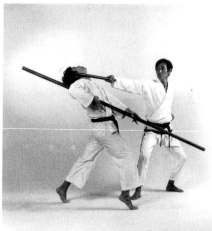

D: Execute a baton strike against A's Adam's apple.

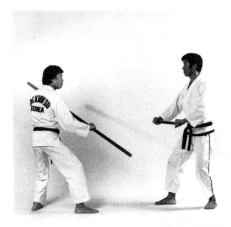

A: Hold pole facing D.
D: Hold baton facing A.

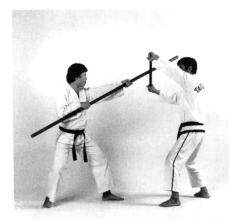

A: Move left foot forward while striking the pole diagonally downward toward D's shoulder.

D: Move right foot backward while blocking the pole with baton.

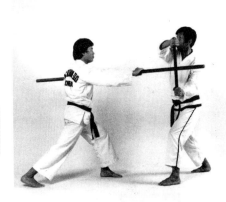

A: Strike the pole horizontally toward D's ribs.

D: Block the pole with baton.

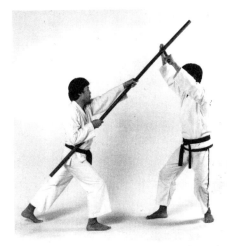

A: Move right foot forward while striking the pole vertically downward toward D's head.

D: Move left foot backward while blocking the pole with baton.

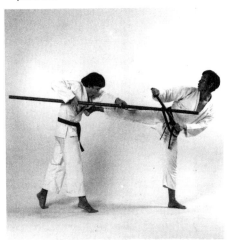

D: Execute a right side-snapping kick against A's epigastrium.

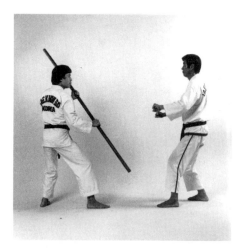

A: Hold pole facing D.
D: Hold baton facing A.

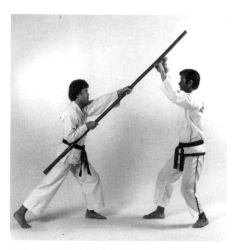

A: Move left foot forward while striking the pole vertically downward toward D's head.
D: Move left foot backward while blocking the pole with baton.

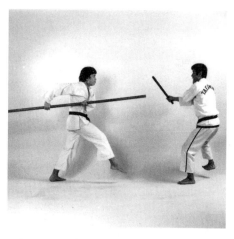

A: Prepare to thrust while moving right foot forward.
D: Hold baton in right hand while moving right foot backward and prepare to block.

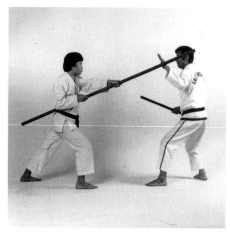

A: Thrust the pole toward D's solar plexus.
D: Block the pole with left knife hand.

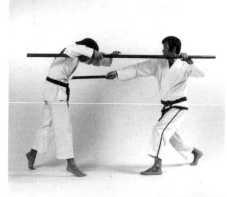

D: Grab the pole with left hand while executing baton thrust against A's umbilicus.

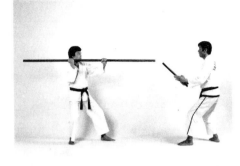

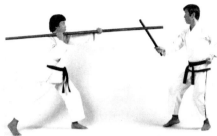

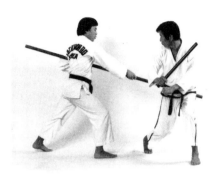

A: Point pole at D.
D: Hold baton facing A.

A: Thrust pole toward D's face while sliding forward.

D: Move left foot backward while blocking the pole with baton.

A: Move right foot forward while striking the pole vertically downward toward D's head.

D: Move left foot to the left while preparing the baton strike.

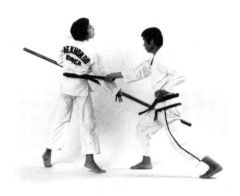

D: Execute a baton strike against A's kidney.

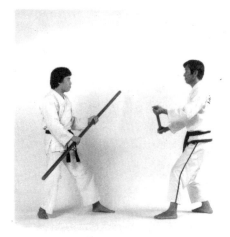

A: Hold pole facing D.
D: Hold baton facing A.

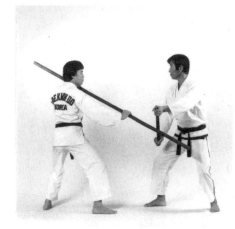

A: Move right foot forward while striking the pole diagonally upward toward D's leg.

D: Move left foot backward while blocking the pole with baton.

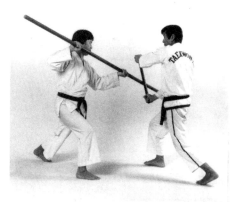

A: Strike the pole diagonally upward toward D's leg.

D: Block the pole with baton.

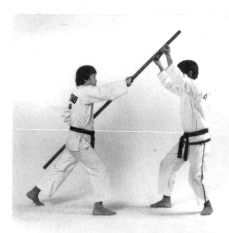

A: Strike the pole vertically downward toward D's head.

D: Block the pole with baton.

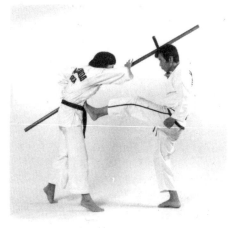

D: Execute a left front snap kick against A's umbilicus.

Defense Against a Pole Attack

In a pole attack, lengthen your strike during the dodge so the attacker will find it necessary to take an extra step for a combination movement.

Block with the palm in the event the attacker is at close range and is attacking with a half-strike. When the attacker thrusts with the pole, use a palm-block to push aside the pole. However, when the attacker strikes with the pole, never block a full strike with the palms.

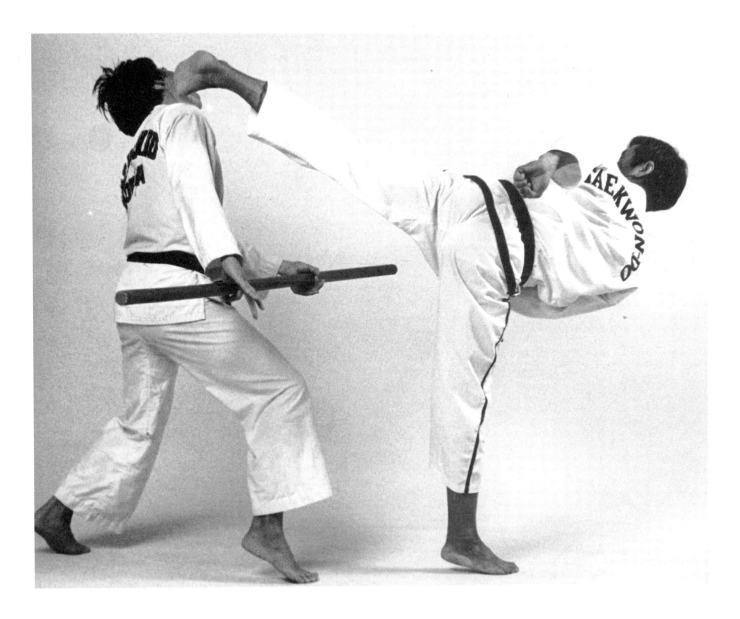

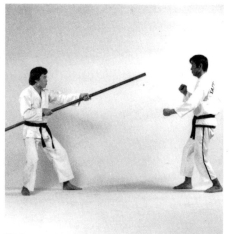

A: Point pole at D.

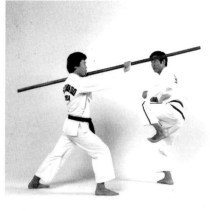

A: Move right foot forward while striking the pole vertically upward toward D's scrotum.

D: Step to the right with the right foot and raise left leg.

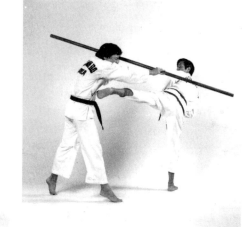

D: Execute left turning kick against A's epigastrium.

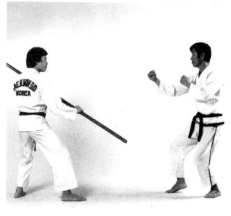

A: Hold pole facing D.

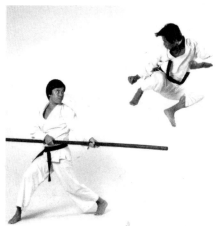

A: Move left foot forward while striking the pole horizontally inward toward D's knee.

D: Jump up to dodge the pole.

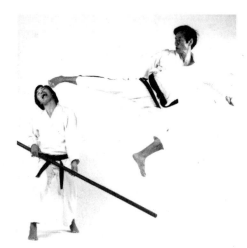

D: Execute a right flying side-snapping kick against A's face.

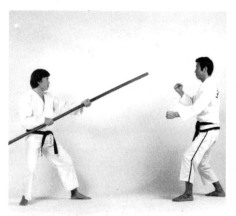

A: Hold pole facing D.

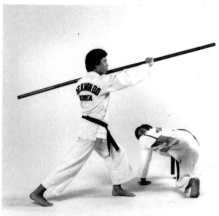
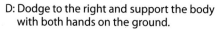

A: Move left foot forward while striking the pole diagonally upward toward D's ribs.

D: Dodge to the right and support the body with both hands on the ground.

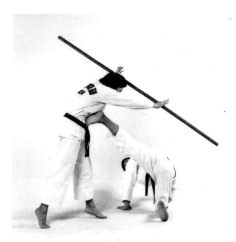

D: Execute a left turning kick against A's stomach.

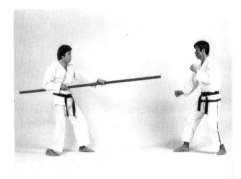

A: Point pole at D.

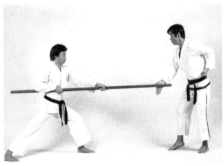

A: Move left foot forward while thrusting the pole toward D's umbilicus.

D: Slide backward while blocking the pole with right palm.

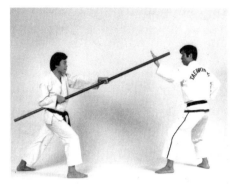

A: Move right foot forward while thrusting the pole toward D's face.

D: Move right foot backward while blocking the pole with left knife hand.

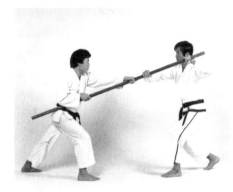

D: Grab the pole with both hands and prepare to kick.

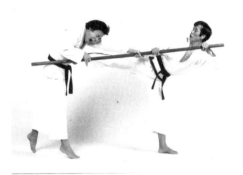

D: Pull the pole while executing right pushing kick against A's floating ribs.

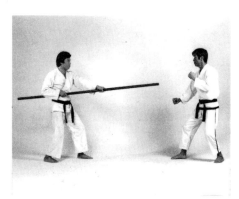

A: Point pole at D.

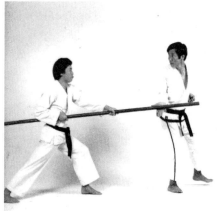
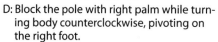

A: Move left foot forward while thrusting the pole toward D's umbilicus.

D: Block the pole with right palm while turning body counterclockwise, pivoting on the right foot.

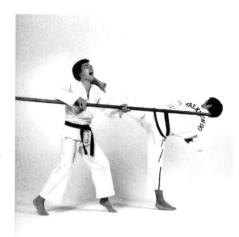

D: Execute a left reverse turning kick against A's post-auricular muscle.

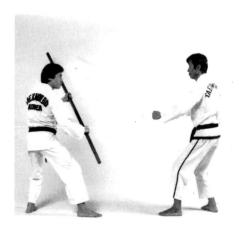

A: Hold pole facing D.

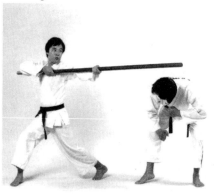

A: Move left foot forward while striking the pole horizontally inward toward D's neck.

D: Move left foot backward while bending over to dodge the pole.

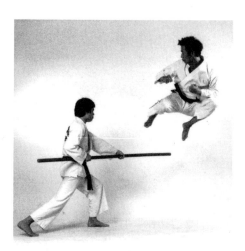

A: Strike the pole horizontally toward D's knee.

D: Jump up to dodge the pole.

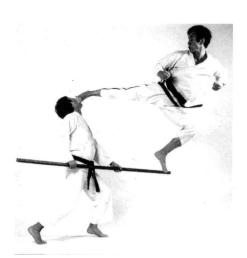

D: Execute a right flying side-snapping kick against A's jaw.

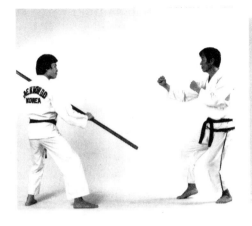

A: Hold pole facing D.

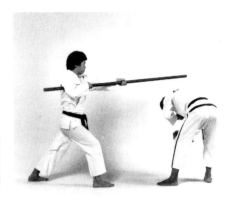

A: Move left foot forward while striking the pole horizontally inward toward D's neck.

D: Move the right foot backward while dodging the pole.

A: Move right foot forward while striking the pole horizontally toward D's neck.

D: Bend over to dodge the pole.

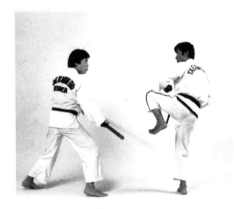

A: Prepare to strike horizontally.
D: Raise the left leg.

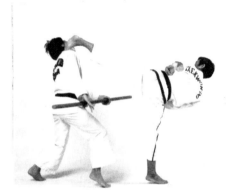

D: Execute a left turning kick against A's jaw.

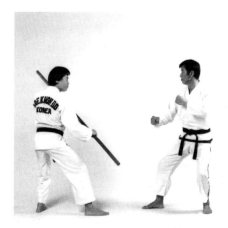

A: Hold pole facing D.

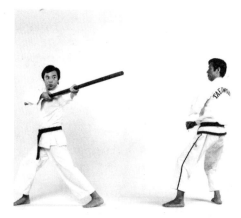

A: Move left foot forward while striking the pole horizontally toward D's head.

D: Move right foot backward while dodging the pole.

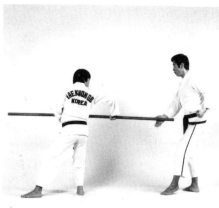

A: Move right foot backward and turn body clockwise, pivoting on left foot while thrusting the pole toward D's umbilicus.

D: Slide backward while blocking the pole with the right palm.

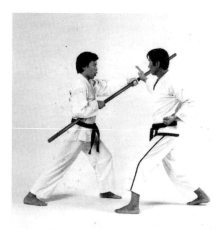

A: Move left foot forward and turn body clockwise pivoting on right foot while striking the pole diagonally downward toward D's shoulder.

D: Move right foot backward while blocking the pole with right palm.

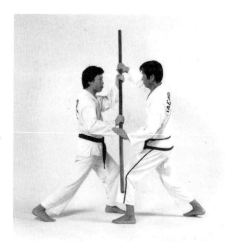

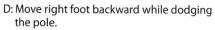

A: Strike with the pole diagonally upward toward D's ribs.

D: Grab the pole with the right hand while blocking the pole with the left arc-hand.

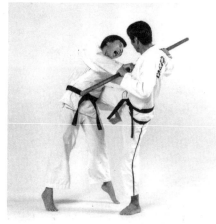

D: Execute a right knee kick against A's floating ribs.

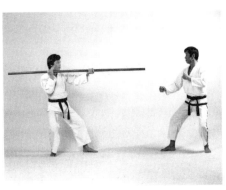

A: Point pole at D.

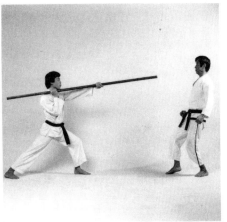

A: Move left foot forward while thrusting the pole toward D's face.

D: Slide backward while dodging the pole.

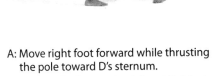

A: Move right foot forward while thrusting the pole toward D's sternum.

D: Move right foot to the right while blocking the pole with left palm.

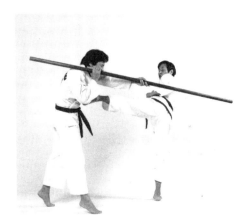

D: Execute a left turning kick against A's solar plexus.

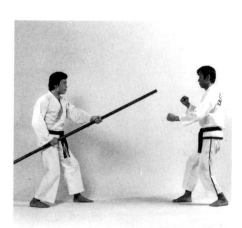

A: Point pole at D.

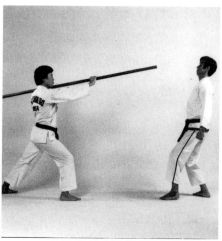

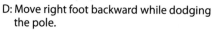

A: Move right foot forward while striking the pole vertically upward toward D's chin.

D: Move right foot backward while dodging the pole.

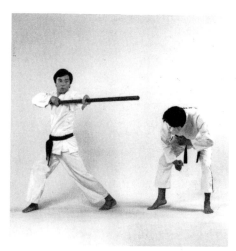

A: Move left foot forward while striking the pole horizontally toward D's neck.

D: Move the left foot backward while bending over to dodge the pole.

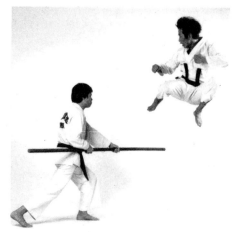

A: Strike with the pole horizontally toward D's knee.

D: Jump up to dodge the pole.

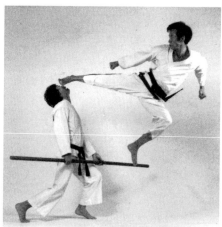

D: Execute a right flying side-snapping kick against A's face.

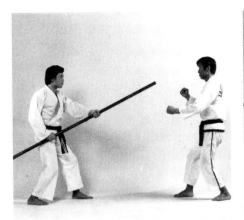

A: Point pole at D.

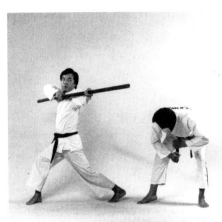

A: Move right foot forward while striking the pole vertically upward toward D's scrotum.

D: Move right foot backward while dodging the pole.

A: Move left foot forward while striking the pole horizontally inward toward D's neck.

D: Move left foot backward while bending body to dodge the pole.

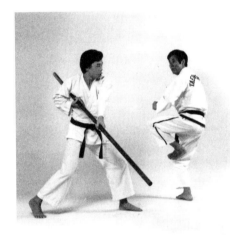

A: Prepare to strike diagonally upward.

D: Step to the right with right foot and raise left leg.

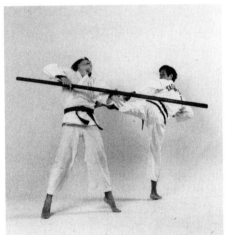

D: Execute a left side-snapping kick against A's kidney.

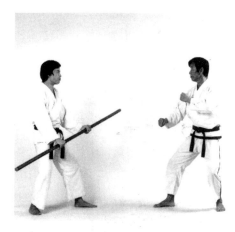

A: Hold pole facing D.

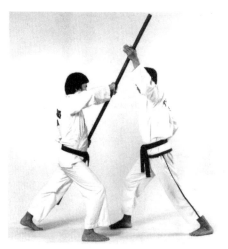

A: Move right foot forward while striking the pole diagonally downward toward D's shoulder.

D: Move right foot forward while blocking the pole with left arc-hand.

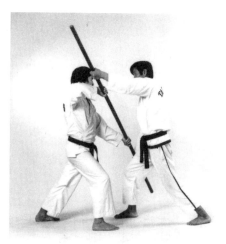

A: Strike diagonally upward with the pole toward D's knee.

D: Grab the pole with left hand while blocking the pole with right arc-hand.

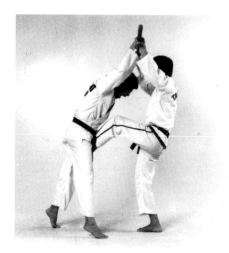

D: Pull up the pole while executing a left front snap kick against A's scrotum.

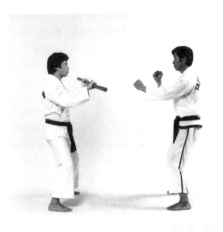

A: Hold pole facing D.

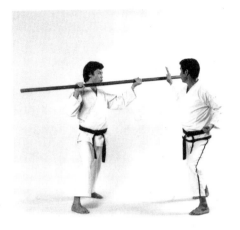

A: Strike horizontally inward with the pole toward D's neck while turning body clockwise pivoting on both feet.

D: Block the pole with right palm while turning body counterclockwise, pivoting on both feet.

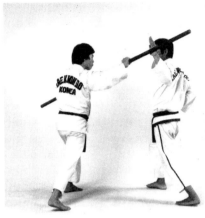

A: Strike horizontally inward with the pole toward D's neck while turning body counterclockwise, pivoting on both feet.

D: Block the pole with left palm while turning body clockwise pivoting on both feet.

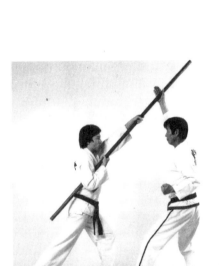

A: Move left foot forward while striking the pole vertically downward toward D's shoulder.

D: Move right foot backward while blocking the pole with right palm.

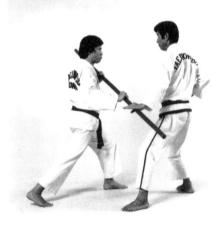

A: Strike diagonally upward with the pole toward D's ribs.

D: Move left foot to the left while blocking the pole with left palm.

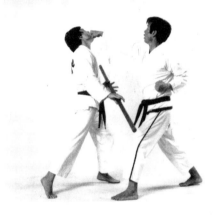

D: Execute a right punch against A's jaw.

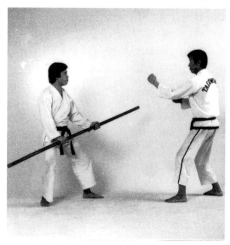

A: Hold pole facing D.

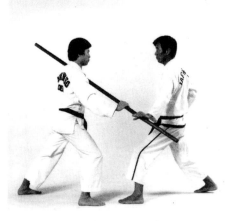

A: Move right foot forward while striking the pole diagonally upward toward D's ribs.

D: Move right foot backward while blocking the pole with left palm.

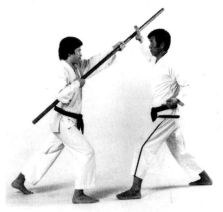

A: Strike diagonally downward with the pole toward D's shoulder.

D: Block the pole with right palm.

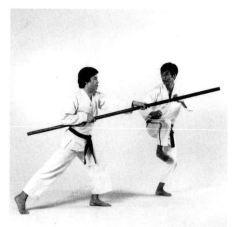

A: Move left foot forward while thrusting the pole toward D's epigastrium.

D: Move left foot backward while turning body counterclockwise, and raise the right leg.

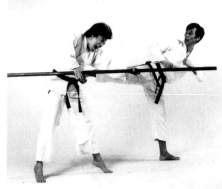

D: Execute a right side-snapping kick against A's floating ribs.

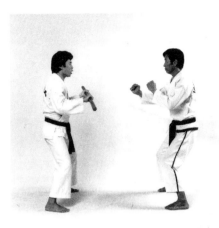

A: Hold pole facing D.

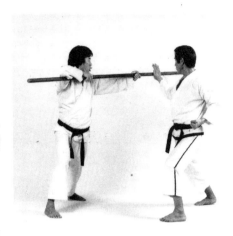

A: Strike the pole horizontally inward toward D's neck while turning body clockwise pivoting on both feet.

D: Block the pole with right palm while turning body counterclockwise, pivoting on both feet.

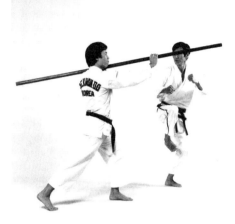

A: Move left foot forward while striking the pole vertically upward toward D's scrotum.

D: Move left foot backward while turning body counterclockwise, and raise the right leg.

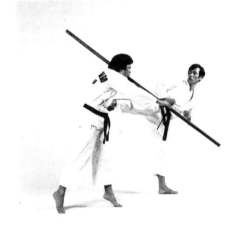

D: Execute a right side-snapping kick against A's floating ribs.

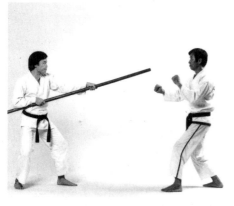

A: Point pole at D.

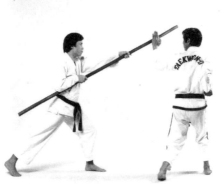

A: Move left foot forward while thrusting the pole toward D's face.

D: Block the pole with the left palm while turning body clockwise, pivoting on both feet.

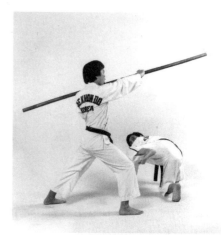

A: Move right foot forward while striking the pole diagonally upward toward D's kidney.

D: Dodge to the right and then support the body with both hands on the ground.

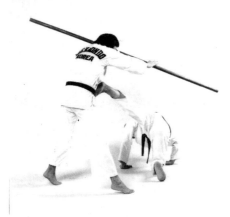

D: Execute a left side-snapping kick against A's floating ribs.

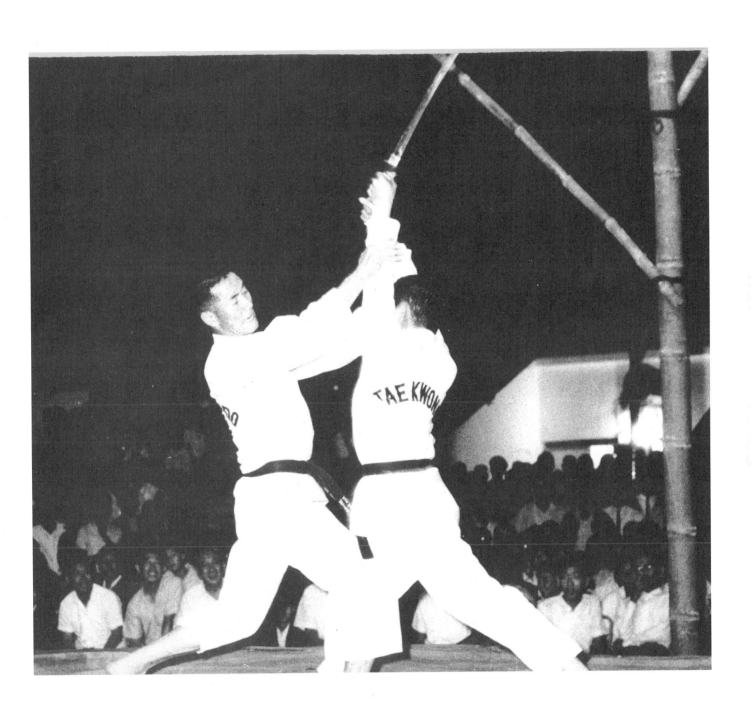

Defense Against a Sword Attack

The defender should use the same techniques when combating an attacker with a sword as for a knife attack or pole attack. However, the defender should keep a little more distance between himself and the attacker because it is more difficult to dodge a sword when it is in a sweeping motion. Sharp swords can be wielded easily by an attacker and they can cause more serious slashing wounds than a small knife, so the defender must show extra caution and judge his distance correctly.

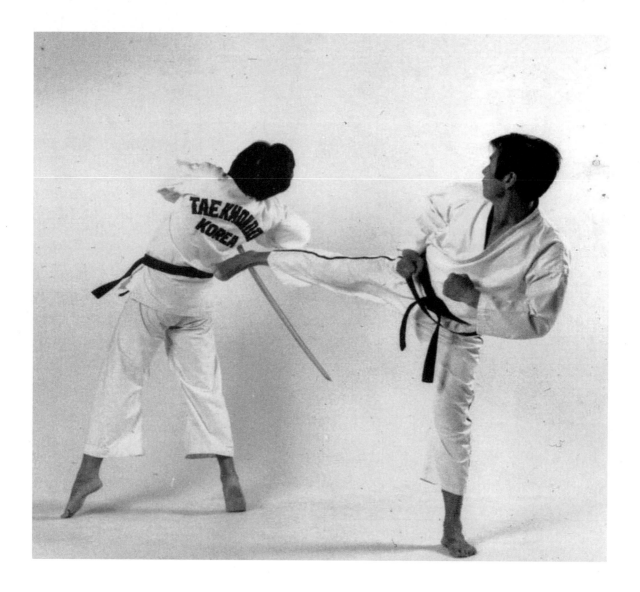

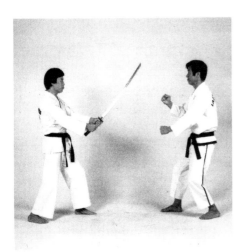

A: Point sword at D.

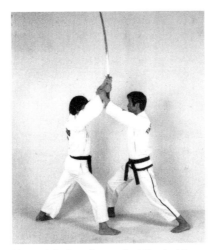

A: Move right foot forward while slashing the sword vertically downward toward D's head.

D. Move right foot forward while blocking A's arm with arc-hands.

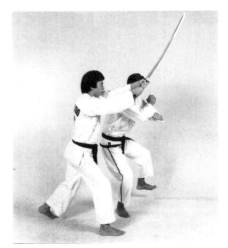

D. Prepare to strike while turning body counterclockwise, pivoting on right foot.

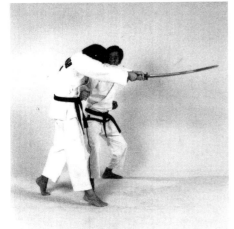

D. Execute a right back-fist strike against A's epigastrium.

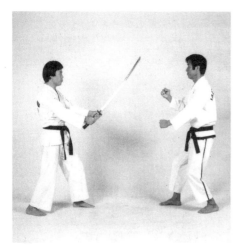

A: Point sword at D.

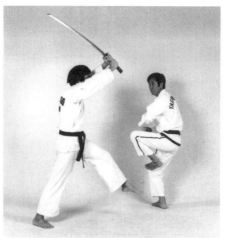

A: Move left foot forward while slashing the sword vertically downward toward D's head.

D: Step to the right with right foot and raise left leg.

D. Execute a left side-snapping kick against A's floating ribs.

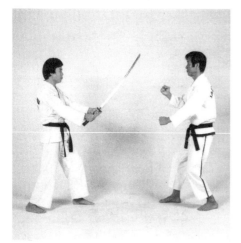

A: Point sword at D.

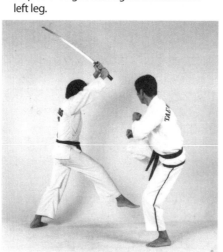

A: Move right foot forward while slashing the sword vertically downward toward D's head.

D: Step to the left with the left foot and raise the right leg.

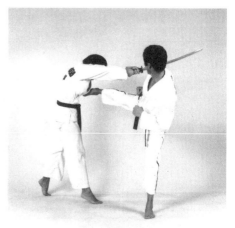

D. Execute a right turning kick against A's umbilicus.

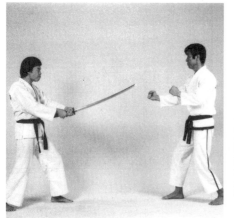

A: Point sword at D.

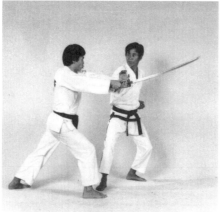

A: Move right foot forward while stabbing the sword toward D's face.

D: Exert a pushing block against A's arm with right palm while turning body counter-clockwise, pivoting on the right foot.

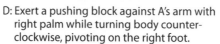

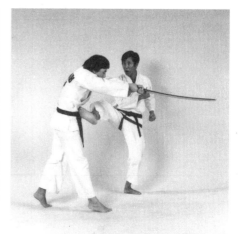

D: Execute a right twisting kick against A's umbilicus.

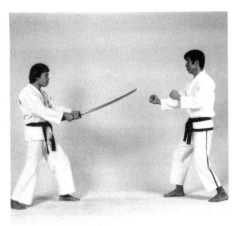

A: Point sword at D.

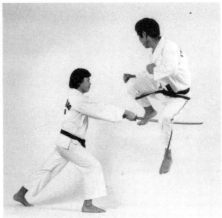

A: Move right foot forward while stabbing the sword toward D's umbilicus.

D: Jump to the left while dodging the sword.

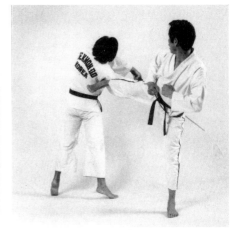

D: Land on left foot while executing right side-snapping kick against A's ribs.

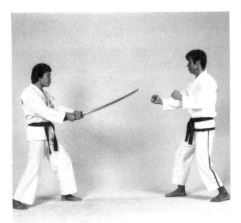

A: Point sword at D.

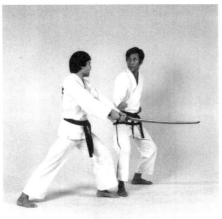

A: Move left foot forward while stabbing the sword toward D's sternum.

D: Exert strike-block against A's wrist with right side-fist while turning body counter-clockwise, pivoting on right foot.

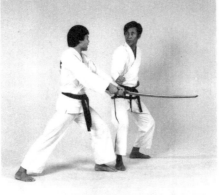

D: Execute a right back-fist strike against A's jaw.

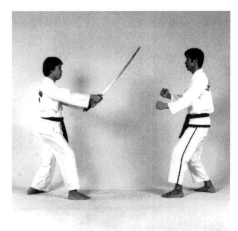

A: Point sword at D.

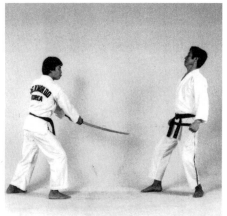

A: Slide forward while slashing the sword vertically downward toward D's head.

D: Move left foot backward while dodging the sword.

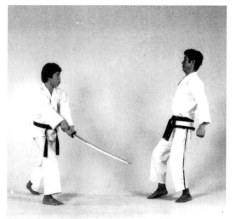

A: Slide forward while slashing the sword diagonally downward toward D's shoulder.

D: Slide backward while dodging the sword.

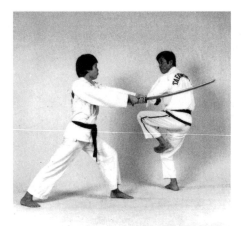
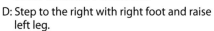

A: Move left foot forward while stabbing the sword toward D's umbilicus.

D: Step to the right with right foot and raise left leg.

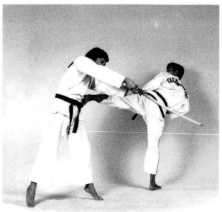

D: Execute a left side-snapping kick against A's floating ribs.

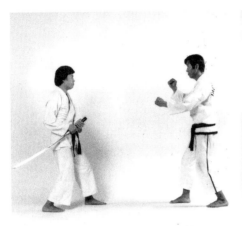

A: Hold sword facing D.

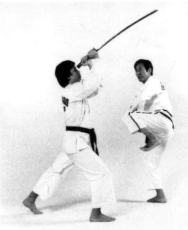
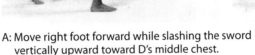

A: Move right foot forward while slashing the sword vertically upward toward D's middle chest.

D: Step to the right with right foot and raise left leg.

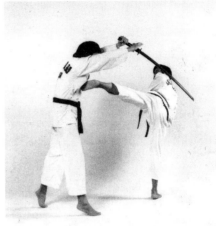

D: Execute a left turning kick against A's umbilicus.

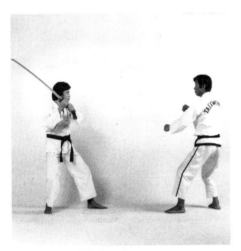

A: Hold sword facing D.

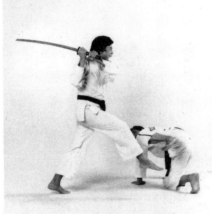
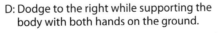

A: Move right foot forward while slashing the sword diagonally downward toward D's shoulder.

D: Dodge to the right while supporting the body with both hands on the ground.

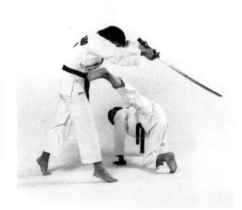

D: Execute a left turning kick against A's stomach.

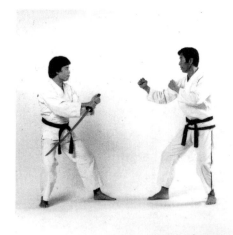

A: Hold sword facing D.

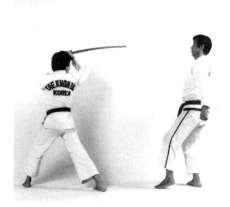

A: Move right foot forward while slashing the sword diagonally upward toward D's body.

D: Move right foot backward while dodging the sword.

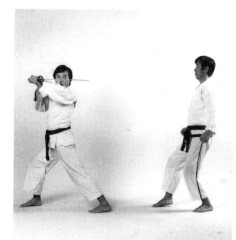

A: Move left foot forward while slashing the sword horizontally toward D's body.

D: Move left foot backward while dodging the sword.

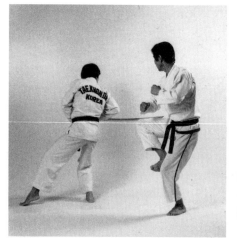

A: Move right foot backward while stabbing the sword toward D's stomach.

D: Step to the left with left foot and raise right leg.

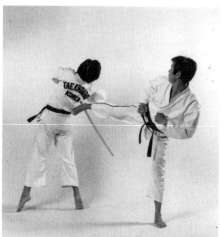

D: Execute a right side-snapping kick against A's kidney.

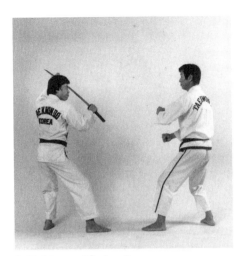

A: Hold sword facing D.

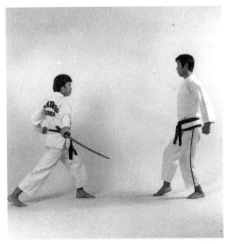

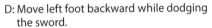

A: Move left foot forward while slashing the sword diagonally downward toward D's shoulder.

D: Move left foot backward while dodging the sword.

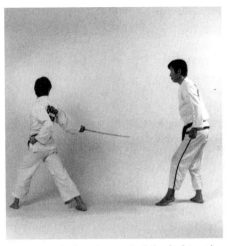

A: Move right foot forward while slashing the sword diagonally downward toward D's shoulder.

D: Move right foot backward while dodging the sword.

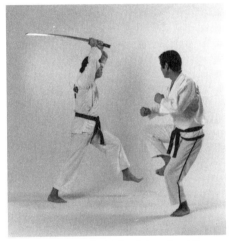

A: Hold the sword with both hands while moving left foot forward and slashing the sword vertically downward.

D: Step to the left with left foot and raise right leg.

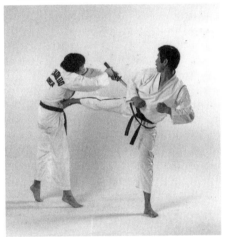

D: Execute a right side-snapping kick against A's floating ribs.

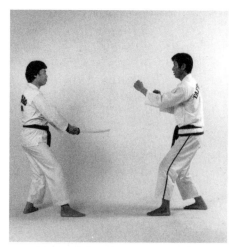

A: Hold sword facing D.

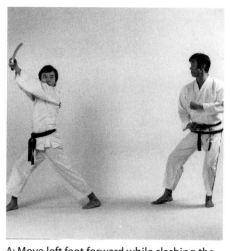

A: Move left foot forward while slashing the sword diagonally upward toward D's body.

D: Move left foot backward while dodging the sword.

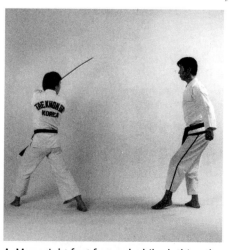

A: Move right foot forward while slashing the sword diagonally upward toward D's body.

D: Move right foot backward while dodging the sword.

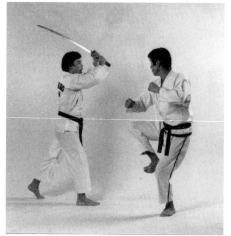

A: Prepare to slash downward.

D: Step to the left with left foot and raise right leg.

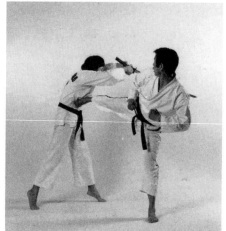

D: Execute a right side-snapping kick against A's floating ribs.

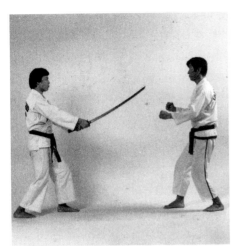

A: Hold sword facing D.

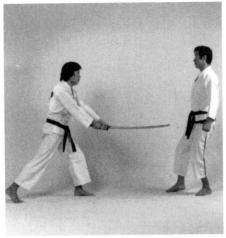

A: Slide forward while slashing the sword vertically downward toward D's head.

D: Slide backward while dodging the sword.

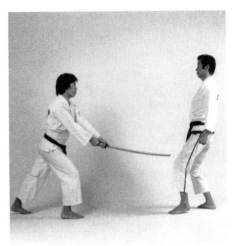

A: Move right foot forward while slashing the sword vertically downward toward D's head.

D: Move right foot backward while dodging the sword.

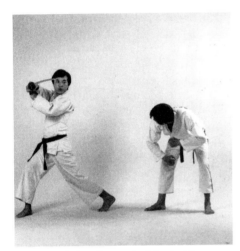

A: Move left foot forward while slashing the sword horizontally inward toward D's neck.

D: Move left foot backward while bending body to dodge the sword.

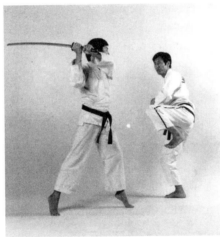

A: Prepare to slash downward.

D: Step to the right with right foot and raise left leg.

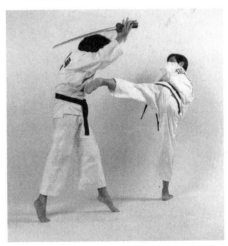

D: Execute a left turning kick against A's solar plexus.

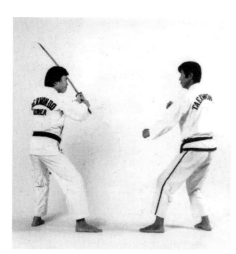

A: Hold sword facing D.

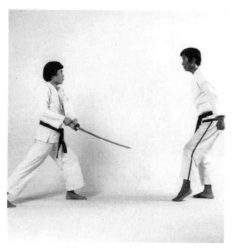

A: Move left foot forward while slashing the sword diagonally downward toward D's shoulder.

D: Slide backward while dodging the sword.

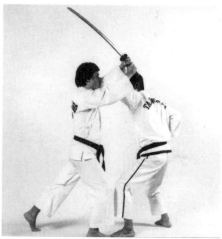

A: Move right foot forward while slashing the sword diagonally downward toward D's shoulder.

D: Move right foot to the right while blocking A's upper arm with left outer forearm.

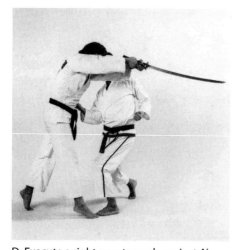

D: Execute a right upset punch against A's floating ribs.

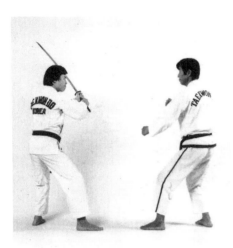

A: Hold sword facing D.

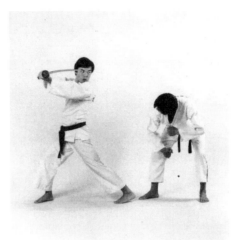

A: Move left foot forward while slashing the sword horizontally inward toward D's neck.

D: Move left foot backward while bending body to dodge the sword.

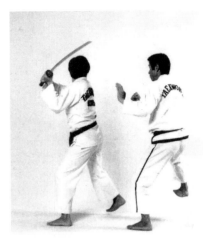

A: Turn body clockwise pivoting on left foot while preparing to slash.

D: Move right foot backward while preparing to block.

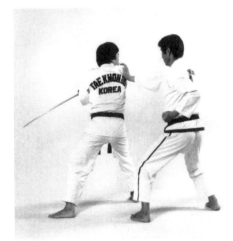

A: Slash with the sword diagonally upward toward D's body.

D: Push A's under shoulder with right palm.

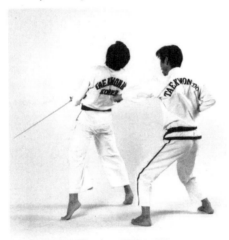

D: Execute a left fist-punch against A's kidney.

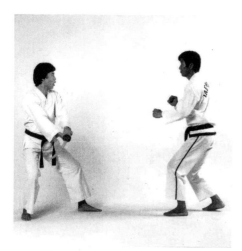

A: Hold sword facing D.

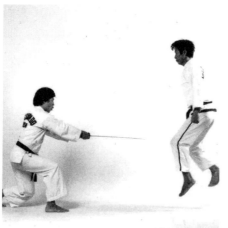

A: Move right foot forward while slashing the sword horizontally toward D's upper leg.

D: Jump backward while dodging the sword.

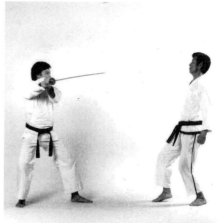

A: Move left foot forward while slashing the sword horizontally toward D's neck.

D: Move left foot backward while dodging the sword.

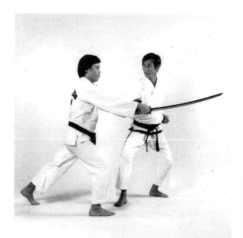

A: Move right foot forward while stabbing the sword toward D's epigastrium.

D: Exert pushing-block against A's arm with right palm while turning body counter-clockwise, pivoting on right foot.

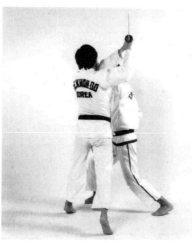

A: Move left foot to the left while slashing the sword diagonally toward D's body.

D: Move right foot to the right while blocking against A's upper arm with left outer forearm.

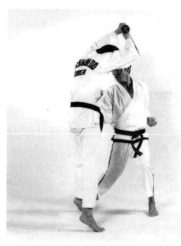

D: Execute a right upset punch against A's floating ribs.

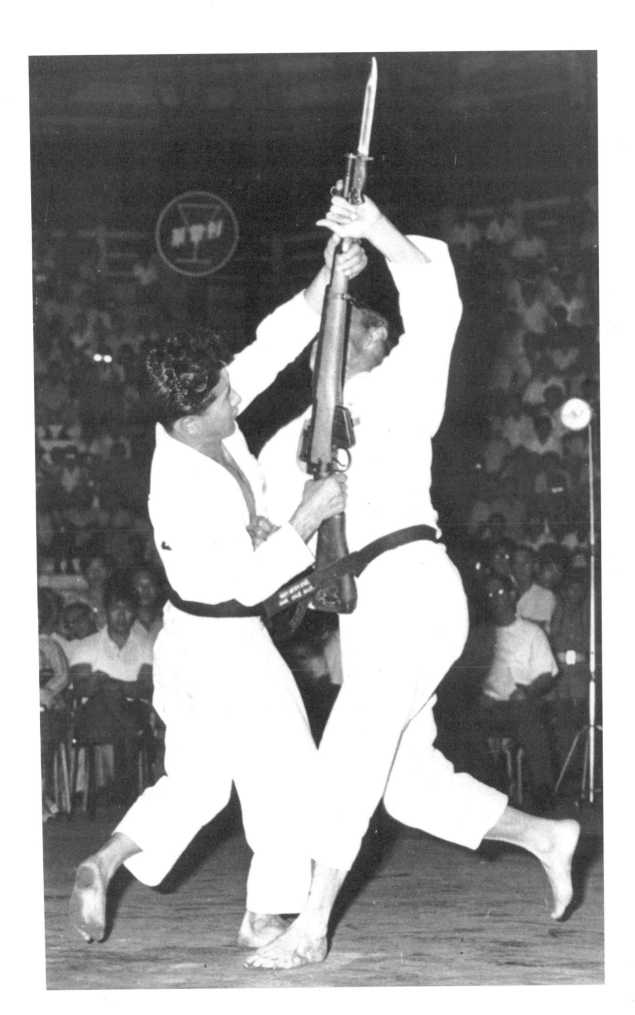

Defense Against a Bayonet Attack

Use of the bayonet is the sole dominion of the armed forces, but the defense techniques are generally identical to those defense techniques previously described in this book.

The palm-block or knife-hand block is an effective technique against the attacker who swings or thrusts his bayonet. Dodge sideways or away from the bayonet and block instantly with a palm-block or knife-hand, and then counterattack.

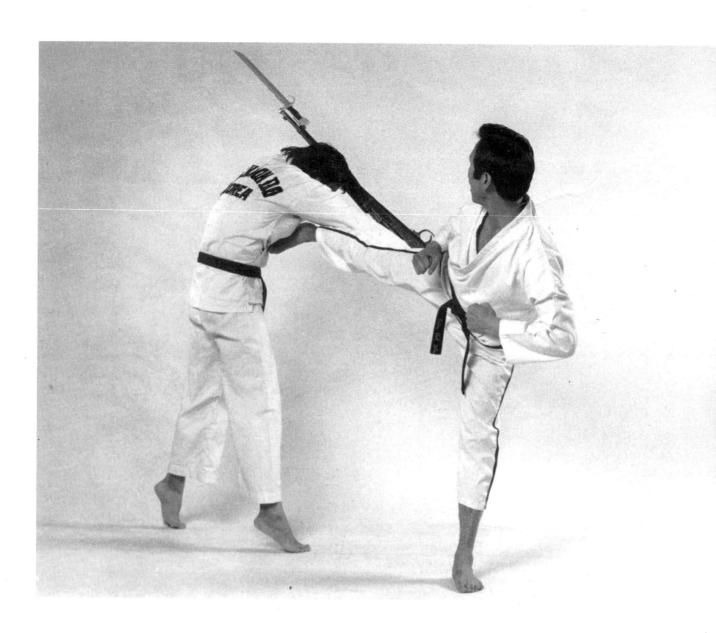

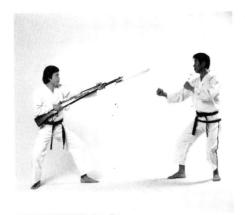

A: Point bayonet at D.

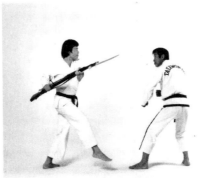
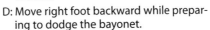

A: Move right foot forward while preparing to slash.

D: Move right foot backward while preparing to dodge the bayonet.

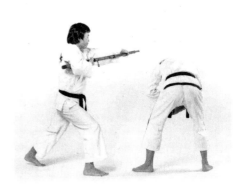

A: Slash the bayonet horizontally toward D's neck.

D: Bend body over to dodge the bayonet.

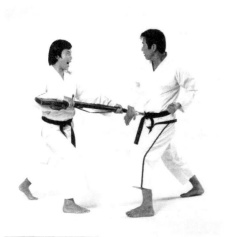

A: Slash the bayonet horizontally toward D's body.

D: Move left foot to the left while blocking barrel with right palm.

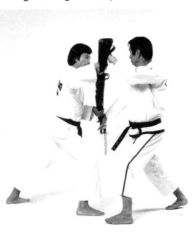

A: Strike with the butt end diagonally toward D's jaw.

D: Block the stack with left palm.

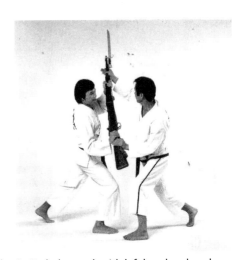

D: Grab the stock with left hand and push up with right hand while turning the rifle counterclockwise.

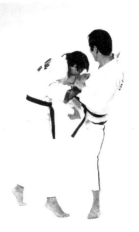

D: Execute a right knee kick against A's floating ribs.

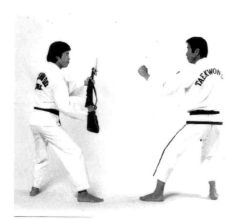

A: Hold rifle facing D.

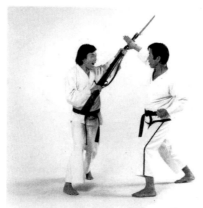

A: Slash the bayonet diagonally downward toward D's shoulder while turning body clockwise, pivoting on both feet.

D: Block the barrel with right palm while moving right foot backward.

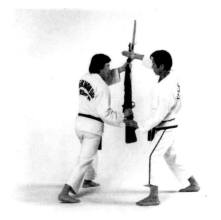

A: Strike with the butt end diagonally upward toward D's ribs.

D: Block the stack with the left palm.

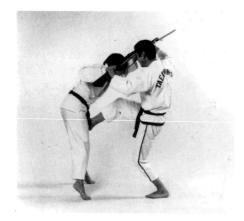

D: Execute a right front kick against A's groin.

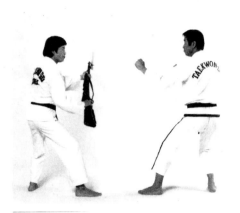

A: Hold rifle facing D.

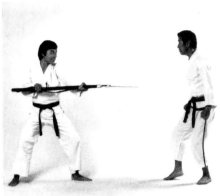

A: Move left foot forward while slashing the bayonet horizontally toward D's ribs.

D: Move left foot backward while dodging the bayonet.

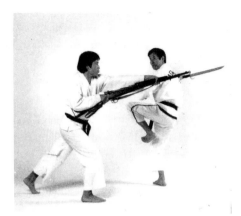

A: Move right foot forward while lunging the bayonet toward D's solar plexus.

D: Step to the right with right foot and raise left leg.

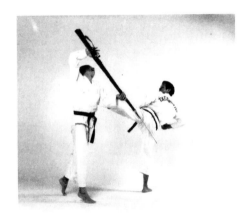

D: Execute a left side-snapping kick against A's armpit.

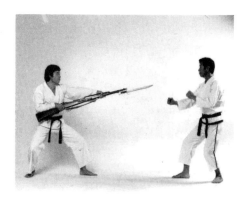

A: Point bayonet at D.

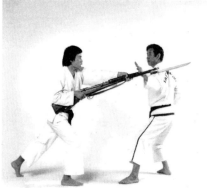

A: Move right foot forward while lunging the bayonet toward D's sternum.

D: Move right foot to the right while blocking the barrel with the left knife-hand.

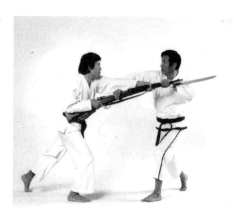

D: Grab the barrel with left hand and grab the stalk with right hand while preparing to kick.

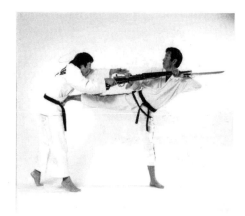

D: Pull the rifle backward while executing a right pushing kick against A's sternum.

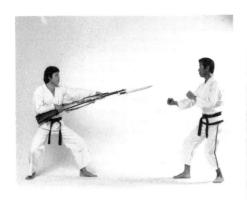

A: Point bayonet at D.

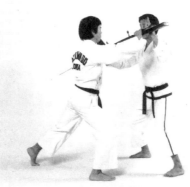

A: Move right foot forward while striking the butt end horizontally toward D's jaw.

D: Move right foot to the right while blocking the barrel with right palm and block the stalk with left palm.

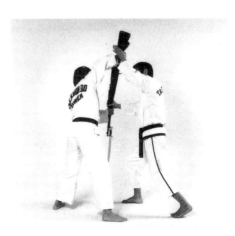

D: Grab the rifle with both hands and turn it clockwise.

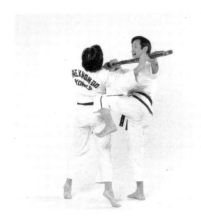

D: Execute a left knee kick against A's kidney.

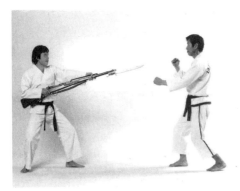

A: Point bayonet at D.

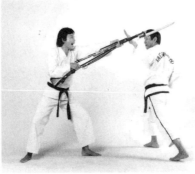

A: Slide forward while preparing to lunge.
D: Prepare to dodge backward.

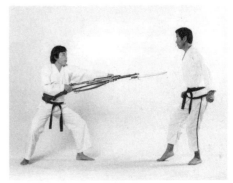

A: Slide forward while lunging the bayonet toward D's epigastrium.
D: Slide backward while dodging the bayonet.

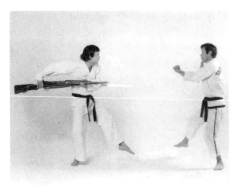

A: Slide forward while preparing to lunge.
D: Prepare to dodge to the right.

A: Slide forward while lunging the bayonet toward D's windpipe.
D: Move right foot to the right while blocking the barrel with left knife-hand.

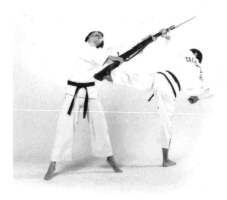

D: Grab the barrel with left hand while executing a left side-snapping kick against A's ribs.

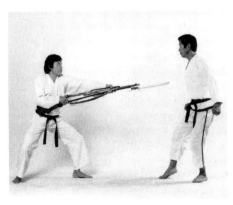

A: Point bayonet at D.

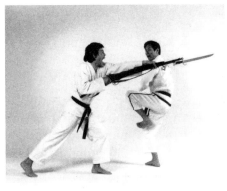

A: Move left foot forward while lunging the bayonet toward D's solar plexus.

D: Step to the right with right foot and raise left leg.

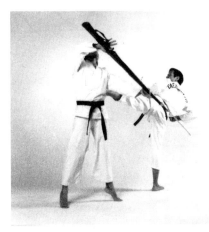

D: Execute a left side-snapping kick against A's ribs.

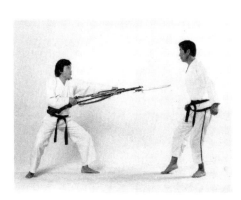

A: Point bayonet at D.

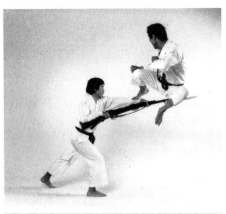

A: Move right foot forward while lunging the bayonet toward D's solar plexus.

D: Jump to the left to dodge the bayonet.

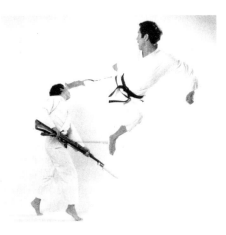

D: Execute a right flying side-snapping kick against A's jaw.

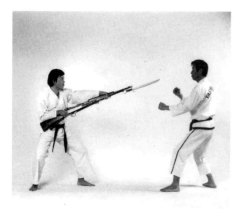

A: Point bayonet at D.

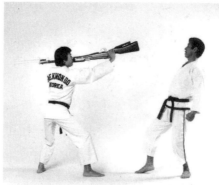

A: Move right foot forward while striking the butt end diagonally upward toward D's jaw.

D: Move left foot backward while dodging the butt end.

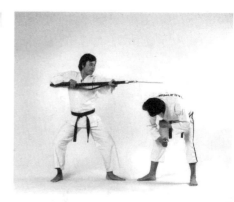

A: Move left foot forward while slashing the bayonet horizontally inward toward D's neck.

D: Bend body to dodge the bayonet.

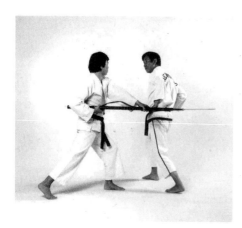

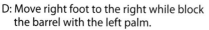

A: Slash horizontally outward toward D's body.

D: Move right foot to the right while block the barrel with the left palm.

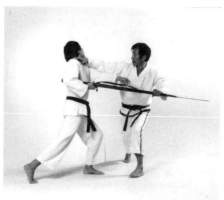

D: Grab and pull the barrel with the left hand and hold A's neck with right hand.

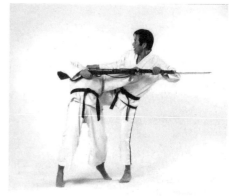

D: Pull A's neck with right hand while executing a right knee kick against A's ribs.

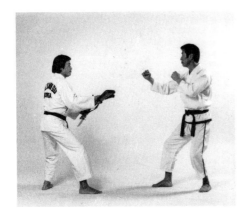

A: Hold rifle facing D.

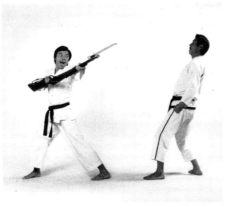

A: Move left foot forward while slashing the bayonet diagonally inward toward D's ribs.

D: Move right foot backward while dodging the bayonet.

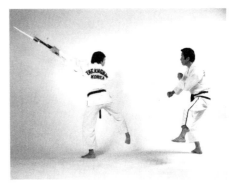

A: Turn body clockwise, pivoting on left foot and prepare to strike with the butt end.

D: Move left foot to the left while preparing to dodge to the left.

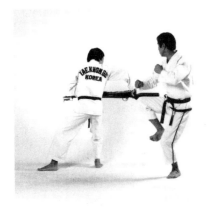

A: Move right foot backward while striking the butt end toward D's solar plexus.

D: Step to the left with left foot and raise right leg.

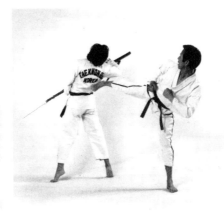

D: Execute a right side kick against A's kidney.

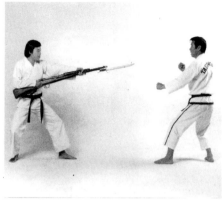

A: Point rifle facing D.

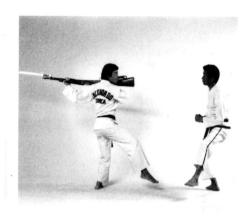

A: Move right foot forward while striking the butt end vertically upward toward D's chin.

D: Slide backward while dodging the butt end.

A: Raise right leg and prepare to strike with the butt end.

D: Prepare to dodge to the left.

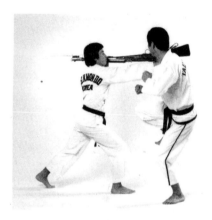

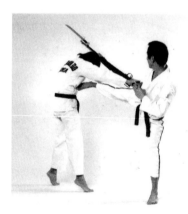

A: Slide forward while striking the butt end toward D's face.

D: Step to the left with left foot and raise right leg.

D: Execute a right turning kick against A's epigastrium.

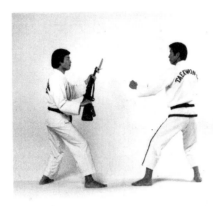

A: Hold bayonet facing D.

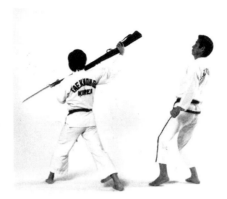

A: Move right foot forward while striking the butt end diagonally upward toward D's ribs.

D: Slide backward while dodging the butt end.

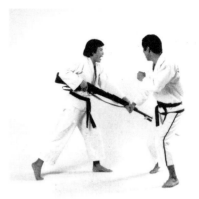

A: Move left foot forward while slashing the bayonet vertically downward toward D's head.

D: Shift to the left while dodging the bayonet.

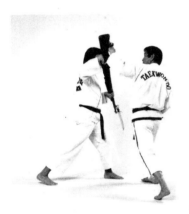

A: Strike with the butt end diagonally inward toward D's neck.

D: Block the stock with the left palm.

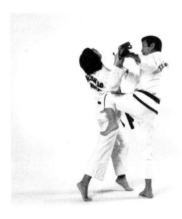

D: Grab rifle with both hands while executing left knee kick against A's ribs.

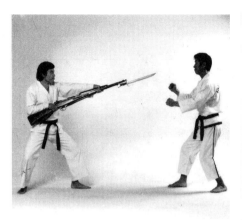

A: Point bayonet at D.

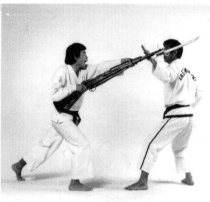

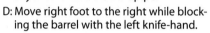

A: Move right foot forward while lunging the bayonet toward D's windpipe.

D: Move right foot to the right while blocking the barrel with the left knife-hand.

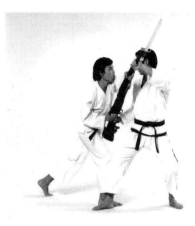

D: Grab and push the barrel with left hand, and grab and pull the stock with right hand while moving right foot forward.

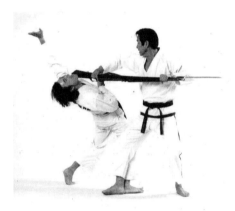

D: Strike with the butt end against A's left armpit.

How to Release an Attacker of a Pistol

Remember that a pistol-wielding attacker is usually very excited and could discharge the weapon even if he only intends to scare the defender. Distraction is a useful method of gaining time for the defender to get into position from which to counterattack. The defender should give the appearance that he is very calm and slowly move his body away from the direction the attacker's pistol is pointing so as to reduce the target area. The defender must be close enough to the attacker to be able to kick or knock the attacker's pistol away: so careful calculation of the distance is very important. To strike the attacker's wrist should be sufficient to make him drop it, or at least it will deflect the direction in which the pistol is pointing, enabling the defender to counterattack with further kicks or blows.

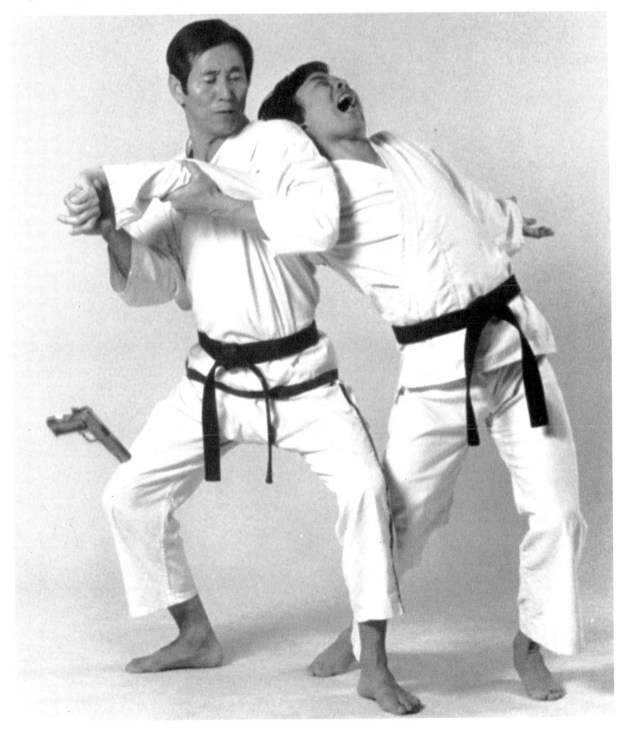

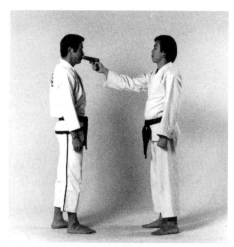

A: Point pistol at D's philtrum.

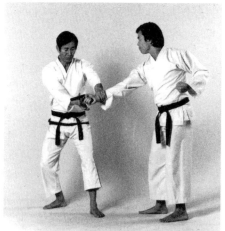

D: Grab A's arm with left hand and move right foot backward while turning body clockwise pivoting on left foot.

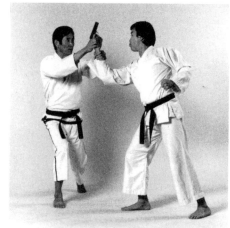

D: Grab A's hand with right hand while moving left foot backward.

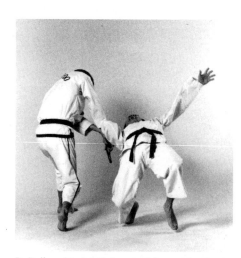

D: Pull and twist A's hand while turning body counterclockwise, pivoting on both feet.

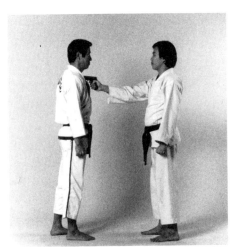

A: Point pistol at D's windpipe.

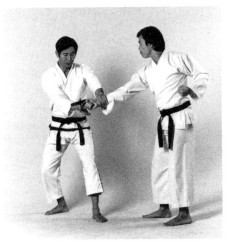

D: Grab A's arm with left hand and move right foot backward while turning body clockwise pivoting on left foot.

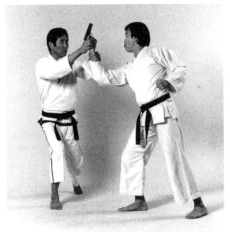

D: Grab A's hand with right hand while moving left foot backward.

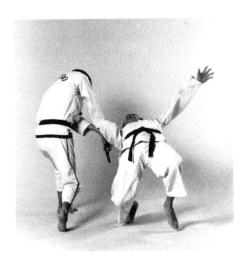

D: Pull and twist A's hand while turning body counterclockwise, pivoting on both feet.

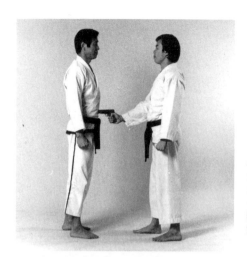

A: Point pistol as D's solar plexus.

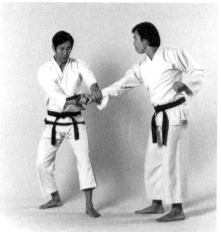

D: Grab A's arm with left hand and move right foot backward while turning body clockwise pivoting on left foot.

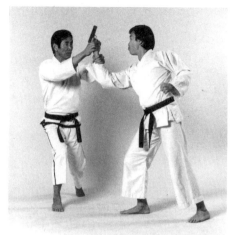

D: Grab A's hand with right hand while moving left foot backward.

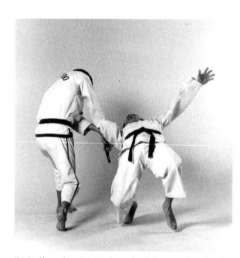

D: Pull and twist A's hand while turning body counterclockwise, pivoting on both feet.

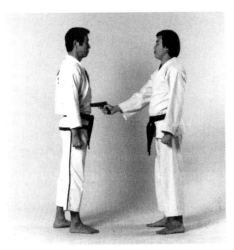

A: Point pistol at D's solar plexus.

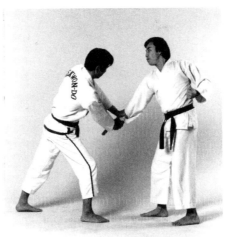

D: Grab A's arm with right hand and move left foot backward while turning body counterclockwise, pivoting on right foot.

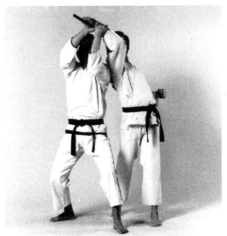

D: Grab A's arm with both hands and raise A's arm while moving left foot forward.

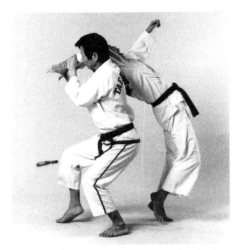

D: Pull and twist A's arm while turning body clockwise pivoting on both feet.

141 / How to Release an Attacker of a Pistol

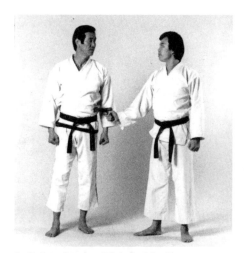

A: Point pistol at D's left side ribs.

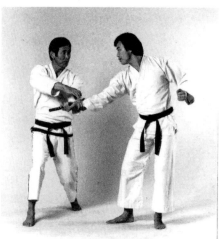

D: Grab A's arm with left hand while moving moving left foot backward.

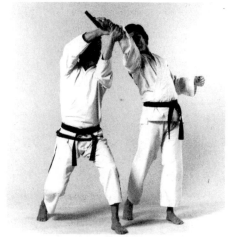

D: Grab and raise A's arm with both hands while moving left foot forward.

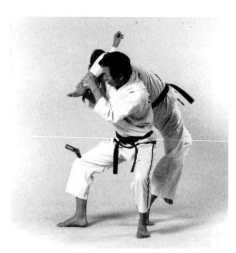

D: Pull A's arm while turning body clockwise, pivoting on both feet.

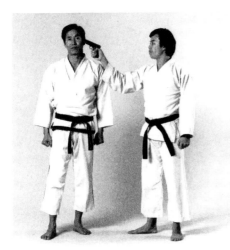

A: Point pistol at D's left temple.

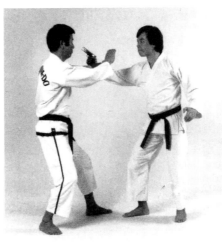

D: Grab A's arm with left hand while moving right foot forward and turn body counter-clockwise.

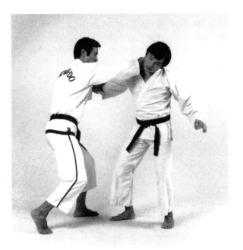

D: Pull A's arm with left hand while holding A's neck with right hand.

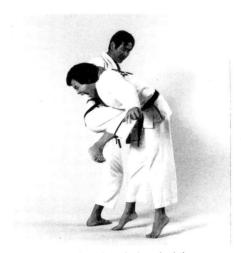

D: Pull A's neck with right hand while executing right knee kick against A's stomach.

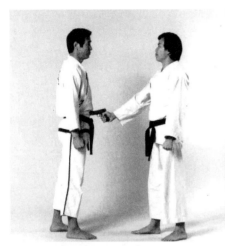

A: Point pistol at D's stomach.

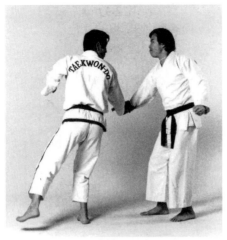

D: Grab and push A's arm with right hand and move left foot backward while turning body counterclockwise, pivoting on right foot.

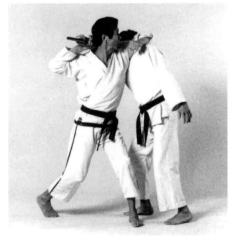

D: Pull A's arm with right hand while executing a left side-elbow strike against A's jaw.

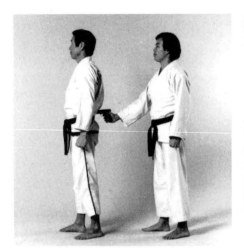

A: Point pistol at D's lower back.

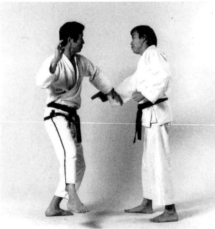

D: Strike block at A's arm with left knife-hand while turning body counterclockwise, pivoting on left foot.

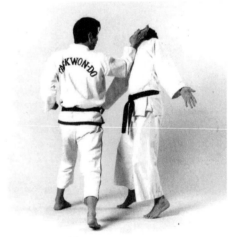

D: Execute a right knife-hand strike against A's neck.

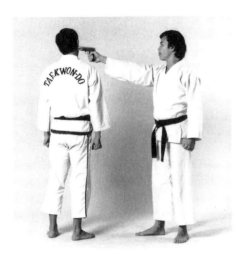

A: Point pistol at D's right temple.

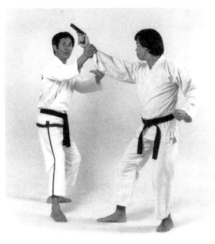

D: Grab and raise A's arm with right hand while moving left foot forward.

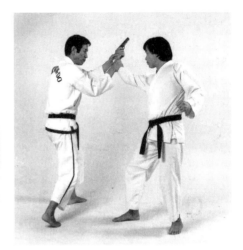

D: Grab A's hand with both hands while moving right foot backward.

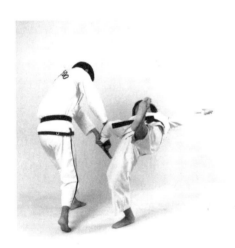

D: Pull and flex A's hand upward and inward.

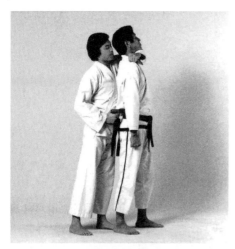

A: Lock D's neck from behind with left arm and point pistol at D's kidney.

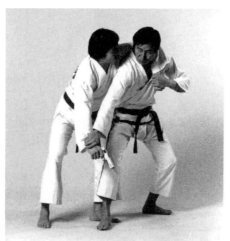

D: Grab and pull downward A's left arm with left hand, and grab and push A's right wrist with right hand while moving left foot to the left.

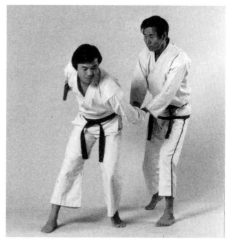

D: Move right foot backward and turn body clockwise, pivoting on left foot while grabbing and twisting A's hand with both hands.

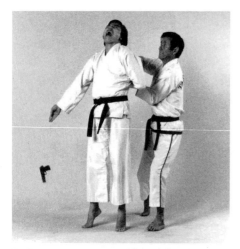

D: Continue to twist and flex A's hand upward and inward.

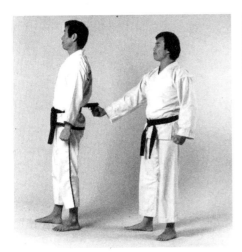

A: Point pistol at D's lower back.

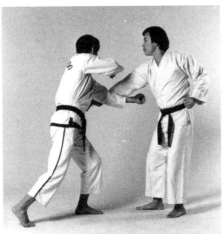

D: Move right foot forward and turn body counterclockwise, pivoting on left foot while blocking A's arm with left forearm.

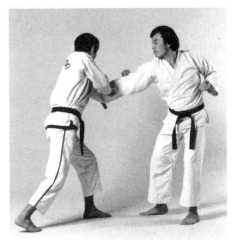

D: Grab A's hand with right hand and lock A's arm with left arm.

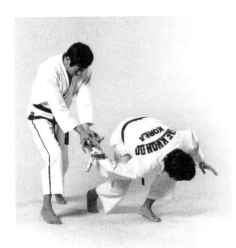

D: Grab and pull A's hand with both hands while moving left foot backward and flex A's hand upward and inward.

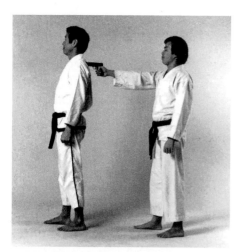

A: Point pistol at D's upper back.

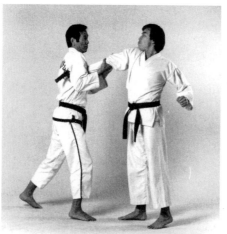

D: Turn body clockwise, pivoting on right foot, and move left foot forward while locking A's arm with right upper arm.

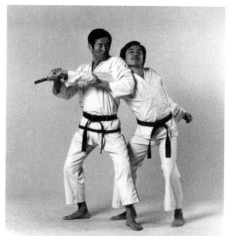

D: Lock A's elbow with left forearm and grab A's hand with right hand while moving left foot forward.

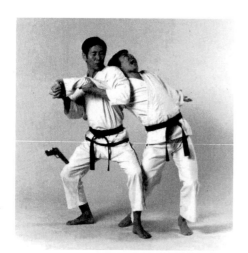

D: Raise A's elbow with left forearm while pulling downward A's hand with right hand.

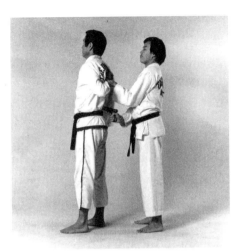

A: Grab and twist D's left arm upward from behind with left hand and point pistol at D's kidney.

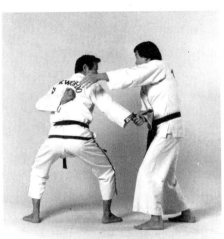

D: Exert pushing block at A's arm with right arc-hand while moving left foot forward and turn body clockwise.

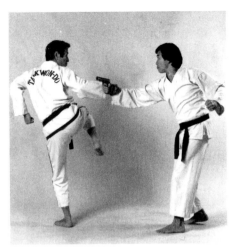

D: Grab and pull A's arm with right hand and raise right leg.

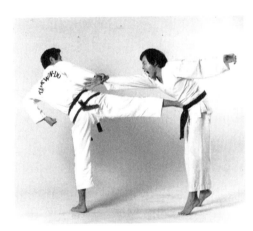

D: Execute a pushing kick against A's stomach.

Defense Against a Pistol

The difficulty in defending against a pistol is enormous, especially when the distance between the gunman and the victim is wide. Thus, we would have to be realistic and cautious in our timing and movements, and to counterattack with the greatest possible speed at the precise moment. To counterattack when two steps away from the gunman is already dangerous. When one step away, only then is it quite possible to, first, steer away from the direction the pistol is pointing, and then either knock the gun from his hand or give powerful kicks or quick blows to his body.

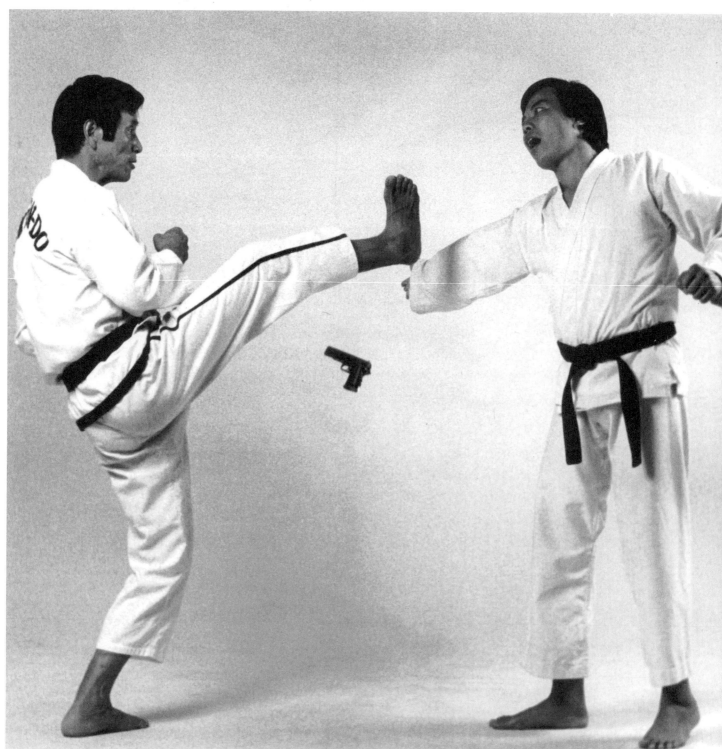

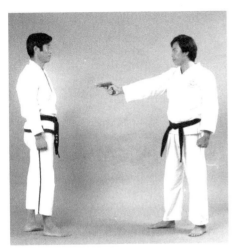

A: Face D and hold pistol in right hand.

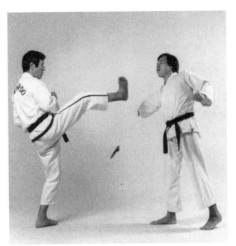

D: Execute a right crescent kick at A's arm.

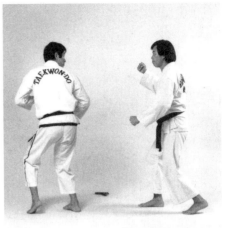

D: Lower the right foot in front of the left foot and prepare to kick.

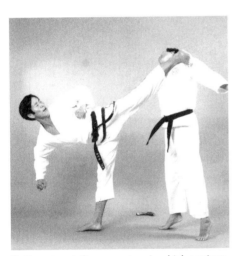

D: Execute a left reverse turning kick against A's neck.

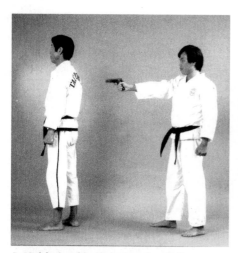

A: Hold pistol in right hand pointing against D's neck.

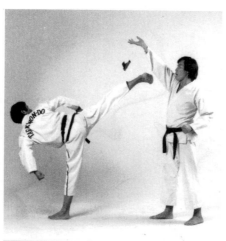

D: Execute a right back side rising kick at A's elbow while turning body clockwise.

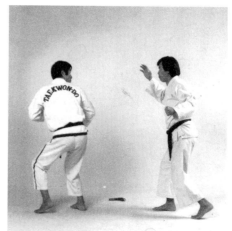

D: Lower the right foot in front of left foot and prepare to kick.

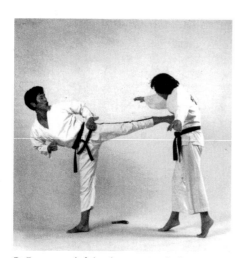

D: Execute a left back snapping kick against A's solar plexus.

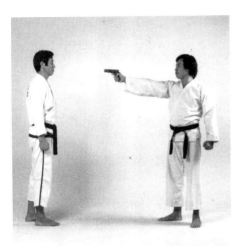

A: Face D and hold pistol in right hand.

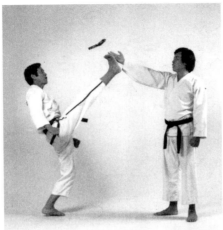

D: Execute a right front snap kick at A's arm.

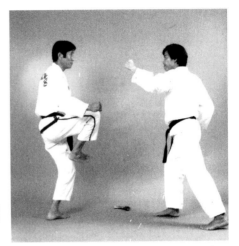

D: Return the right foot to a position beside the left knee and prepare to kick.

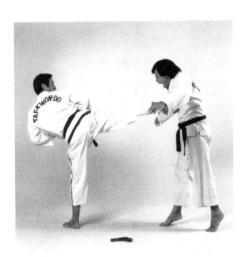

D: Execute a right side-snapping kick against A's solar plexus.

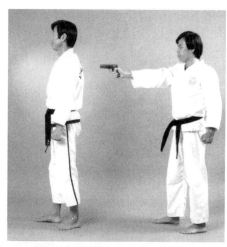

A: Hold pistol in right hand pointing at D's back.

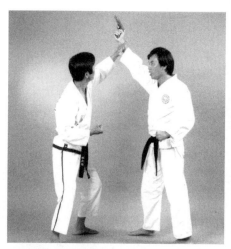

D: Exert pushing block at A's arm with left knife-hand and bend body to the left while turning body counterclockwise, pivoting on left foot.

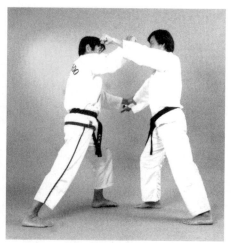

A: Execute a left punch at D's face.
D: Block A's arm with right outer forearm

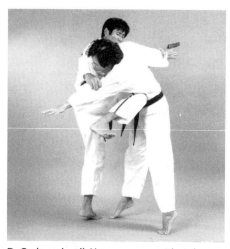

D: Grab and pull A's upper arm with right hand while executing right knee kick against A's floating ribs.

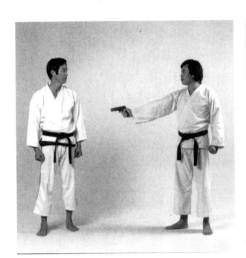

A: Hold pistol in right hand pointing at D's side body.

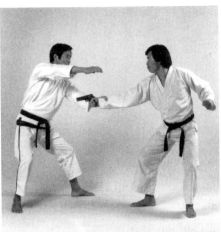

D: Grab and push A's arm with left hand while moving left foot to the left side.

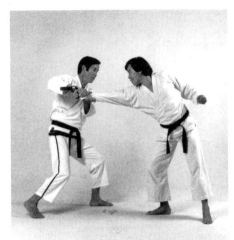

D: Grab A's arm with right hand while pulling A's arm with both hands.

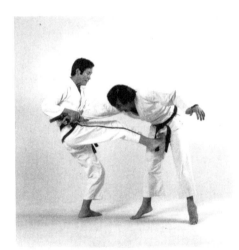

D: Execute a right front snap kick against A's groin.

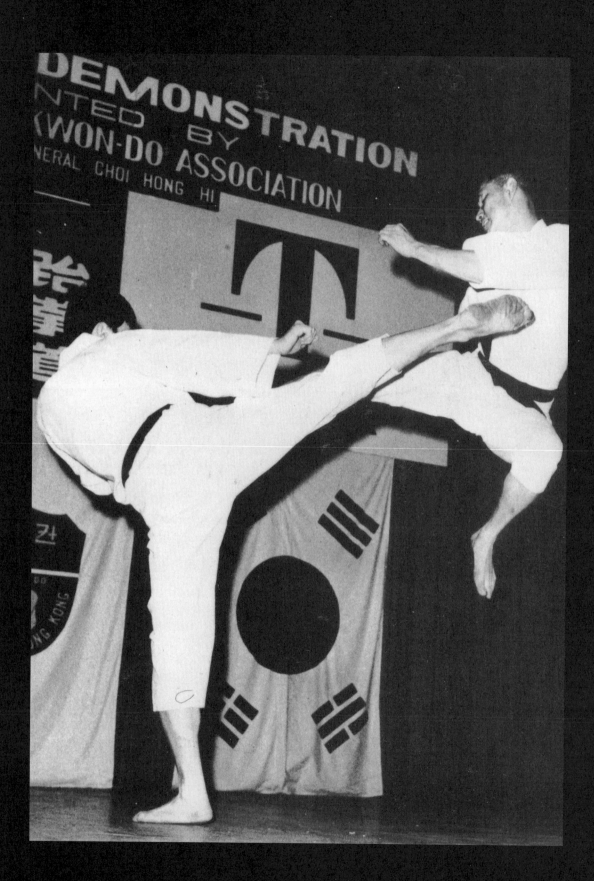

CHAPTER 3
SPARRING

The taekwondo trainee should not move to sparring until he masters the basic taekwondo moves to the point where they can be used instinctively not only to execute simple taekwondo fundamental movements, but also to effectively apply both offensive and defensive moves in sparring.

The sparring position is somewhat different from the fighting positions of boxing, wrestling, or judo, in that it utilizes the fingertips, palm-heel, knife-edge, elbow, and many varied foot techniques. In addition, many defensive techniques are also applied in order to protect the numerous vulnerable parts of the body. Most of all, the combination of powerful hand and foot attacks requires a strong body posture and balance, and the effective use of defensive moves along with offensive moves requires full coordination and exceptional balance to be advantageously executed in sparring.

The offensive-defensive integration is essential for perfect defense because it is difficult to stop a continuous offense with the defensive move alone. Your defensive move combined with your counterattack can easily stop the attacker from succeeding with his continuous attacks and put him into a defensive position.

The exercise is performed under the assumption that the attacker (A) and the defender (D) stand on line EW facing each other.

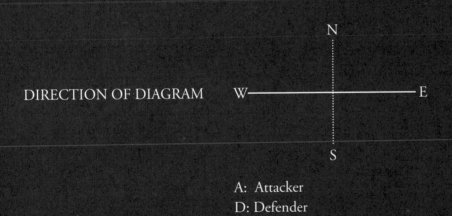

DIRECTION OF DIAGRAM

A: Attacker
D: Defender

For the reader's convenience, each exercise sequence in this chapter begins with a bolded caption.

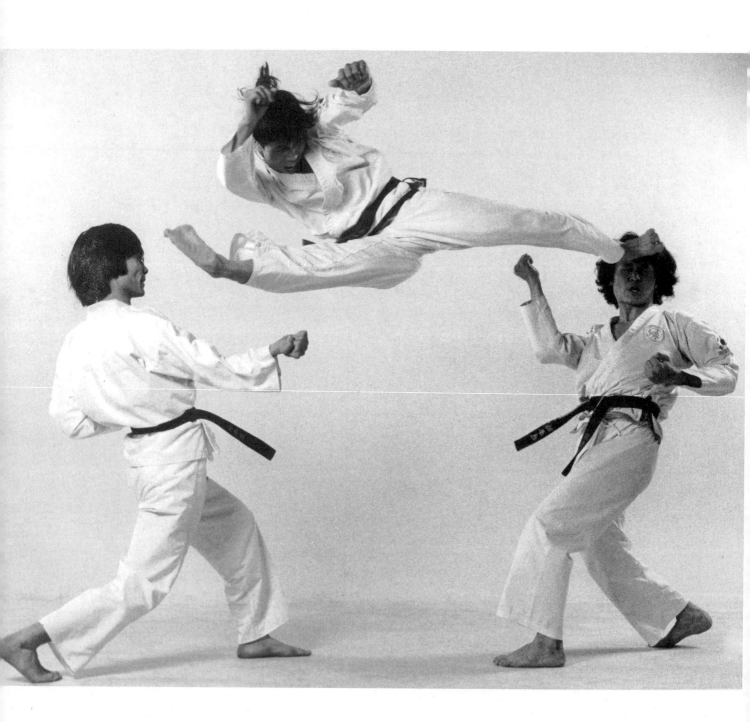

How to Release from a Grab

There are quite a few techniques you can learn so you can release yourself from an attacker's grab, but to effectively apply them requires an understanding of the posture, balance, and mobile forces of the attacker. The defender should endeavor to make use of the attacker's momentum and his instinctive pulling motion by pushing the grabbing hand or any other technique that aims to cancel the attacker's span of control.

With arms and legs moving at the same time, grab with both hands the grabbing hand of the attacker and exert pressure at his hand's weak points. Immediately twist the attacker's hand while executing a truncal twist simultaneously so that that additional strength is added to throw the attacker off balance.

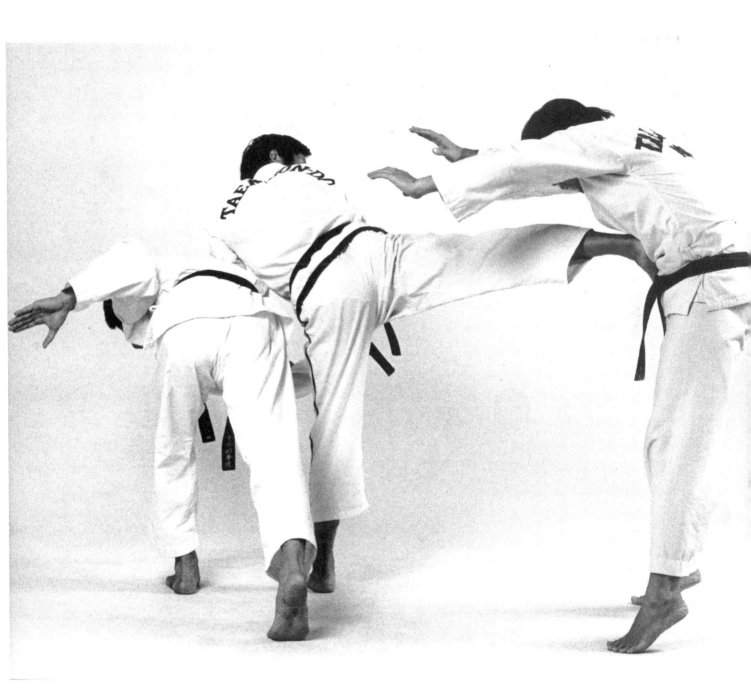

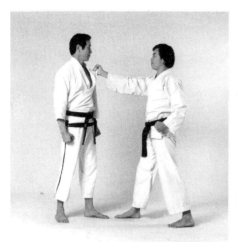

A: Grab D's clothes on left shoulder from front with right hand.

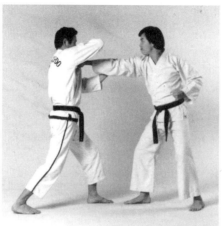

D: Grab A's hand and hold A's elbow with left hand while moving right foot backward.

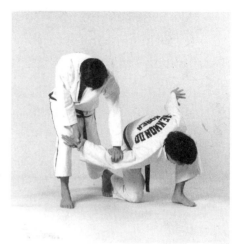

D: Press and twist A's thenar with right thumb while pressing downward A's elbow joint and turn body clockwise pivoting on both feet.

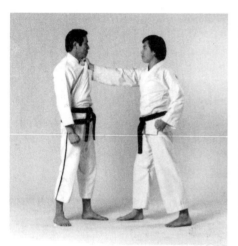

A: Grab D's collar from front with right hand.

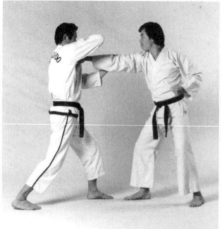

D: Grab A's hand and hold A's elbow with left hand while moving right foot backward.

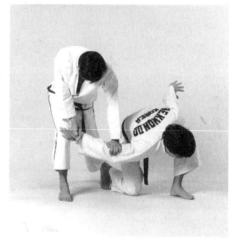

D: Press and twist A's thenar with right thumb while pressing downward A's elbow joint and turn body clockwise pivoting on both feet.

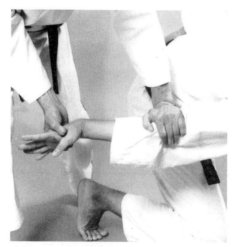

Close-up of press and twist.

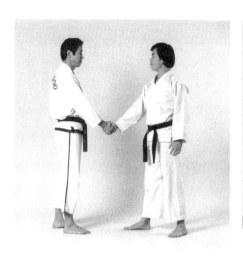

A: Grab D's right hand from front with right hand.

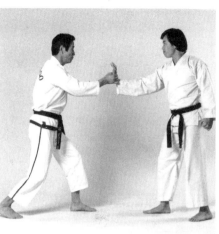

D: Pull and push up right hand and grab A's hand with both hands while moving right foot backward.

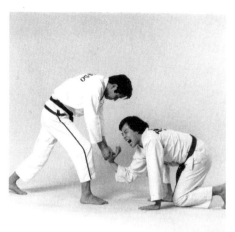

D: Pull and flex A's wrist upward and inward.

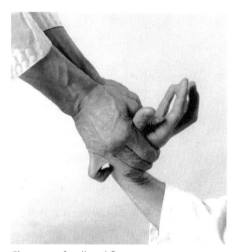

Close-up of pull and flex.

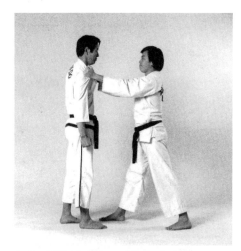

A: Grab D's clothes on both shoulders from front.

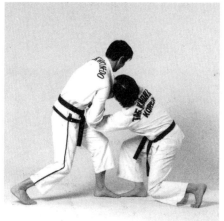

D: Lock A's right elbow joint with left arm and pull while moving right foot backward.

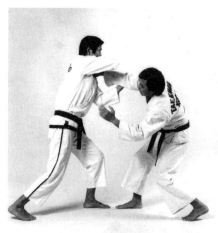

D: Grab A's right hand with right hand and hold A's elbow with left hand.

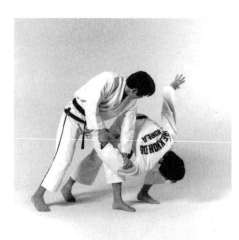

D: Press and twist A's thenar with right thumb while pressing downward A's elbow joint and turn body clockwise, pivoting both feet.

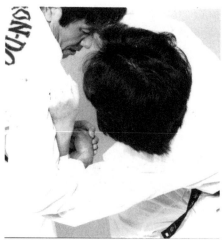

Close-up of lock, pull, and grab.

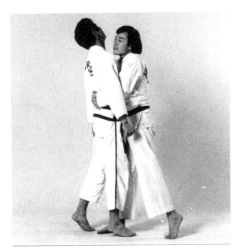

A: Hold D's waist from front with both arms.

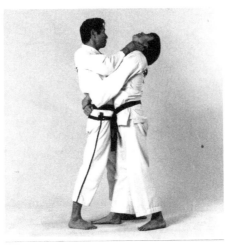

D: Grab A's neck with right arc-hand and hold A's back ribs with left hand.

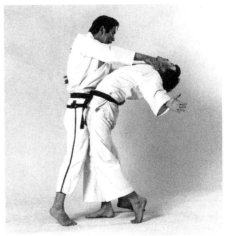

D: Push A's neck with right hand while moving left foot forward.

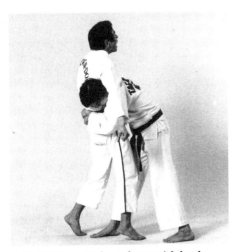

A: Hold D's waist from front with both arms.

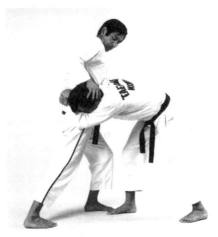

D: Hold A's post-auricular muscle with right middle finger.

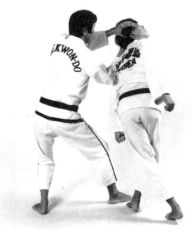

D: Press A's post-auricular muscle and hold A's head with left hand while moving right foot forward.

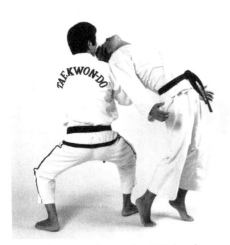

D: Continue pressing and pull A's head downward while turning body counter-clockwise.

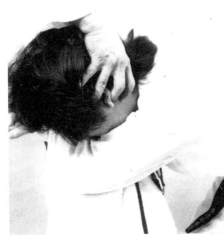

Close-up of press and hold.

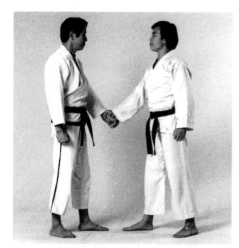

A: Grab D's left hand from front with right hand.

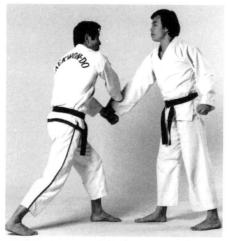

D: Grab A's hand with right hand while moving right foot backward.

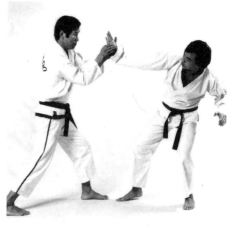

D: Press and twist A's thenar with right thumb and twist and raise left arm.

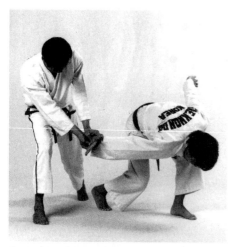

D: Grab and twist A's hand with both hands and flex A's wrist upward and inward while turning body clockwise, pivoting on both feet.

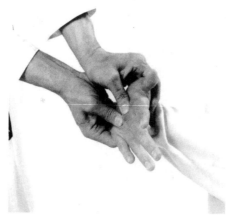

Close-up of grab and twist.

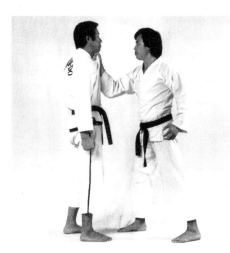

A: Grab D's collar from front with right hand.

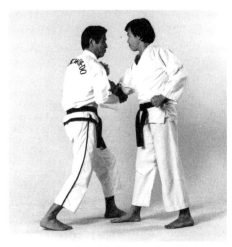

D: Grab A's hand with left hand and hold A's elbow with right hand.

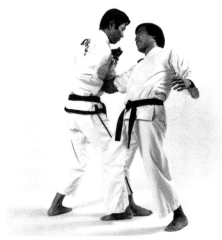

D: Twist and press A's back hand with left thumb and pull A's elbow with right hand while moving right foot forward.

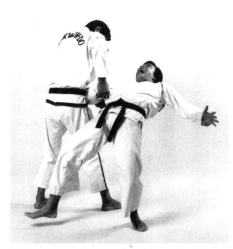

D: Flex A's hand upward and inward while pulling A's elbow.

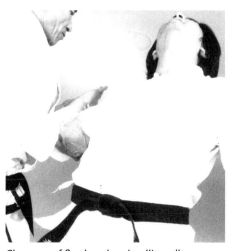

Close-up of flex hand and pulling elbow.

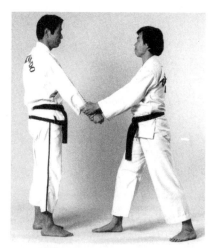

A: Grab D's right arm from front with both hands and pull.

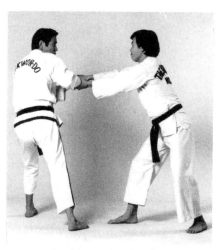

D: Hold and pull the right hand while moving left foot backward.

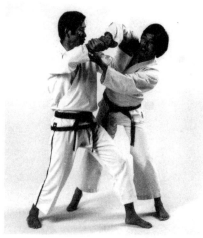

D: Push up A's right elbow joint with left palm and grab A's arm with right hand while moving left foot forward.

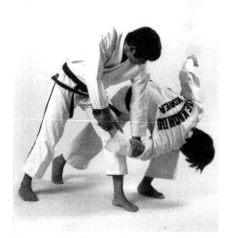

D: Twist and pull A's arm with right hand while pressing A's right elbow joint with left hand.

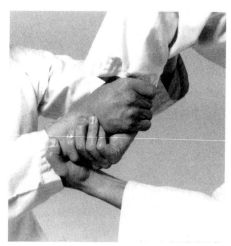

Close-up of push left elbow and grab arm.

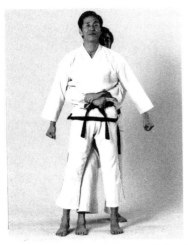

A: Hold D's waist from behind with both arms.

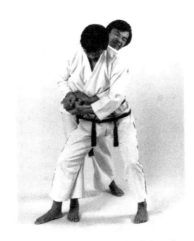

D: Grab A's right hand with both hands and twist clockwise.

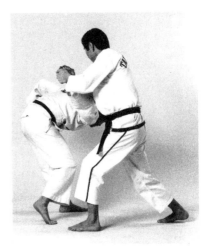

D: Twist A's hand with both hands and press A's arm with right upper arm while turning body clockwise, pivoting on both feet.

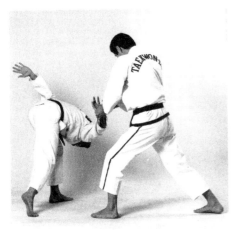

D: Pull and flex A's hand upward and inward while moving right foot backward.

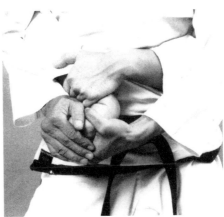

Close-up of twist hand and press arm.

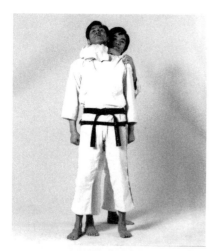

A: Lock D's neck from behind with right arm and grab D's clothes on left shoulder.

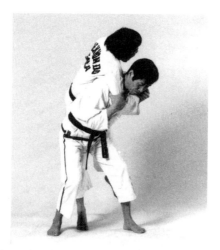

D: Grab A's hand with left hand, and grab A's arm with right hand and pull A's arm with both hands while twisting body counter-clockwise.

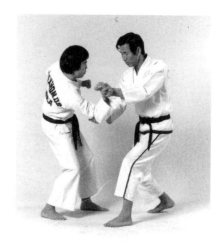

D: Turn body clockwise pivoting on left foot while moving right foot backward.

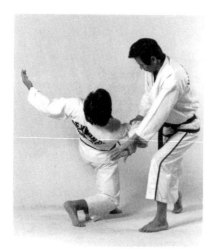

D: Pull A's elbow with right hand and twist A's hand downward with left hand.

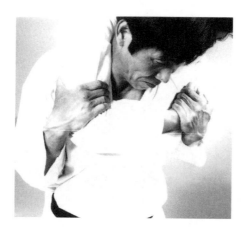

Close-up of turn body clockwise.

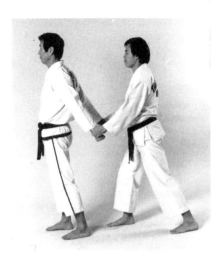

A: Grab D's both arms from behind with both hands.

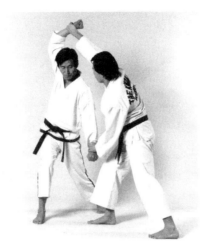

D: Raise the right hand while moving left foot backward and turn body counter-clockwise, pivoting on right foot.

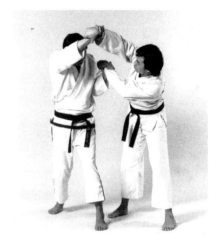

D: Grab and uplift A's left arm with left hand, and grab and pull A's right arm with right hand while moving left foot forward.

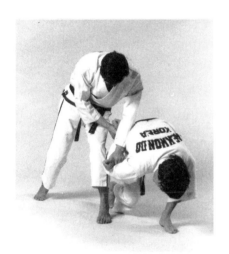

D: Cross and lock A's arms and pull them in opposite directions with both hands.

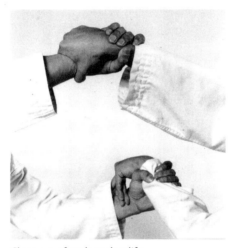

Close-up of grab and uplift.

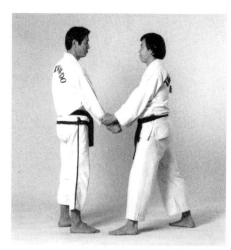

A: Grab D's right arm from front with both hands.

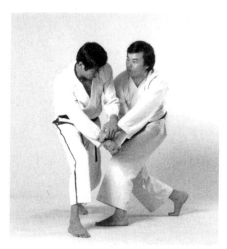

D: Grab A's left hand with left hand and press right arm downward while moving right foot to the right.

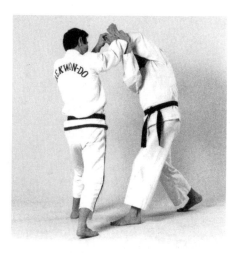

D: Raise right arm and turn body counter-clockwise, pivoting on both feet.

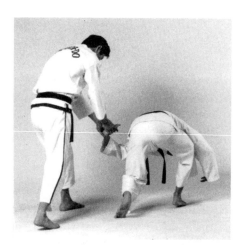

D: Grab A's left hand with both hands while twisting, and flex A's hand inward and upward.

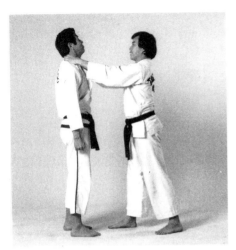

A: Grab D's neck from front with both hands.

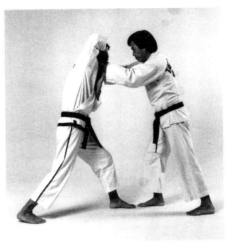

D: Grab A's left hand with both hands while moving right foot backward.

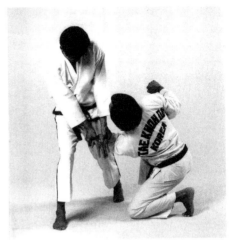

D: Twist and flex A's hand upward and inward while moving left foot backward.

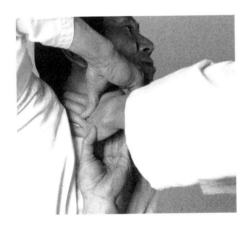

Close-up of the grab.

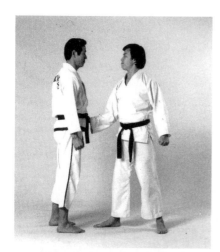

A: Grab D's belt from front with right hand.

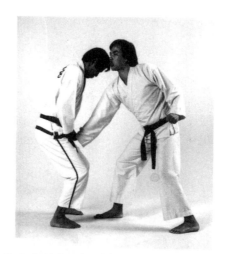

D: Grab A's hand with both hands and flex A's hand downward.

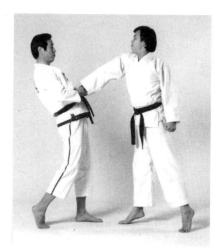

D: Flex A's hand upward while moving right foot backward.

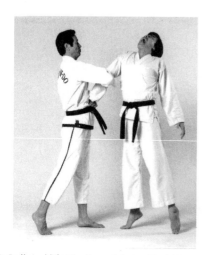

D: Pull and lift A's elbow joint with right forearm.

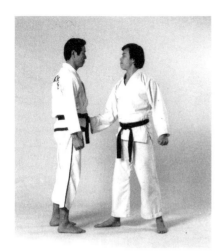

A: Grab D's belt from front with right hand.

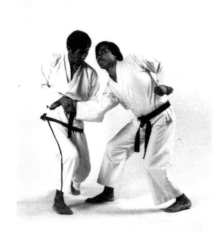

D: Grab and twist A's hand with both hands and twist body clockwise.

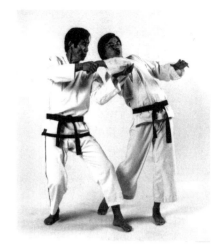

D: Hold and raise A's elbow with left hand and turn body clockwise while moving left foot forward.

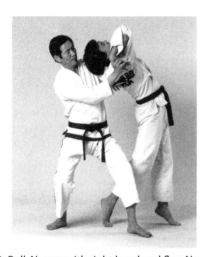

D: Pull A's arm with right hand and flex A's hand upward and inward with right hand.

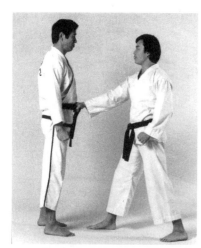

A: Grab D's belt from front with right hand.

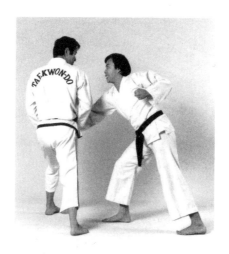

D: Grab and pull A's hand with both hands and slide left foot to the left while twisting body counterclockwise.

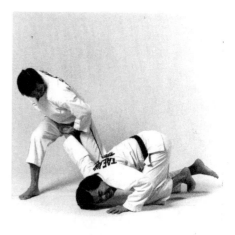

D: Pull and turn body clockwise while moving right foot to the right, and press A's wrist joint with left reverse knife-hand.

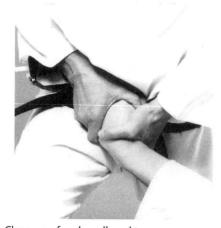

Close-up of grab, pull, and turn.

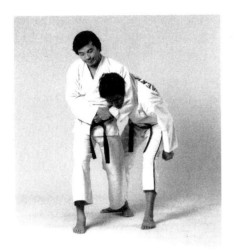

A: Lock D's neck from behind side with left arm and grab the arm with right hand.

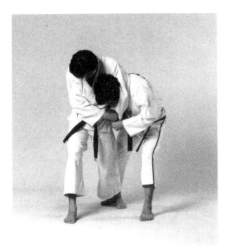

D: Grab A's right hand with both hands and twist A's hand.

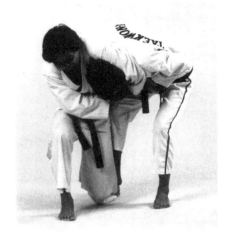

D: Exert pressing kick at A's left back of the knee (fossa) with right leg and twist A's hand.

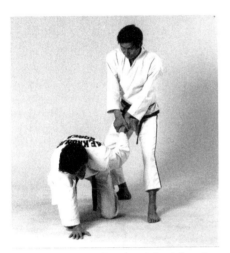

D: Twist and pull A's hand with both hands while moving right foot backward.

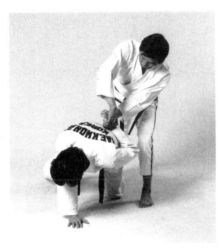

D: Twist and uplift A's hand with both hands.

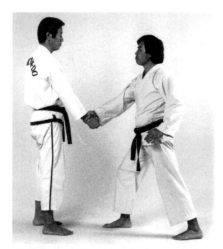

A: Grab D's right arm from front with right hand.

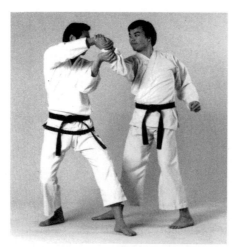

D: Grab A's arm with left hand and raise A's arm while moving left foot forward.

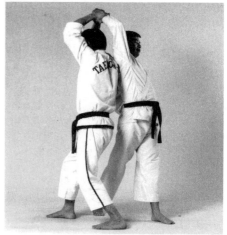

D: Twist and grab A's hand with right hand while turning body clockwise pivoting on right foot.

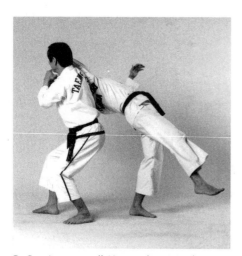

D: Continue to pull A's arm downward.

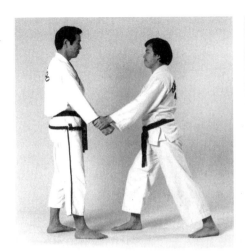

A: Grab D's both arms from front with both hands.

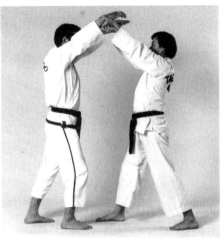

D: Move both arms outward and then inward while raising and twisting both arms.

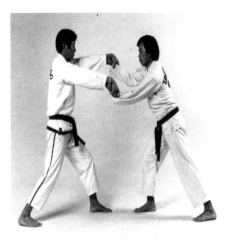

D: Grab and pull A's both arms while moving right foot backward.

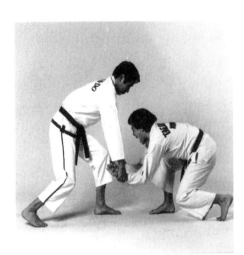

D: Pull and twist A's both arms.

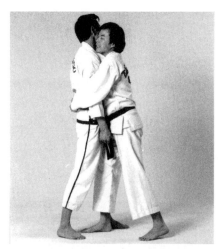

A: Grab D's waist from front with both arms.

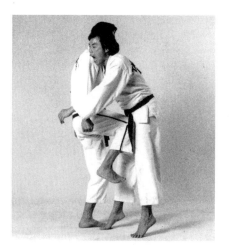

D: Kick to A's scrotum with right knee.

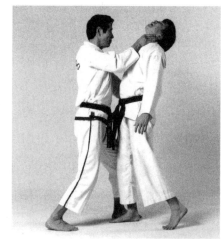

D: Lower the right foot backward and grab A's neck with right arc-hand and hold A's back ribs with left hand.

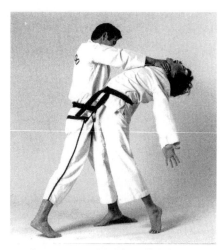

D: Pull A's waist with left hand while pushing A's neck downward with right hand.

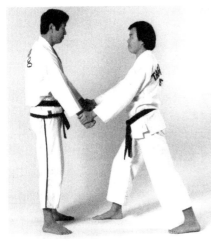

A: Grab D's both arms from front with both hands.

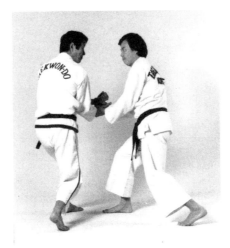

D: Grab A's right hand with right hand while turning body counterclockwise, pivoting on both feet.

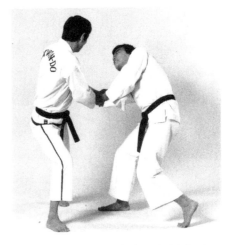

D: Twist and grab A's right hand with both hands while turning body clockwise, pivoting on both feet.

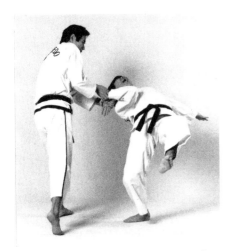

D: Continue to twist A's hand downward.

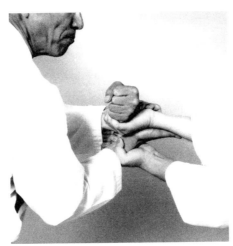

Close-up of grabbing and pivoting.

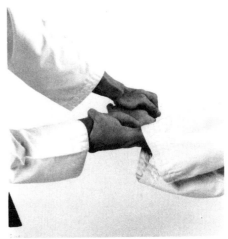

Close-up of twist and grab.

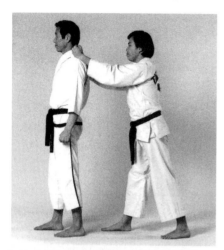

A: Grab D's clothes on both shoulders from behind with both hands.

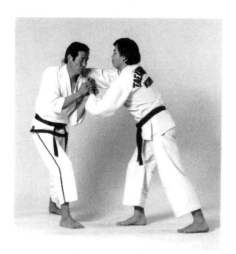

D: Grab A's left hand with both hands while moving left foot backward and turn body counterclockwise.

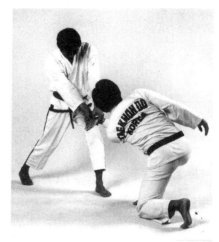

D: Pull and flex A's hand downward and inward while moving right foot backward.

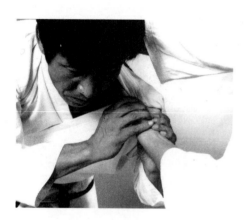

Close-up of grab left hand.

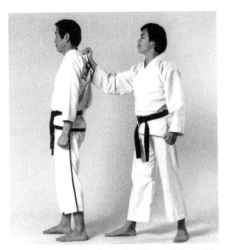

A: Grab D's collar from behind with right hand.

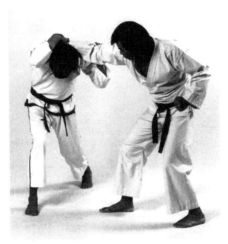

D: Grab A's hand with right hand and hold A's elbow with left hand while moving left foot backward and turn body counterclockwise.

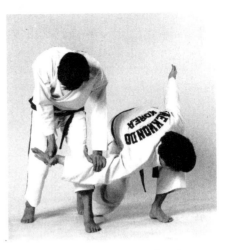

D: Press and twist A's thenar with right thumb while pressing downward A's elbow joint and moving left foot forward.

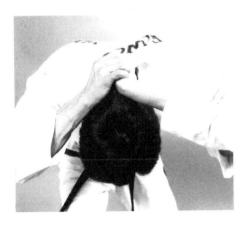

Close-up of grab and hold.

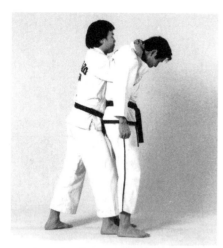

A: Lock D's neck with both arms under D's armpits from behind and press D's back neck with both hands.

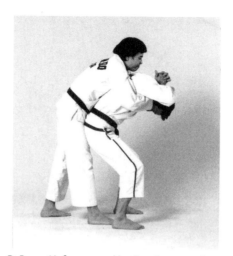

D: Press A's fingers and both palms together while bending body.

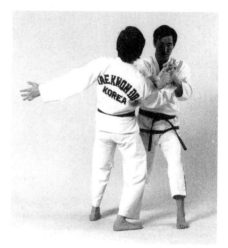

D: Grab and pull A's right finger with right hand and grab A's arm with left hand while moving right foot backward and turning body clockwise.

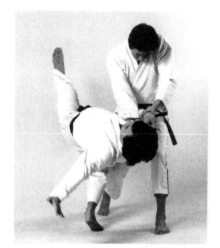

D: Pull A's finger downward with right hand.

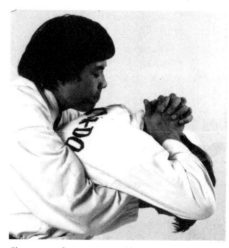

Close-up of pressing and bending.

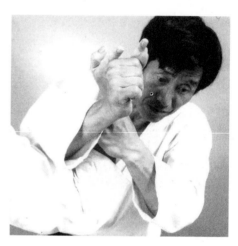

Close-up of grab and pull.

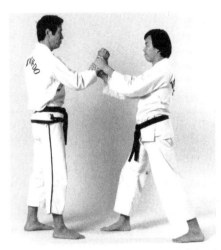

A: Grab D's right arm from front with both hands.

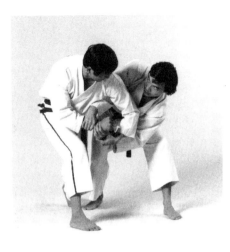

D: Grab A's left hand with left hand while moving right foot to the right.

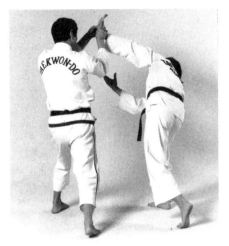

D: Twist and grab A's left hand with both hands while turning body counterclockwise, pivoting on both feet.

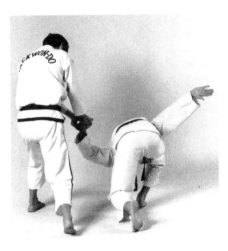

D: Twist and flex A's hand inward and upward.

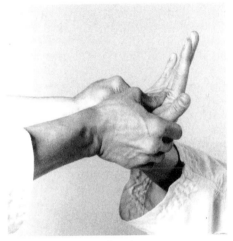

Close-up of twist and grab.

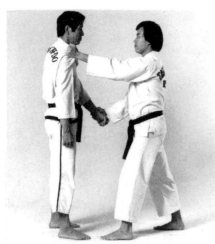

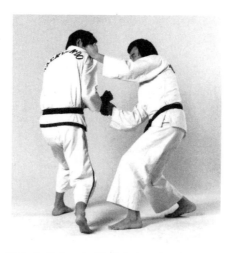

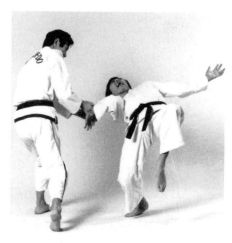

A: Grab D's clothes on right shoulder with left hand and grab D's left arm from front with right hand.

D: Grab A's hand with right hand and turn body counterclockwise, pivoting on both feet.

D: Grab and twist downward A's right hand with both hands while turning body clockwise, pivoting on both feet.

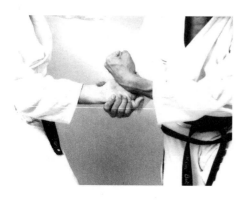

Close-up of hand grab.

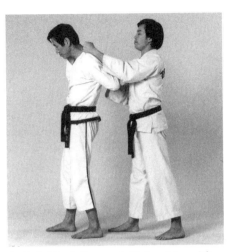

A: Grab D's clothes on left shoulder with left hand and grab and twist D's left arm upward from behind with right hand.

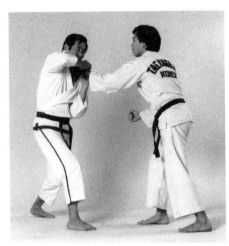

D: Grab A's left hand with right and twist body counterclockwise while moving left foot backward.

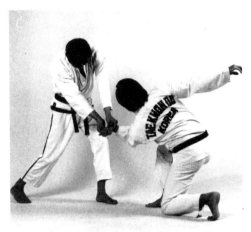

D: Grab A's hand with both hands, and pull and flex A's hand downward and inward while moving right foot backward.

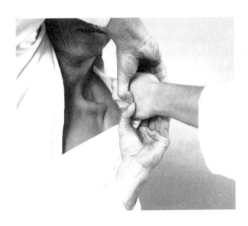

Close-up of hand grab.

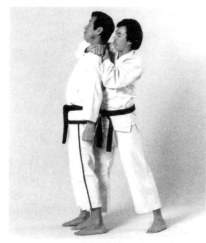

A: Lock D's neck from behind with right arm and hold it with left hand.

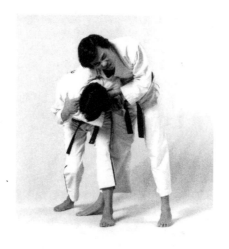

D: Grab and pull A's arm with both hands and twist body counterclockwise.

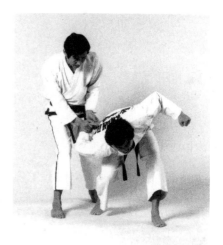

D: Pull and grab A's hand with both hands while moving left foot backward.

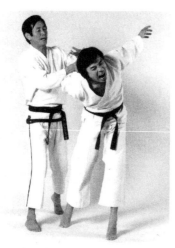

D: Twist A's hand upward.

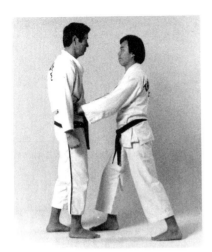

A: Grab D's side belts from front with both hands.

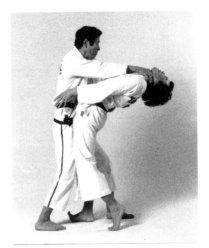

D: Grab A's throat with the right arc-hand while pushing the lower back with the left palm and moving the left foot forward.

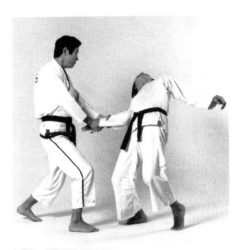

D: Grab A's arm with left hand and grab A's hand with right hand while moving left foot backward.

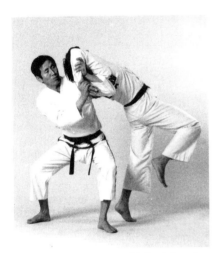

D: Twist and pull A's arm with both hands while turning body clockwise pivoting on right foot.

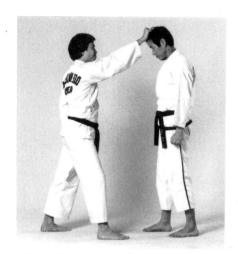

A: Grab D's hair from front with right hand.

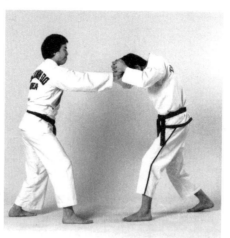

D: Hold and pull A's fist with both hands while moving right foot backward.

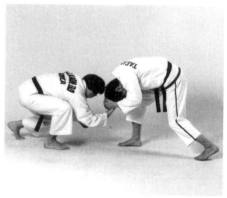

D: Pull and flex A's fist upward and inward while moving left foot backward and bend body forward.

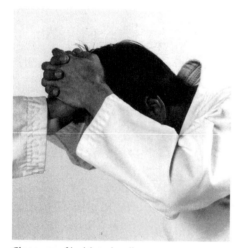

Close-up of hold and pull.

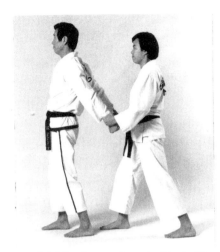

A: Grab D's both arms from behind with both hands.

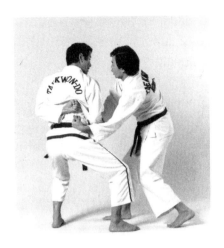

D: Move right foot backward while turning body clockwise and press A's arm with right arm.

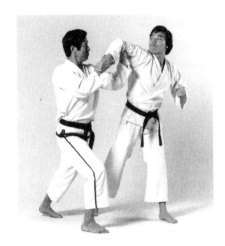

D: Grab A's right arm with right hand hold and raise A's elbow with left hand while turning body clockwise.

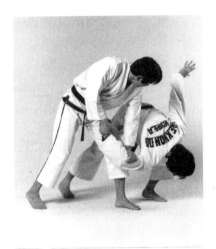

D: Press A's elbow with left hand while moving left foot forward.

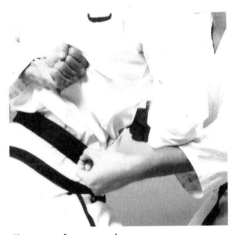

Close-up of move and press.

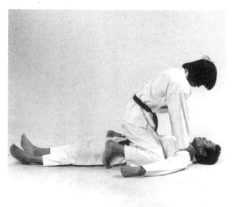

A: Press D's neck from above with both hands.

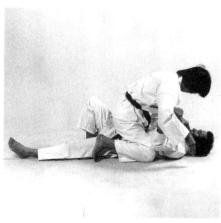

D: Execute a wedging block to A's arm with both inner forearms.

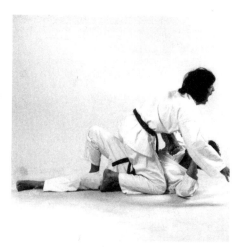

D: Execute a right elbow strike against A's ribs.

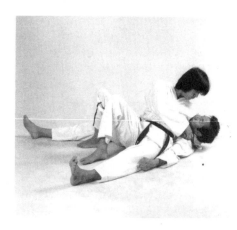

A: Lock D's neck from side with the left arm and hold his arm with the right hand.

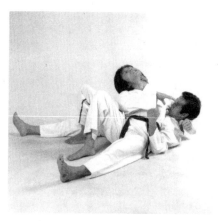

D: Press and push A's upper neck with the right press finger.

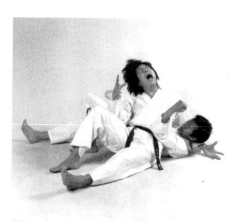

D: Execute a left elbow trust against A's ribs.

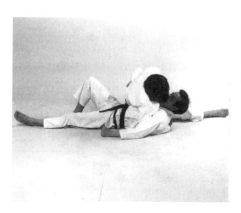

A: Lock D's neck with right arm and hold his arm with the left hand.

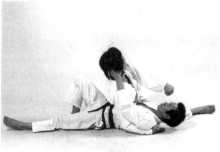

D: Press A's post-auricular muscle with the left finger.

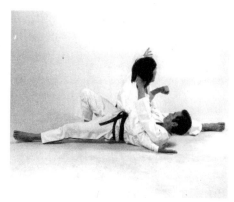

D: Execute a right elbow thrust against A's solar plexus.

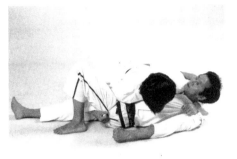

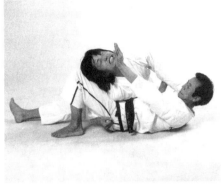

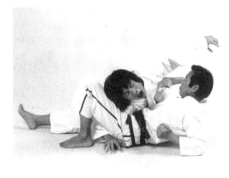

A: Lock D's neck and right upper leg with left and right hand respectively.

D: Push A's chin with left open fist.

D: Execute a right elbow trust against A's ribs

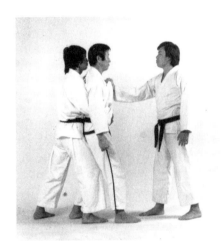

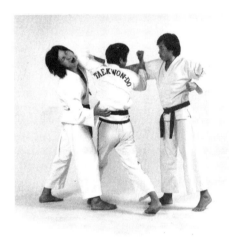

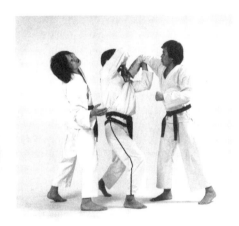

Back-A: Hold D's waist from behind with both hands.
Front-A: Grab D's collar from front with right hand.

D: Block to Front-A's elbow with the right arm and exert left elbow strike to Back-A's jaw while turning body counterclockwise, pivoting on both feet.

D: Grab Front-A's hand with the right hand, and hold Front-A's elbow upward with left hand.

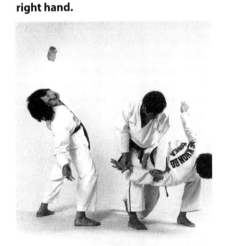

D: Twist and pull Front-A's arm with the right hand while pressing Front-A's elbow joint with left hand.

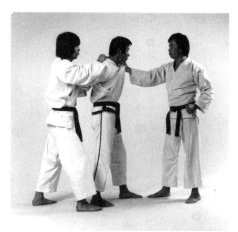

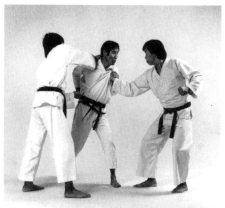

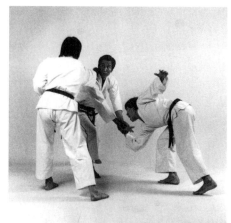

Right-A: Grab D's clothes with right hand, and grab and twist D's right arm upward with left hand.
Left-A: Grab D's collar with right hand.

D: Grab Left-A's hand with left hand while turning body clockwise pivoting on left foot.

D: Grab Left-A's hand with both hands, and flex Left-A's hand upward and inward while moving left foot backward.

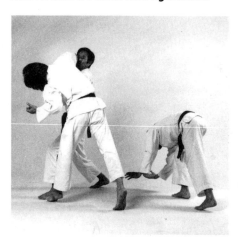

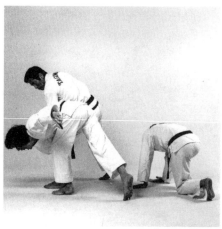

D: Grab Right-A's arm with right hand, and hold Right-A's elbow upward while moving left foot forward.

D: Twist and pull Right-A's arms with right hand while pressing Right-A's elbow joint with left hand.

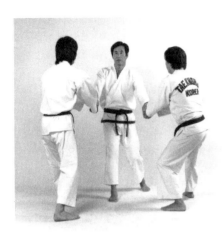

A: Grab and pull D's arms with both hands from front.

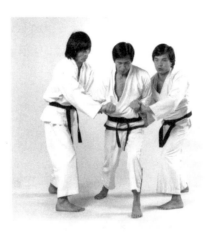

D: Move left foot forward while pushing and twisting both arms.

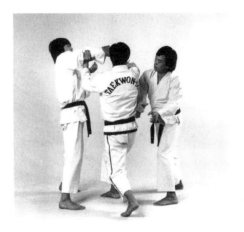

D: Grab Right-A's arm with right hand, and hold Right-A's elbow upward with left hand while turning body clockwise pivoting on both feet.

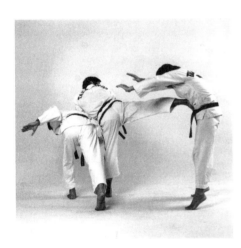

D: Move left foot forward while twisting Right-A's arm with right hand, and push elbow with left hand simultaneously, execute a side pushing kick against Left-A's ribs.

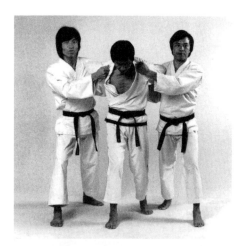

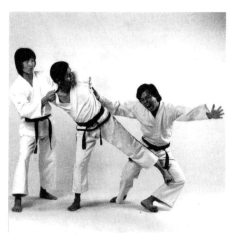

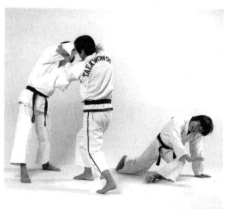

Right-A: Grab D's clothes with right hand and grab and twist D's right arm upward with left hand.

Left-A: Grab D's clothes with left hand, and grab and twist D's left arm upward with right hand.

D: Exert left side pressing kick to Left-A's knee joint.

D: Grab Right-A's arm with right hand, and hold Right-A's elbow upward with left hand while lowering the left foot forward and turn body clockwise, pivoting on right foot.

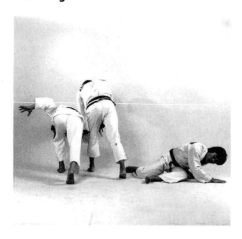

D: Twist and pull Right-A's arm with right hand, and press Right-A's elbow joint with left hand while moving left foot forward.

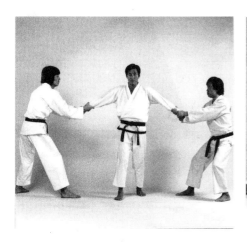

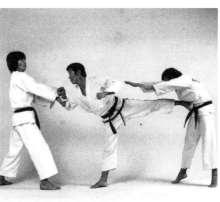

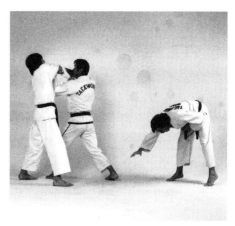

A: Grab and pull D's arm with both hands from both sides.

D: Execute left side thrusting kick to Left-A's epigastrium.

D: Grab Right-A's arm with right hand, and hold Right-A's elbow upward with left hand while lowering left foot forward and turning body clockwise pivoting on right foot.

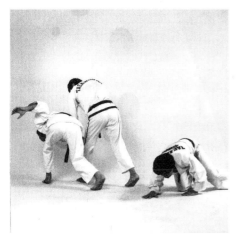

D: Twist and pull Right-A's arm with right hand while pressing Right-A's elbow joint with left hand.

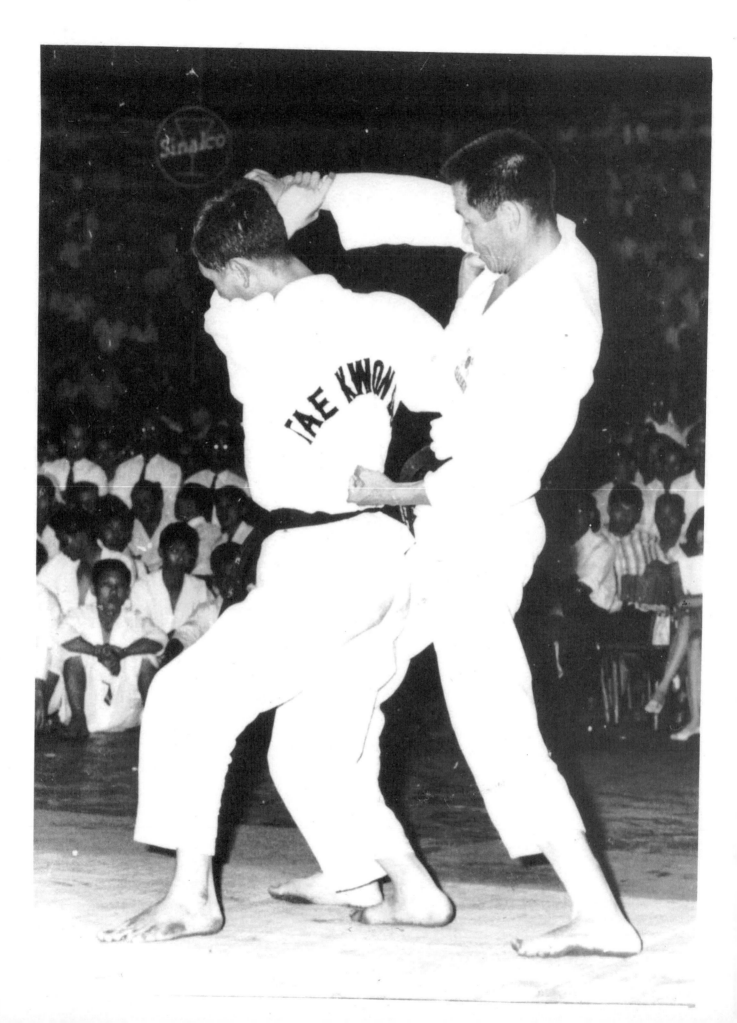

Throwing and Falling Techniques

The basic factor for effective mobilization of physical force depends upon the posture of a person. That is, a balanced and secure posture does not allow for a swift attack while it is good for defense. An unbalanced posture is effective for attack while not favorable for defense. And it is the latter posture which affords maximum advantage for the throw. The throwing technique is used only when you aim to not inflict grievous bodily harm on an attacker, but merely to counter an attack.

Falling could be practiced either from a standing or sitting position, or from a lying down position. Attempt to fall with a rolling motion to the side rather than the flat of the back, and hit the ground with the palm to absorb the shock. In order to prevent a head collision with the ground, press the chin toward the chest.

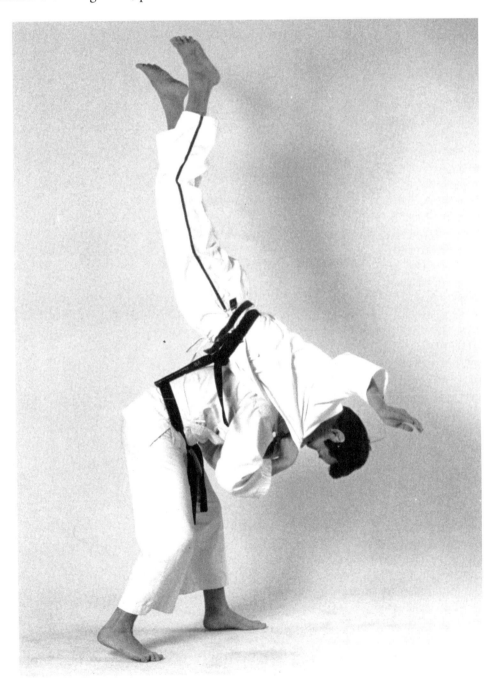

Falling Exercises

The purpose of falling exercises is to learn to control your body when thrown and to break the shock of the fall. The first step is to learn how to fall without getting hurt.

As you fall, keep the chin tucked in by looking down to prevent striking your head against the ground. The legs should be crossed: the right foot falling by side-sole and the left foot by footsword, or vice versa. Falling with crossed legs enables you to act quickly for the counterattack and to be ready for the standing position.

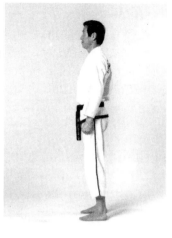

Ready stance.

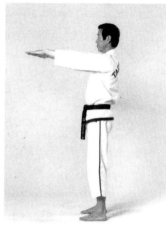

Prepare for backward falling down.

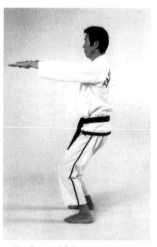 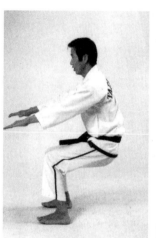 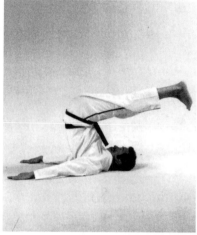 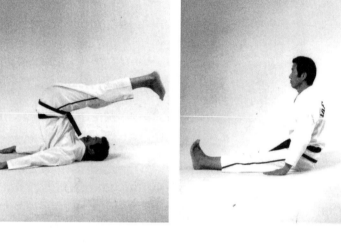

1. Backward falling sequence.

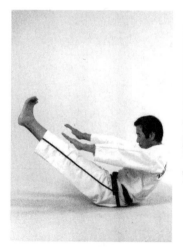 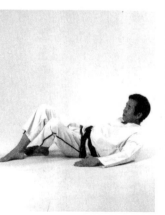 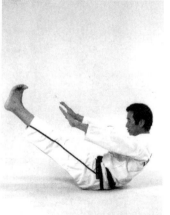 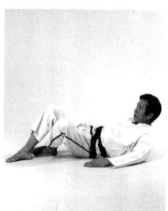

2. Sideways falling sequence.

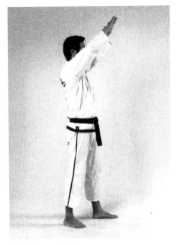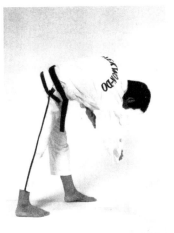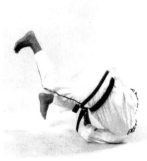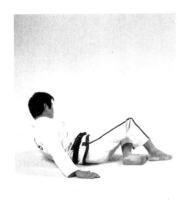

3. Forward falling sequence.

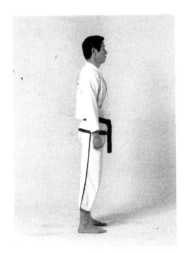

Ready stance.

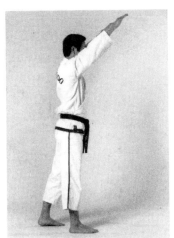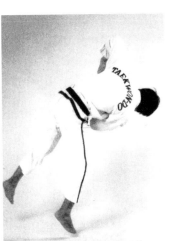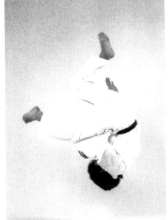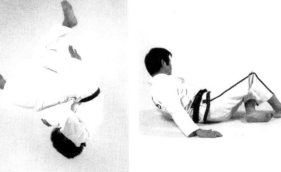

4. Flying falling sequence.

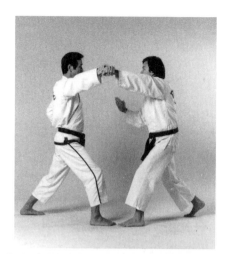

A: Grab D's right arm with left hand.

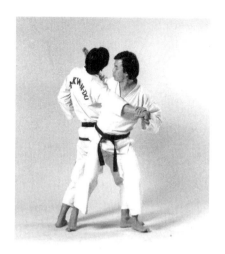

A: Hold D's angle of mandible with right palm while moving right foot forward.

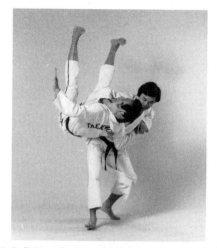

A: Pull D's right arm with left hand and push D's angle of mandible with right palm while twisting hip.

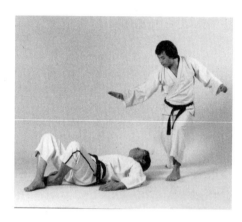

A: Prepare to punch.
D: Fall by placing both palms against the ground and cross the leg to prepare to kick.

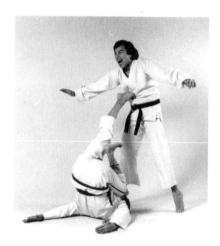

D: Execute a right counterattack with ball of foot against A's solar plexus.

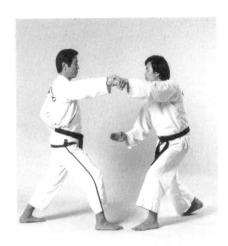

A: Grab D's right arm with left hand.

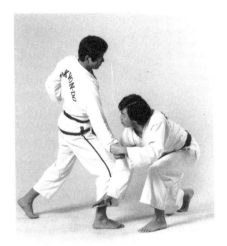

A: Pull and twist downward D's right arm with left hand while striking D's leg with right knife-hand.

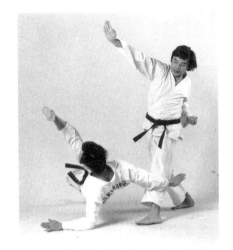

D: Grab and pull D's right leg to the right with the right hand.

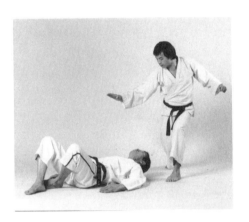

A: Prepare to kick.
D: Fall by placing both palms against the ground and cross the legs to prepare to kick.

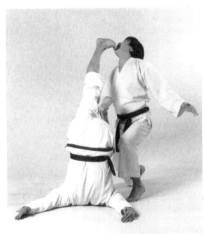

D: Execute a right counterattack with ball of foot against A's face.

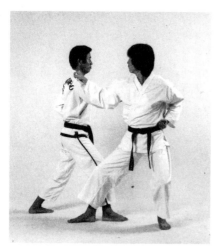

A: Grab D's clothes at right shoulder with right hand.

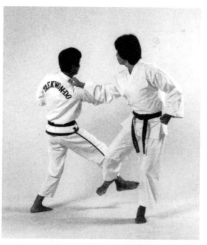

A: Pull D's clothes at shoulder with right hand and exert a reverse hooking kick at A's right leg with right back heel.

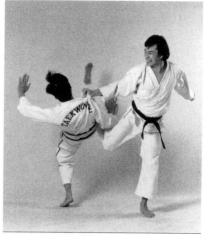

A: Continue pulling D's clothes at shoulder and twist counterclockwise.

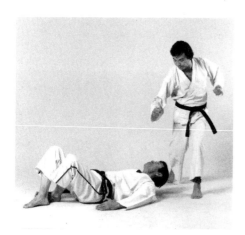

A: Prepare to punch.

D: Fall by placing both palms against the ground and cross the legs to prepare to kick.

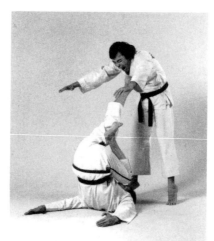

D: Execute a right counterattack with ball of foot against A's solar plexus.

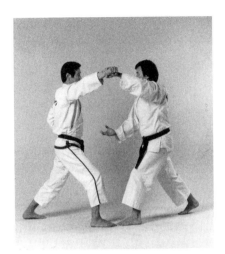

A: Grab D's right arm with left hand.

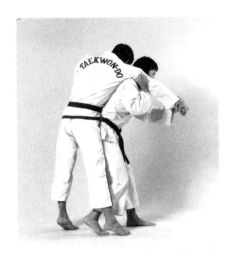

A: Hold D's armpit upward with right hand while moving right foot forward.

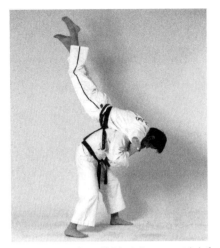

A: Simultaneously pull D's right arm with left hand, lift D's armpit with right hand, and move left foot to the left while turning body counterclockwise.

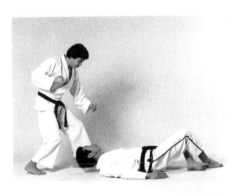

A: Prepare to punch.
D: Fall by placing both palms against the ground and cross the leg to prepare to kick.

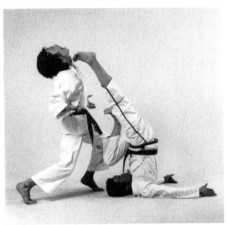

D: Execute a right counterattack with ball of foot against A's face.

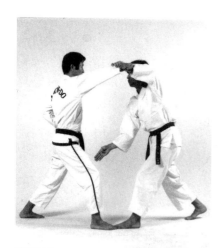

A: Grab D's right arm with left hand.

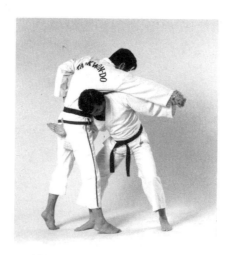

A: Hold D's crotch upward with right arm while moving right foot forward.

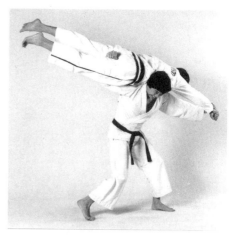

A: Simultaneously pull D's right arm with left hand, lift D's crotch with right arm, and move left foot to the left while turning body counterclockwise.

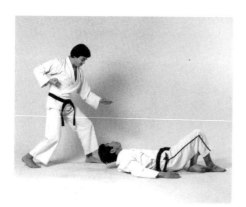

A: Prepare to kick.
D: Fall by placing both palms against the ground and cross the leg to prepare to kick.

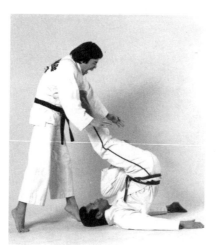

D: Execute a right counterattack with ball of foot against A's solar plexus.

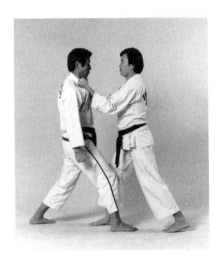

A: Grab D's clothes with both hands.

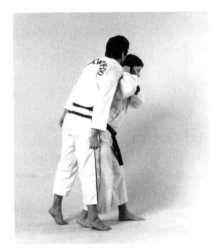

A: Pull D's clothes with both hands and move left foot to the left while turning body counterclockwise.

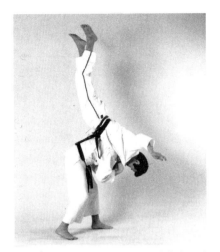

A: Continue pulling D's clothes while bending body.

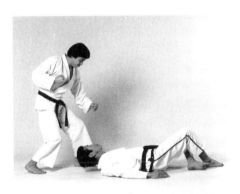

A: Prepare to punch.

D: Fall by placing both palms against the ground and cross the leg to prepare to kick.

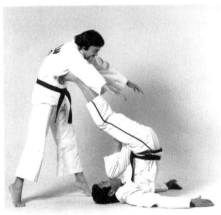

D: Execute a right counterattack with ball of foot against A's solar plexus.

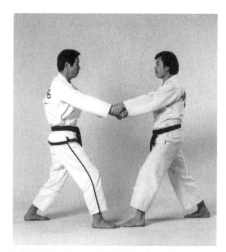

A: Grab D's arms with both hands.

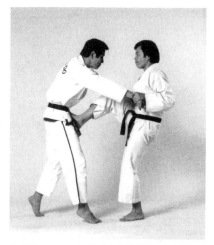

A: Pull D's arm with both hands and exert a pushing kick to D's umbilicus with right foot.

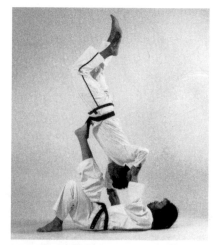

A: Flex an upward pushing kick to D's umbilicus with right foot and pull D's arm while falling to the ground.

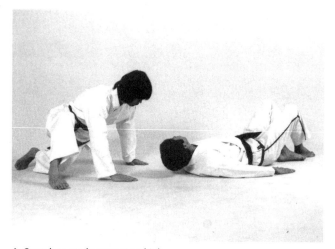

A: Stand up and prepare to kick.
D: Fall by placing both palms against the ground and cross the leg to prepare to kick.

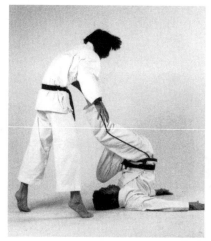

D: Execute a right counterattack with ball of foot against A's solar plexus.

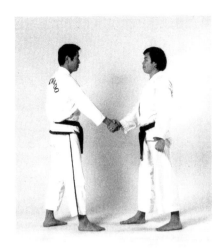

A: Grab D's right hand with right hand.

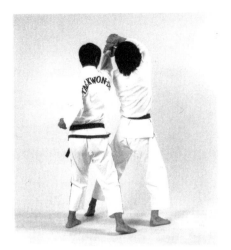

A: Grab D's hand with both hands while moving left foot forward.

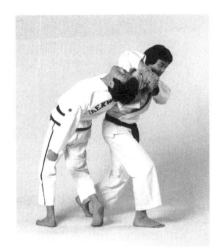

A: Raise and twist D's right hand while turning body clockwise, pivoting on right foot.

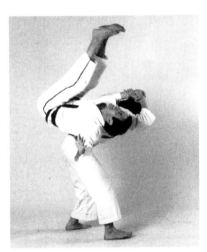

A: Pull D's right hand downward.

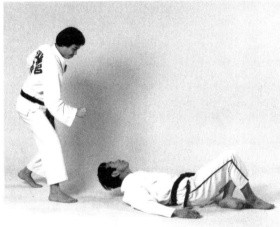

A: Prepare to kick.
D: Fall by placing both palms against the ground and cross the leg to prepare to kick.

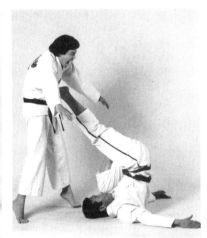

D: Execute a right counterattack with ball of foot against A's solar plexus.

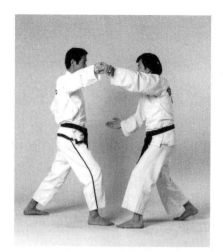

A: Grab D's right arm with left hand.

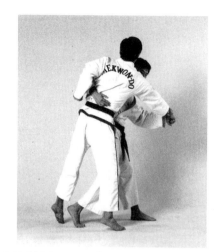

A: Hold D's waist with right hand while moving right foot forward.

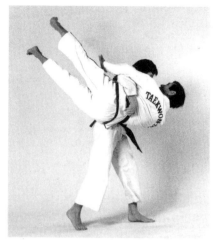

A: Simultaneously pull D's arm with left hand, exert an upward pull at D's waist with right hand and move left foot to the left while twisting hip.

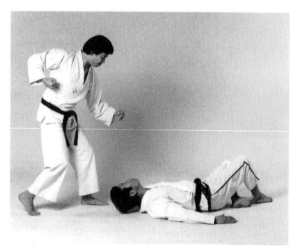

A: Prepare to kick.

D: Fall by placing both palms against the ground and cross the leg to prepare to kick.

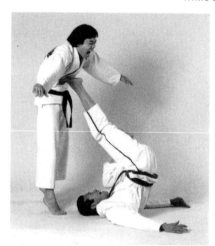

D: Execute a right counterattack with ball of foot against A's solar plexus.

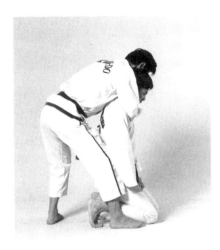

A: Lock D's neck from behind with right arm and grab own arm with left hand.

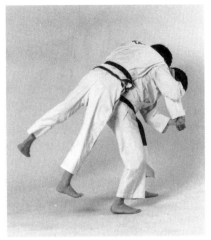

A: Pull D's right arm downward with left hand and pull D's clothes on right shoulder with right hand while moving left foot forward.

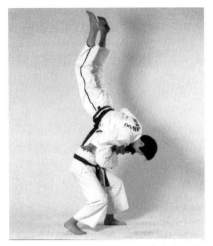

A: Continue to pull D's clothes while bending body.

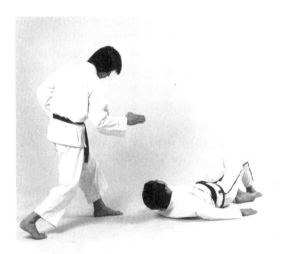

A: Prepare to punch.
D: Fall by placing both palms against the ground and cross the leg to prepare to kick.

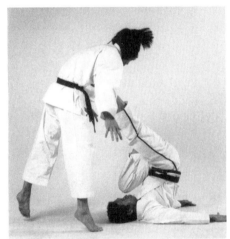

D: Execute a right counterattack with ball of foot against A's solar plexus.

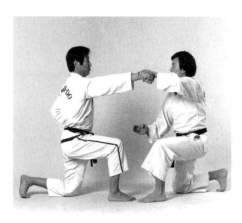

A: Grab D's right arm with left hand.

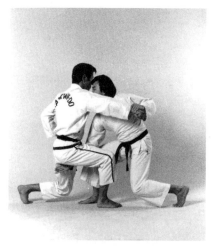

A: Pull and twist downward D's right arm with left hand while striking D's leg with right knife-hand.

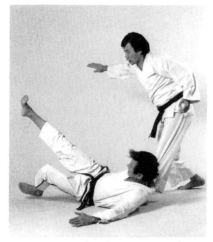

A: Grab and pull D's right leg to the right with right hand.

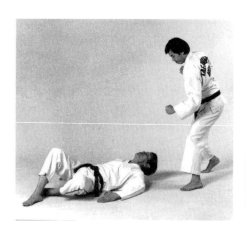

A: Prepare to punch.
D: Fall by placing both palms against the ground and cross the leg to prepare to kick.

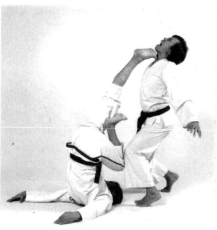

D: Execute a right counterattack with ball of foot against A's face.

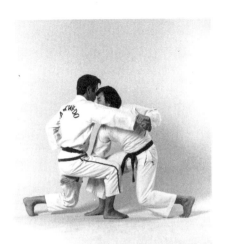

A: Grab D's right arm with left hand.

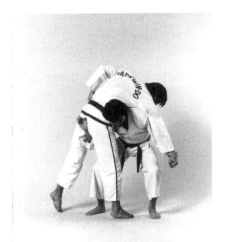

A: Hold D's crotch upward with right arm while puling D's arm with left hand.

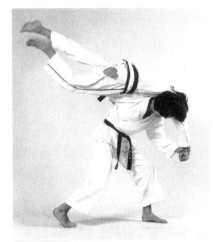

A: Exert an upward pull at D's crotch with right arm and move left foot to the left while turning body counterclockwise.

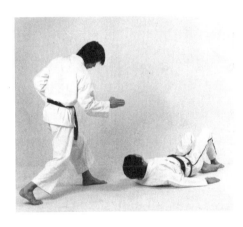

A: Prepare to punch.
D: Fall by placing both palms against the ground and cross the leg to prepare to kick.

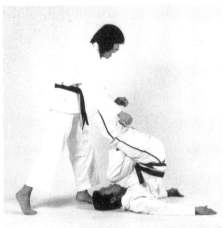

D: Execute a right counterattack with ball of foot against A's solar plexus.

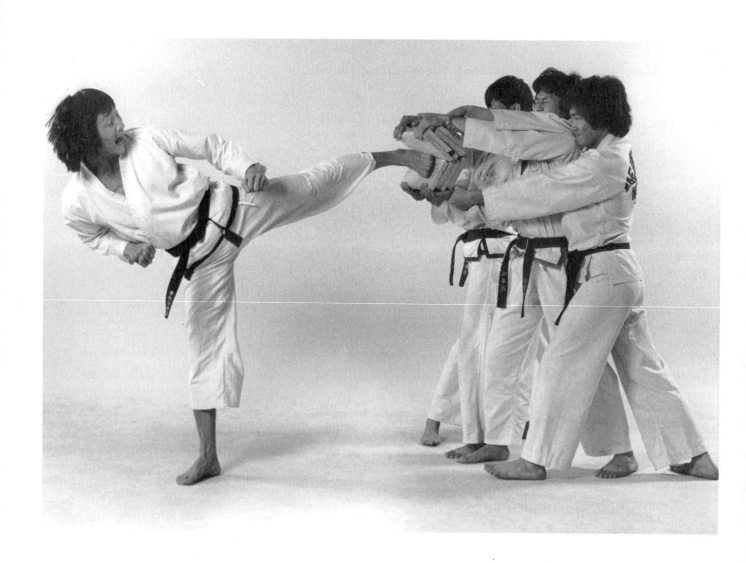

Defense Against Throwing

Being the defender is often more advantageous than being the attacker, for the attacker cannot give serious harm to an opponent. The most important factor for a defense against throwing is using falling techniques, which is to fall without getting hurt and to recover for a counterattack. With the reactionary force, when falling, the defender can counterattack with double or more of the attacker's force.

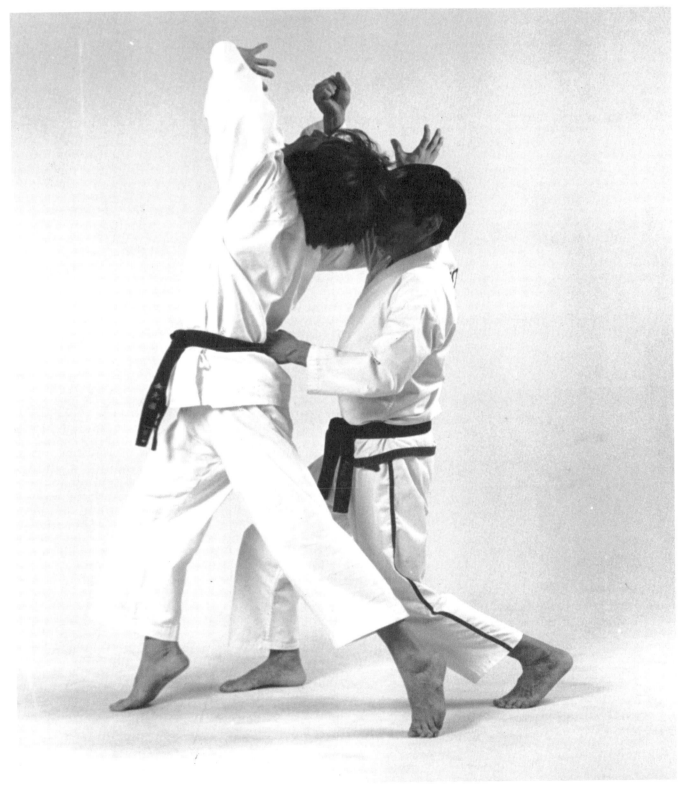

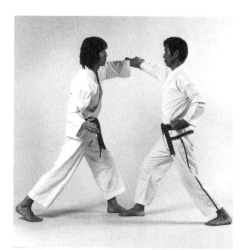

A: Grab D's right arm with left hand.

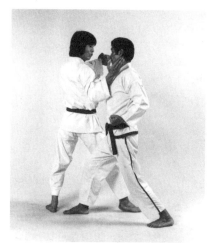

A: Hold D's angle of mandible with the right palm while moving right foot forward.

D: Prepare to punch.

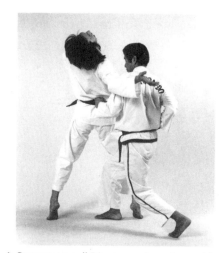

A: Prepare to pull D's arm and exert a pushing at D's angle of mandible while twisting hip.

D: Execute a left vertical punch against A's kidney.

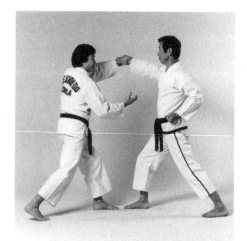

A: Grab D's right arm with left hand.

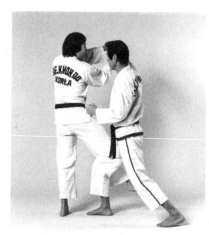

A: Grab and lift D's right arm with both hands and move right foot forward while turning body counterclockwise.

D: Prepare to punch.

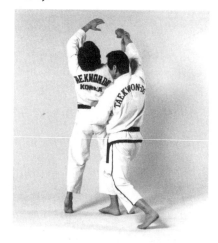

A: Prepare to pull D's arm and turn body counterclockwise while moving right foot forward.

D: Execute a left vertical punch against A's lower back.

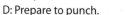

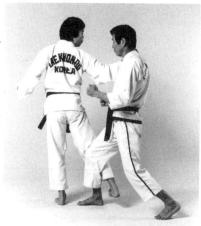

A: Grab D's clothes on right shoulder with right hand.

A: Prepare to exert a reverse hooking kick with right leg.

D: Prepare to punch.

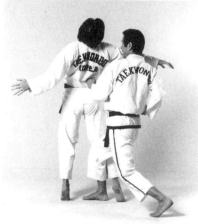

A: Pull D's clothes with right hand and exert a reverse hooking kick to D's right leg with right back heel.

D: Execute a left vertical punch against A's kidney.

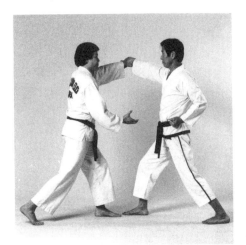

A: Grab D's right arm with left hand.

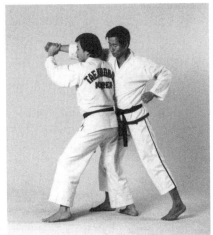
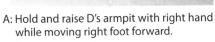

A: Hold and raise D's armpit with right hand while moving right foot forward.

D: Prepare to punch.

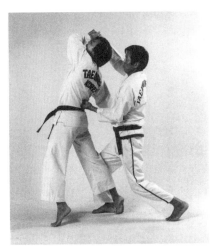

A: Pull D's arm and turn body counterclockwise while moving left foot to the left.

D: Execute a left upset punch against A's lower back.

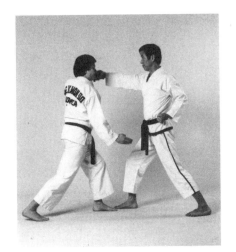

A: Grab D's right arm with left hand.

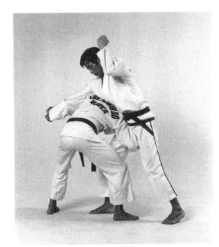
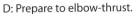

A: Hold and lift D's crotch with right arm while moving right foot forward.

D: Prepare to elbow-thrust.

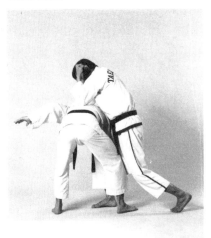

A: Pull D's right arm with left hand and lift D's crotch with right arm while turning body counterclockwise.

D: Execute a left elbow-thrust against A's lower back.

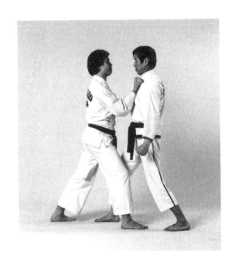

A: Grab D's clothes with both hands.

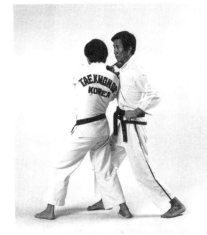

A: Move right foot forward while turning body counterclockwise.

D: Prepare to upset punch.

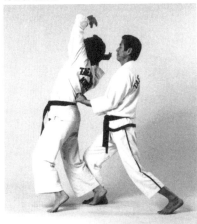

A: Pull D's clothes and turn body counterclockwise while moving left foot to the left.

D: Execute a twin upset punch against A's kidney.

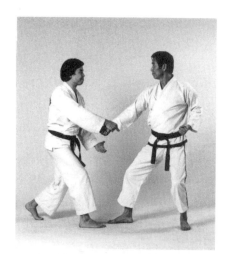

A: Grab D's right arm with right hand.

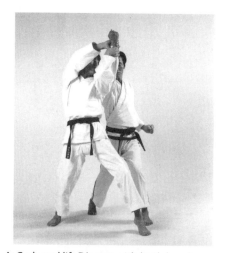

A: Grab and lift D's arm with both hands while moving left foot forward.

D: Prepare to vertical punch.

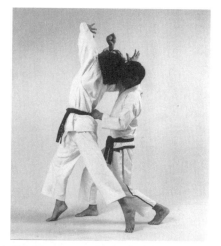

A: Continue to turn body clockwise while pulling D's arm with both hands.

D: Execute a left vertical punch against A's kidney.

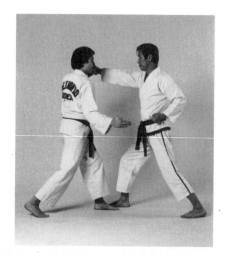

A: Grab D's right arm with left hand.

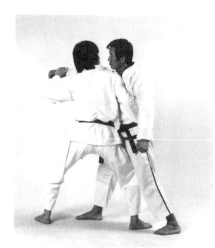

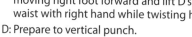

A: Pull D's right arm with left hand while moving right foot forward and lift D's waist with right hand while twisting hip.

D: Prepare to vertical punch.

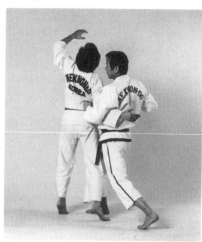

A: Hold D's left side waist with right hand while moving right foot forward.

D: Execute a left vertical punch against A's kidney.

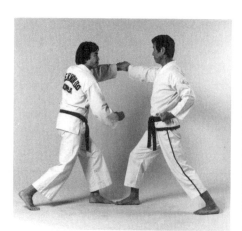

A: Grab D's right arm with left hand.

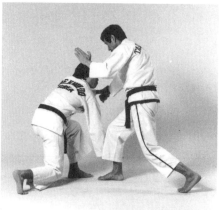

A: Pull and twist downward D's right arm with left hand while preparing to grab D's leg with right hand.

D: Prepare to knife-hand strike.

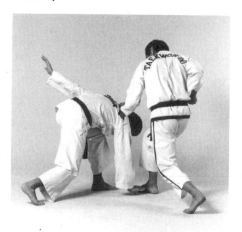

A: Grab and pull D's right leg to the right.

D: Execute a left knife-hand strike against A's neck.

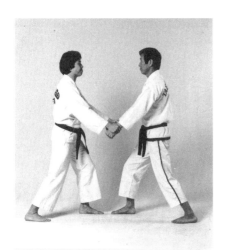

A: Grab D's arm with both hands.

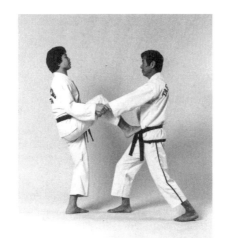

A: Pull D's arm with both hands while exerting a pushing kick to D's umbilicus with right foot.

D: Prepare to twist both arms.

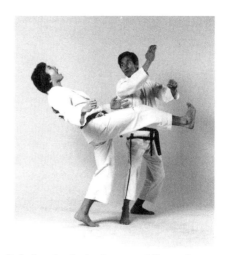

D: Pull and twist both arms while turning body counterclockwise, pivoting on right foot.

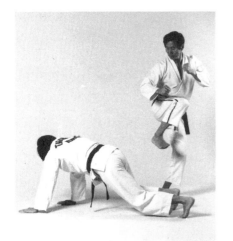

A: Prepare to stand up.
D: Prepare to kick.

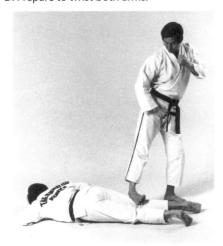

D: Execute right side stomping kick against A's right knee.

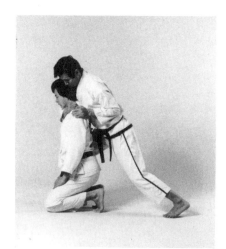

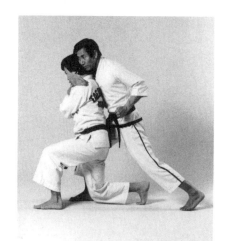

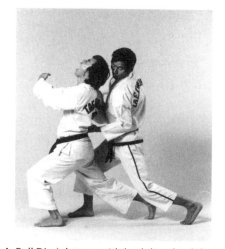

A: Grab D's clothes on right shoulder with right hand and grab D's arm with left hand.

D: Lock A's neck from behind with right arm.

D: Lock A's neck from behind with right arm.
A: Move left foot forward and stand up.
D: Prepare to exert and upset punch.

A: Pull D's right arm with both hands while bending body.
D: Execute a left upset punch against A's lower back.

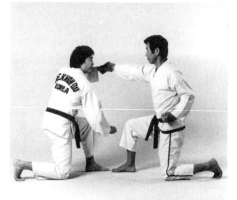

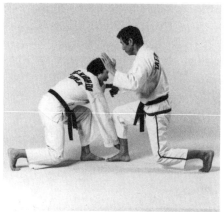

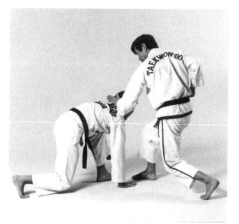

A: Grab D's right arm with left hand.

A: Pull and twist downward D's right arm with left hand while preparing to grab D's leg with right hand.

A: Grab and pull D's right leg to the right.
D: Execute a left knife-hand strike against A's neck.

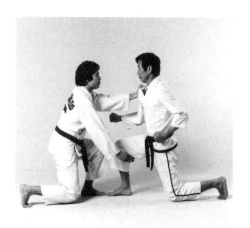

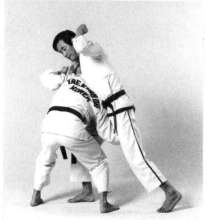

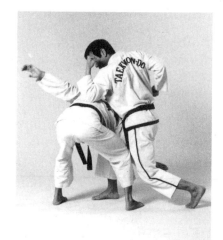

A: Grab D's clothes on shoulder with left hand.

A: Hold and lift D's crotch with right arm while moving right foot forward.
D: Prepare to elbow-thrust.

A: Pull D's right arm with left hand and lift D's crotch with right arm while turning body counterclockwise.
D: Execute left elbow thrust against A's middle back.

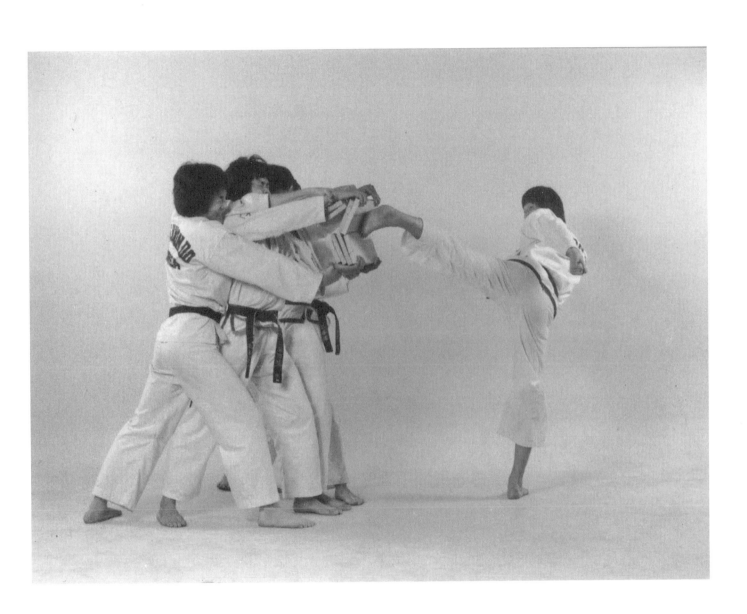

Defense Techniques in Free Sparring

Both the hands and legs should be used in defense, and when coordinated with the correct body movements, accurate and precisely timed hand and foot movements can block any attack. The defender must keep his eyes on his attacker if he is going to interpret his attacker's next move and be able to automatically take a defending position or counterattacking position. The defender should note his attacker's weak points and be ready to take advantage of them. Furthermore, a defender should capitalize on his attacker's momentum and direction of attack in order to gain the upper hand. Balance and confidence cannot be overemphasized, and the defender's movements should be controlled, yet smooth, quick, and accurate.

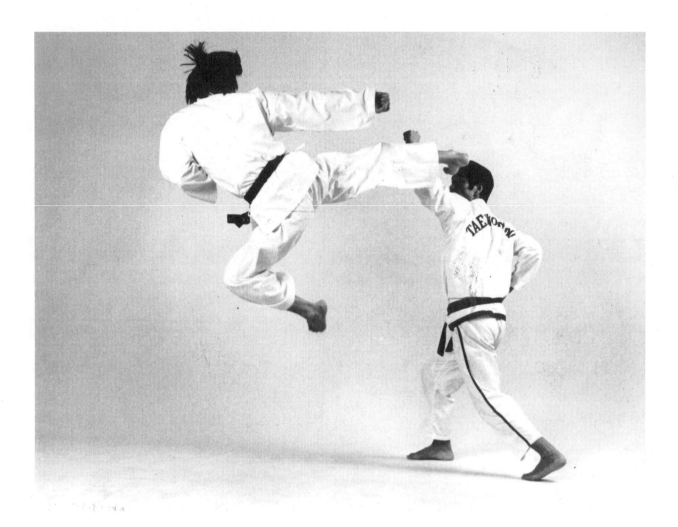

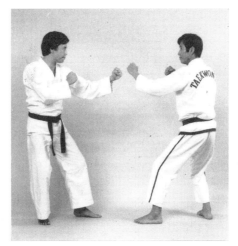

A: Face D in left L-stance with a fist guarding block.

D: Face A in left L-stance with a fist guarding block.

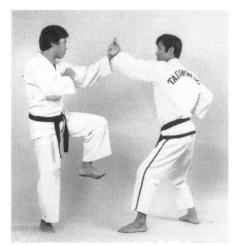

A: Fake strike to D's arm with the left knife-hand while preparing to execute turning kick.

D: Block A's arm with the left outer forearm.

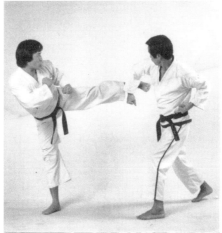

A: Execute a turning kick to D's lower abdomen with the left foot.

D: Block A's leg with the right outer forearm.

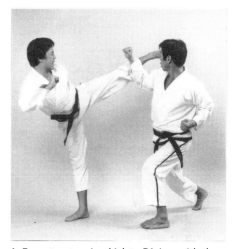

A: Execute a turning kick to D's jaw with the left foot.

D: Block A's leg with the right outer forearm while slipping the left foot.

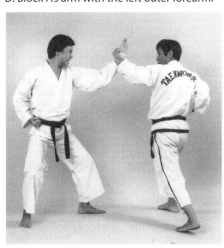

A: Execute a knife hand strike to D's neck.

D: Block A's arm with the left outer forearm.

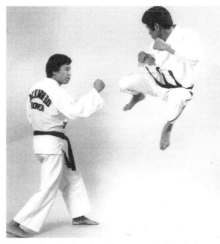

A: Punch to D's solar plexus with the right fist.

D: Jump to dodge to the left while preparing to execute turning kick.

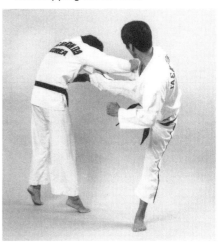

D: Land on the left foot while executing a right turning kick against A's umbilicus.

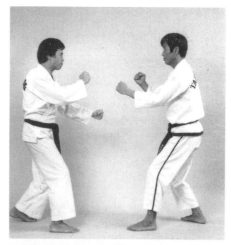

A: Face D in right walking stance with a fist guarding block.

D: Face A in left walking stance with a fist guarding block.

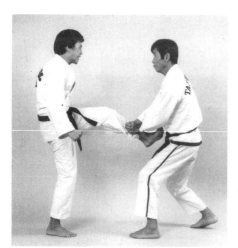

A: Execute front snap kick to D's scrotum with left instep.

D: Execute pressing block at A's leg with X-fist.

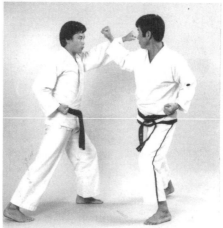

A: Lower the left foot forward and then left punch to D's philtrum.

D: Block A's arm with the right outer forearm while slipping the left foot.

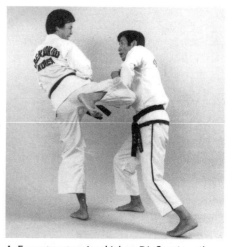

A: Execute a turning kick to D's floating ribs with the right knee.

D: Block A's upper leg with both side fists while turning body clockwise.

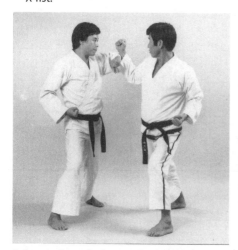

A: Lower the right foot to the right and execute a left side elbow strike to D's jaw.

D: Block A's arm with the right outer forearm while turning body counterclockwise.

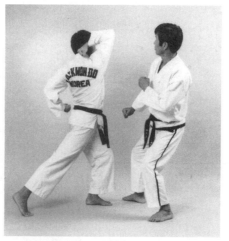

A: Execute an upward elbow strike to D's chin while moving left foot forward.

D: Dodge to the left while preparing to right knee kick.

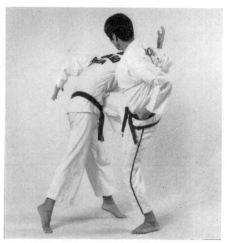

D: Execute a right knee kick against A's epigastrium.

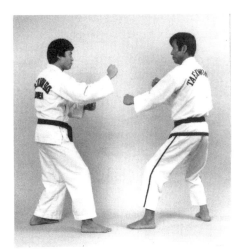

A: Face D in right natural stance with a fist guarding block.

D: Face A in left L-stance with a fist guarding block.

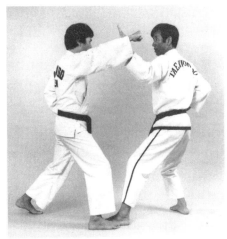

A: Punch to D's face with the right fist while slipping the right foot.

D: Block A's arm with the left knife-hand.

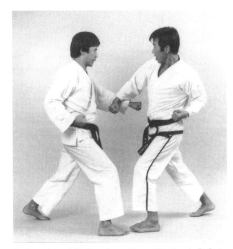

A: Punch to D's floating ribs with the left fist.

D: Block A's arm with right outer forearm.

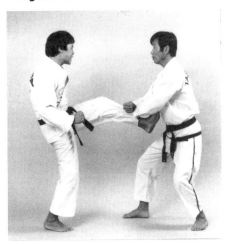

A: Execute a front snap kick to D's lower abdomen with the left foot.

D: Exert pressing block to A's leg with X-fist while moving left foot backward.

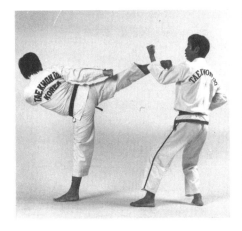

A: Lower the left foot to a position in front of the right foot and execute a side pushing kick to D's sternum with the right foot.

D: Block A's leg with left outer forearm while moving right foot backward.

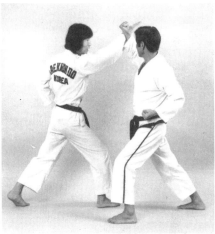

A: Lower the right foot to right and execute right back-fist strike to D's jaw.

D: Block A's arm with the right outer forearm while slipping the left foot.

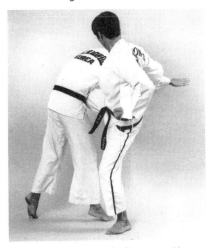

D: Execute a right knee kick against A's epigastrium.

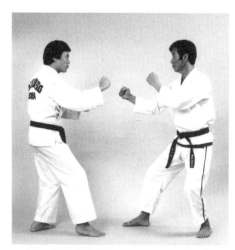

A: Face D in right natural stance with a fist guarding block.

D: Face A in right L-stance with a fist guarding block.

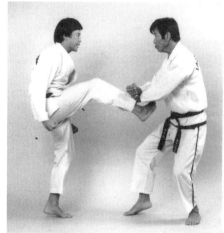

A: Execute a front snap kick to D's umbilicus with the right foot.

D: Block A's leg with X-fist.

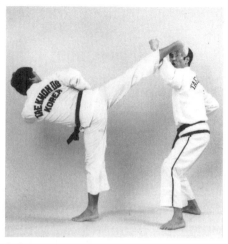

A: Execute a turning kick to D's jaw with the right foot.

D: Block A's leg with left outer forearm while moving the right foot to the right.

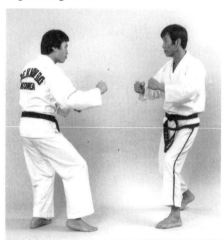

A: Lower the right foot to a position in front of the left foot and prepare to front snap kick.

D: Prepare to block.

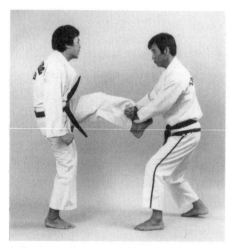

A: Execute a front snap kick to D's umbilicus with the left foot.

D: Exert pressing block to A's leg with X-fist.

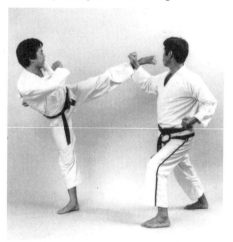

A: Execute a turning kick to D's jaw with the left foot.

D: Block A's leg with the right outer forearm while turning body counterclockwise.

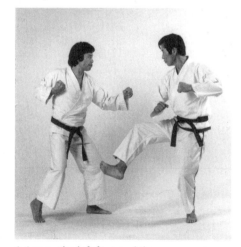

A: Lower the left foot and then prepare to execute right punch.

D: Prepare to execute twisting kick.

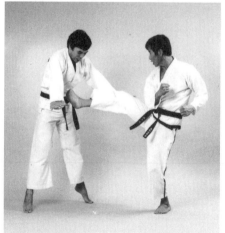

D: Execute a right twisting kick against A's lower abdomen.

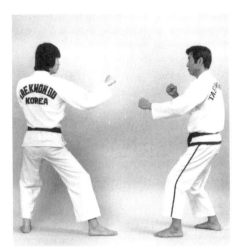

A: Face D in right L-stance with a fist guarding block.

D: Face A in left natural stance with a fist guarding block.

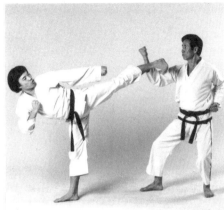

A: Execute a side-snapping kick to D's face with the left foot.

D: Block A's leg with the right outer forearm while moving the left foot backward.

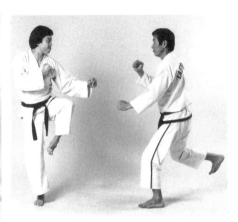

A: Bring the left foot to a position beside the right knee joint while preparing to jump side kick.

D: Prepare to dodge.

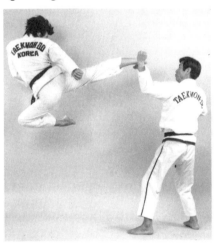

A: Execute a jumping side pushing kick to D's face with the right foot.

D: Block A's leg with the left outer forearm while moving the right foot backward.

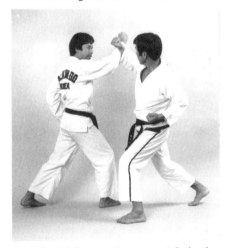

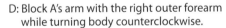

A: Land at D's front and execute right back-fist strike to D's jaw.

D: Block A's arm with the right outer forearm while turning body counterclockwise.

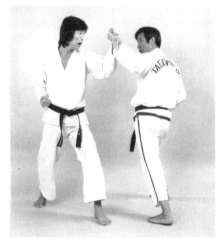

A: Strike D's jaw with the left back-fist and turn body counterclockwise while moving the left foot backward.

D: Block A's arm with the left outer forearm.

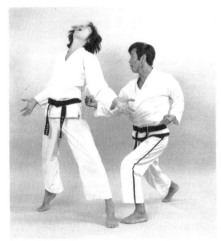

D: Execute a right punch against A's kidney.

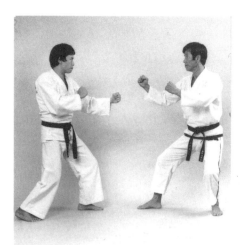

A: Face D in left natural stance with a fist guarding block.

D: Face A in right L-stance with a fist guarding block.

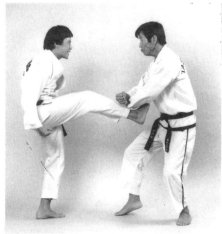

A: Execute a front snap kick to D's scrotum with the right foot.

D: Block A's leg with X-fist while pulling the right foot.

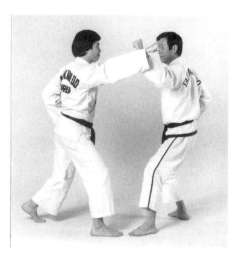

A: Lower the right foot forward and then execute right punch to D's chin.

D: Block A's arm with the left outer forearm while moving the right foot backward.

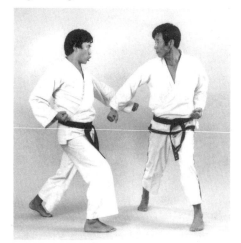

A: Punch to D's solar plexus with the left fist.

D: Block A's arm with the right outer forearm.

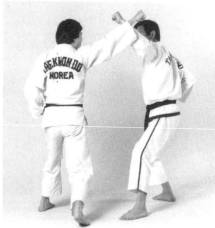

A: Punch to D's jaw with the right fist.

D: Exert rising block to A's arm with the left outer forearm.

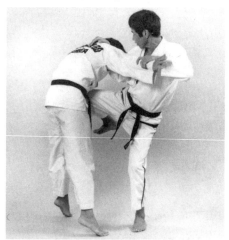

D: Execute a right knee kick against A's umbilicus.

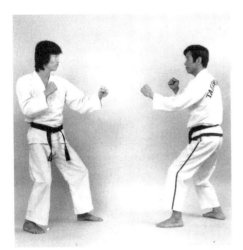

A: **Face D in left natural stance with a fist guarding block.**
D: **Face A in left L-stance with a fist guarding block.**

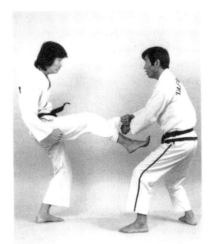

A: Execute a front snap kick to D's umbilicus with the right foot.
D: Exert pressing block to A's leg with X-fist.

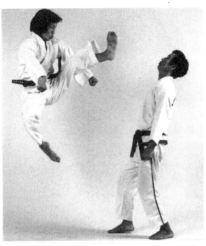

A: Execute a jumping crescent kick to D's jaw with the left foot.
D: Move left foot backward while dodging A's leg.

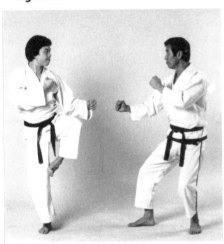

A: Land with right foot while preparing to side kick.
D: Prepare to block.

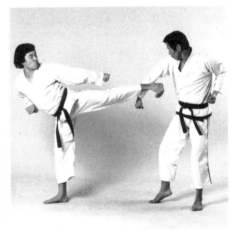

A: Execute a side-snapping kick to D's floating ribs with the left foot.
D: Block A's leg with the right inner forearm while pulling the right foot.

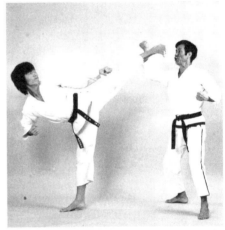

A: Execute a side-snapping kick to D's face with the left foot.
D: Block A's leg with the right outer forearm while moving the right foot to the right.

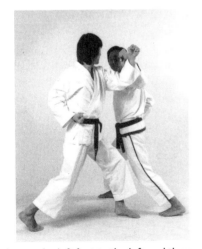

A: Lower the left foot to the left and then execute left back-fist strike to D's jaw.
D: Block A's arm with the left outer forearm while turning body clockwise.

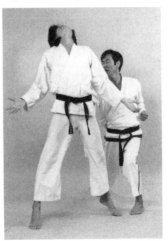

D: Execute a right punch against A's kidney.

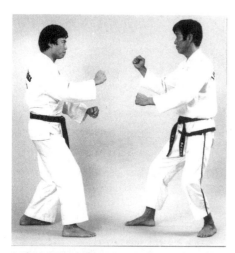

A: Face D in right natural stance with a fist guarding block.

D: Face A in right L-stance with a fist guarding block.

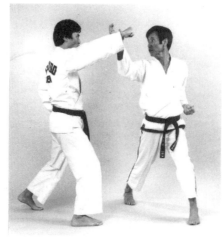

A: Fake punch to D's face with the right fist while sliding the right foot.

D: Block A's arm with the right palm while moving right foot to the right.

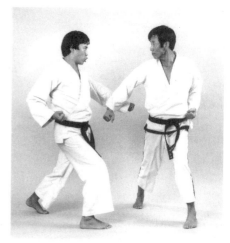

A: Punch to D's floating ribs with the left fist while turning body clockwise.

D: Block A's arm with the right outer forearm.

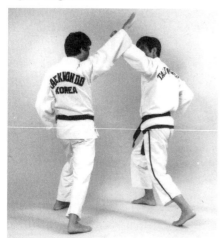

A: Thrust to D's eyeball with the right flat fingertip.

D: Block A's arm with the left outer forearm while turning body clockwise.

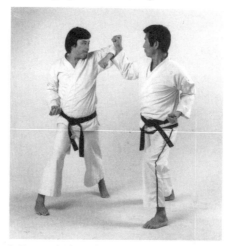
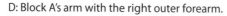

A: Execute side strike to D's jaw with the left elbow while slipping the left foot.

D: Block A's arm with the right outer forearm.

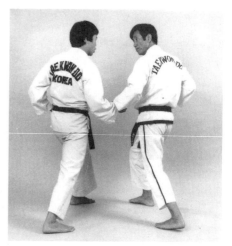

A: Execute vertical punch to D's epigastrium with the right fist.

D: Block A's arm with the left outer forearm.

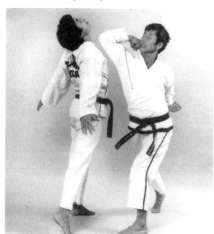

D: Execute a right upward elbow strike against A's chin.

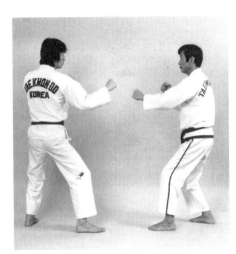

A: **Face D in right L-stance with a fist guarding block.**
D: **Face A in left natural stance with a fist guarding block.**

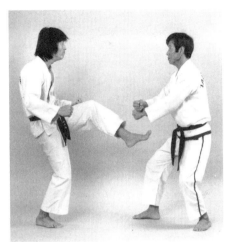

A: Fake a front snap kick to D's epigastrium with the left foot.
D: Move left foot backward while exerting pressing block to A's leg with X-fist.

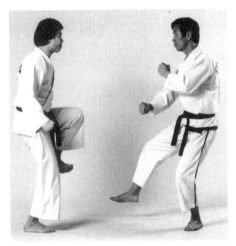

A: Bring the left foot to a position in front of the right knee joint while preparing to execute a jumping turning kick.
D: Prepare to block.

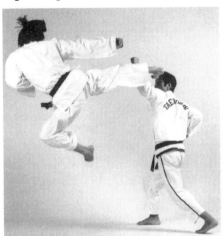

A: Execute a jumping turning kick to D's jaw with the right foot.
D: Block A's leg with left outer forearm while moving the right foot to the right and turn body clockwise.

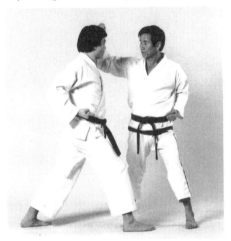
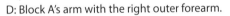

A: Land at D's side and then execute left punch to D's face.
D: Block A's arm with the right outer forearm.

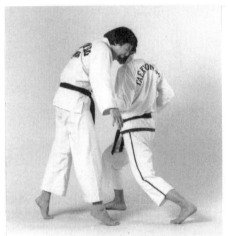

D: Execute a left punch against A's epigastrium.

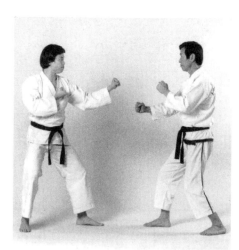

A: **Face D in left L-stance with a fist guarding block.**
D: **Face A in right natural stance with a fist guarding block.**

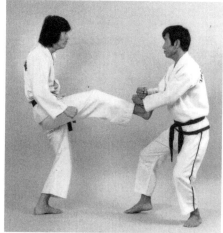

A: Fake a front snap kick to D's lower abdomen with the right foot.
D: Block A's leg with X-fist while pulling the right foot.

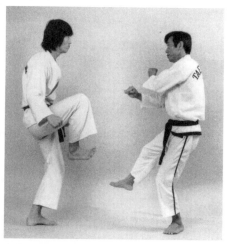

A: Prepare to execute a turning kick.
D: Prepare to block.

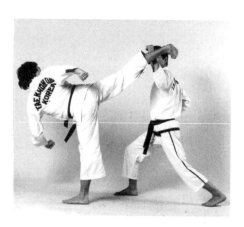

A: Execute a turning kick to D's jaw with the right foot.
D: Block A's leg with the left outer forearm while shifting to right with right foot.

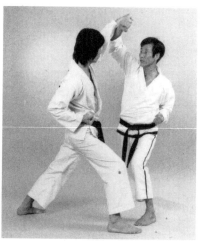

A: Lower the right foot forward and then execute left punch to D's face.
D: Block A's arm with the right outer forearm.

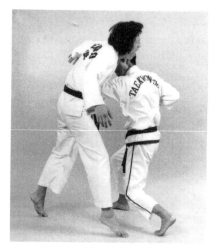

D: Execute a left side elbow strike against A's solar plexus.

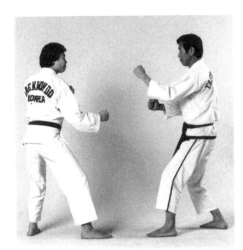

A: Face D in right L-stance with a fist guarding block.

D: Face A in left natural stance with a fist guarding block.

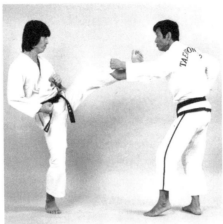

A: Execute a crescent kick to D's arm with the left foot.

D: Pull the left hand while pulling the left foot.

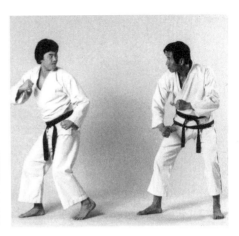

A: Lower the left foot beside the right foot while preparing to execute a reverse turning kick.

D: Prepare to move left foot backward.

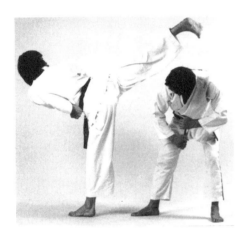

A: Execute a reverse turning kick to D's neck with the right back heel.

D: Move left foot backward while bending body to dodge the leg.

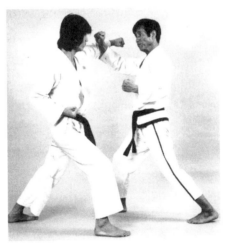
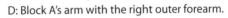

A: Lower the right foot to the right and then execute a left punch to D's face.

D: Block A's arm with the right outer forearm.

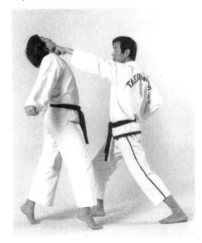

D: Execute a left punch against A's philtrum.

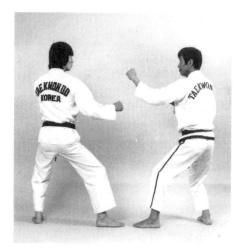

A: Face D in right L-stance with a fist guarding block.

D: Face A in left L-stance with a fist guarding block.

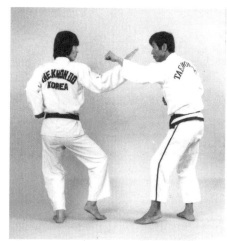

A: Execute a fake strike to D's arm with the right knife-hand while preparing to execute a twisting kick.

D: Prepare to execute right punch.

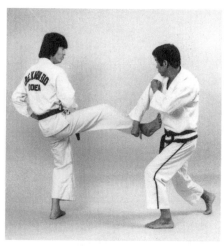

A: Execute a twisting kick to D's lower abdomen with the right foot.

D: Block A's leg with the right outer forearm while moving the left foot to the left.

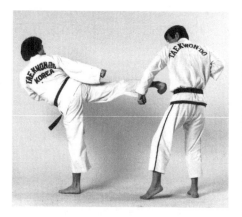

A: Execute a side-snapping kick to D's umbilicus with the right foot.

D: Block D's leg with the left inner forearm while pulling the left foot.

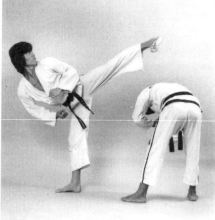

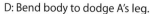

A: Lower the right foot to right and then execute a right reverse turning kick to D's neck.

D: Bend body to dodge A's leg.

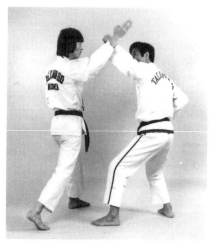

A: Lower the left foot to the left and then execute a right knife-hand strike to D's neck.

D: Block A's arm with the left outer forearm.

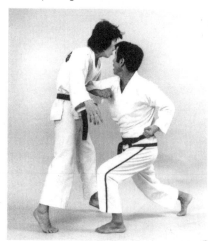

D: Execute a right side-elbow strike against A's solar plexus.

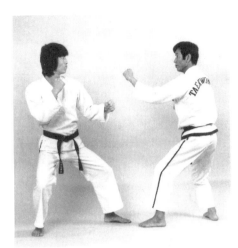

A: Face D in left L-stance with a fist guarding block.
D: Face A in left L-stance with a fist guarding block.

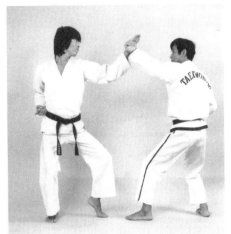

A: Execute a fake strike to D's neck with the left knife-hand while preparing to execute a side kick.
D: Block A's arm with the left outer forearm.

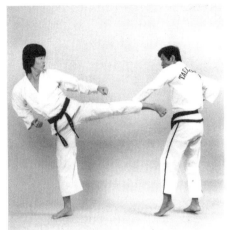

A: Execute a side-snapping kick to D's floating ribs with the left foot.
D: Block A's leg with the left outer forearm while pulling the left foot.

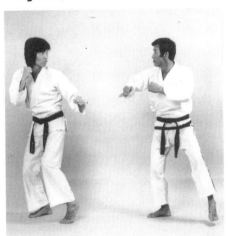

A: Lower the left foot beside the right foot while preparing to execute back side kick.
D: Prepare to move left foot backward.

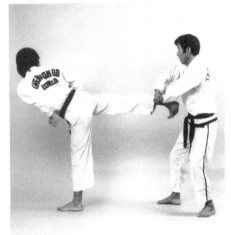

A: Execute a back side thrusting kick to D's solar plexus with the right foot.
D: Block A's leg with both side fists while moving the left foot backward.

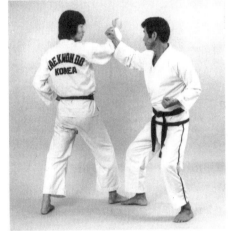

A: Lower the right foot to the right and then execute a right back-fist strike to D's jaw.
D: Block A's arm with the right outer forearm.

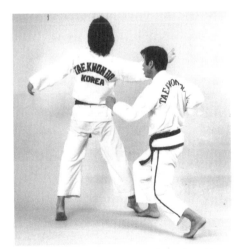

D: Execute a left vertical punch against A's kidney.

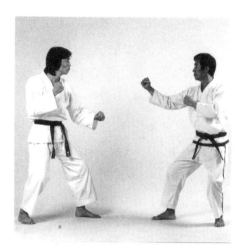

A: Face D in left natural stance with a fist guarding block.

D: Face A in right L-stance with a fist guarding block.

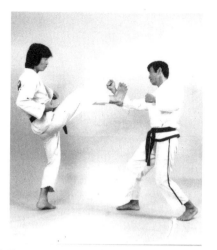

A: Execute a crescent kick to D's arm with the right foot.

D: Pull the right hand while pulling the right foot.

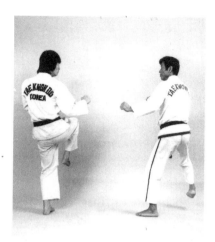

A: Bring the right foot beside the left knee joint while preparing to execute a jumping crescent kick.

D: Prepare to dodge while moving the right foot.

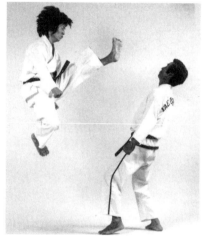

A: Execute a jumping crescent kick to D's jaw with the left foot.

D: Dodge the right foot backward.

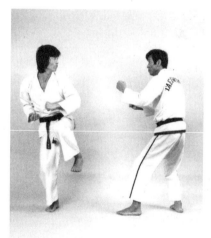

A: Land on the right foot while preparing to execute side kick.

D: Prepare to block.

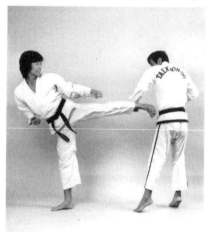

A: Execute a side-snapping kick to D's epigastrium with the left foot.

D: Block A's leg with the left outer forearm while pulling the left foot.

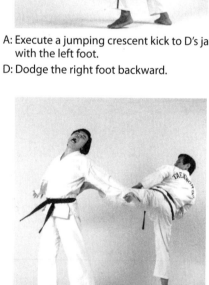

D: Execute a left side-snapping kick against A's kidney.

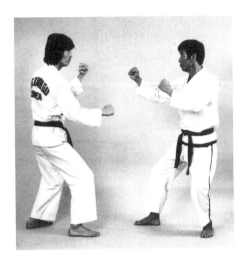

A: **Face D in right natural stance with a fist guarding block.**

D: **Face A in right L-stance with a fist guarding block.**

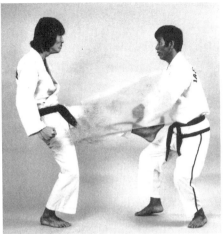

A: Execute a front snap kick to D's umbilicus with the left foot.

D: Block A's leg with X-fist.

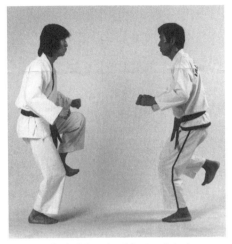

A: Bring the left foot beside the right knee joint while preparing to execute a front snap kick.

D: Move right foot backward while preparing to block.

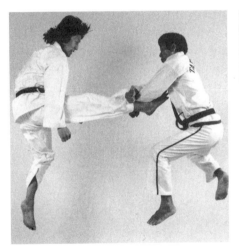

A: Execute a jumping front snap kick to D's chin with the right foot.

D: Block A's leg with X-fist while jumping backward.

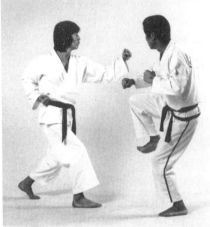

A: Land at D's front while preparing to punch.

D: Land at A's front while preparing to execute turning kick.

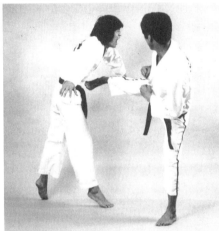

D: Execute a right turning kick against A's epigastrium.

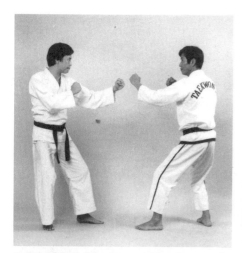

A: Face D in left L-stance with a fist guarding block.

D: Face A in left L-stance with a fist guarding block.

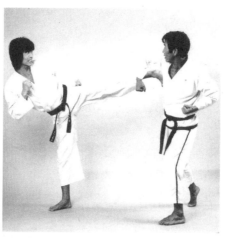

A: Execute a turning kick to D's solar plexus with the left foot.

D: Move left foot to the left while blocking A's leg with right outer forearm.

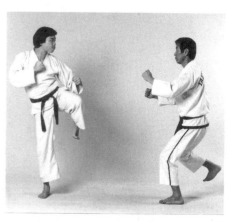

A: Bring the left foot beside the right knee joint while preparing to execute jumping mid-air kick.

D: Move right foot backward while preparing to block.

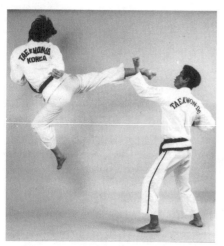

A: Execute a mid-air side kick to D's face with the right foot while spinning clockwise.

D: Block A's leg with the left outer forearm.

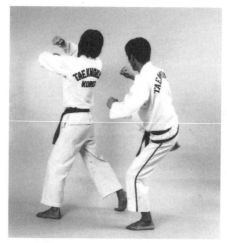

A: Land at D's side while preparing to execute back-fist strike.

D: Move left foot to the left while preparing to execute knee kick.

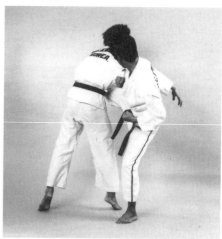

D: Execute a right knee kick against A's ribs.

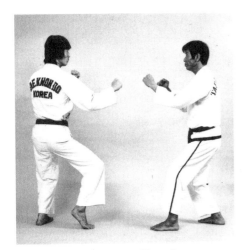

A: Face D in right vertical bending stance with a fist guarding block.

D: Face A in left natural stance with a fist guarding block.

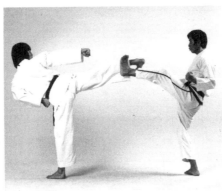

A: Execute a side snapping kick to D's solar plexus with right foot.

D: Block A's leg with the left side sole.

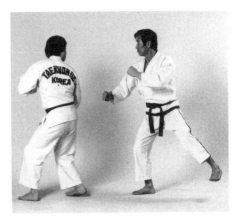

A: Lower the right foot to the right while preparing to execute reverse turning kick.

D: Lower the left foot backward while preparing to block.

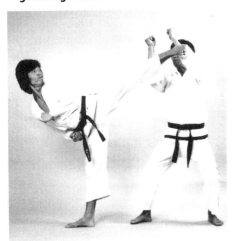

A: Execute a reverse turning kick to D's neck with the left foot.

D: Block A's leg with both outer forearms.

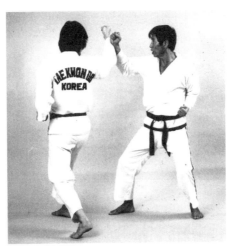

A: Strike at D's jaw with the right back-fist while lowering the left foot forward.

D: Block A's arm with the right outer forearm.

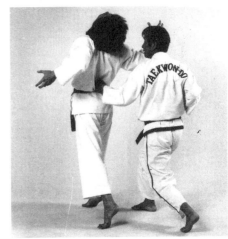

D: Execute a left vertical punch against A's kidney.

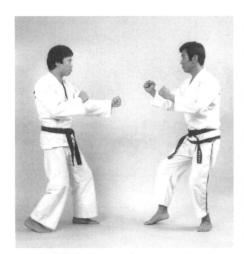

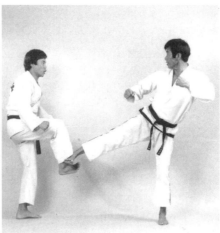

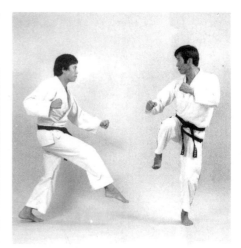

A: Face D in left natural stance with a fist guarding block.

D: Face A in right vertical bending stance with a fist guarding block.

A: Execute a front snap kick to D's umbilicus with the right foot.

D: Execute pressing side kick to A's leg with the right foot.

A: Lower the right foot forward while preparing to right punch.

D: Prepare to side kick.

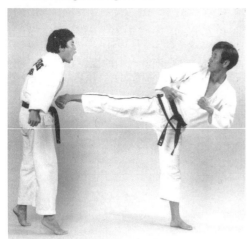

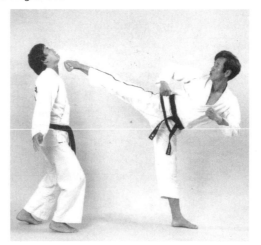

D: Execute a side pushing kick to A's umbilicus with the right foot.

D: Execute a right side-snapping kick against A's neck.

Attacking Techniques in Free Sparring

The student of taekwondo should attack only when there is a chance for a decisive blow. An effective way to score a decisive blow against the attacker is by either breaking through the defense with sheer force or by luring the attacker out of his defense posture by deception. Prior to this, however, the student should position himself securely in an impenetrable guarding posture at all times and attack only after having found or created an opportunity.

Also of vital importance is the proper selection of the weapon for the proper target, such as the use of the knee or elbow, or throw for close range attacks, and use flying kicks, turning kicks, or combination techniques for distant range attacks.

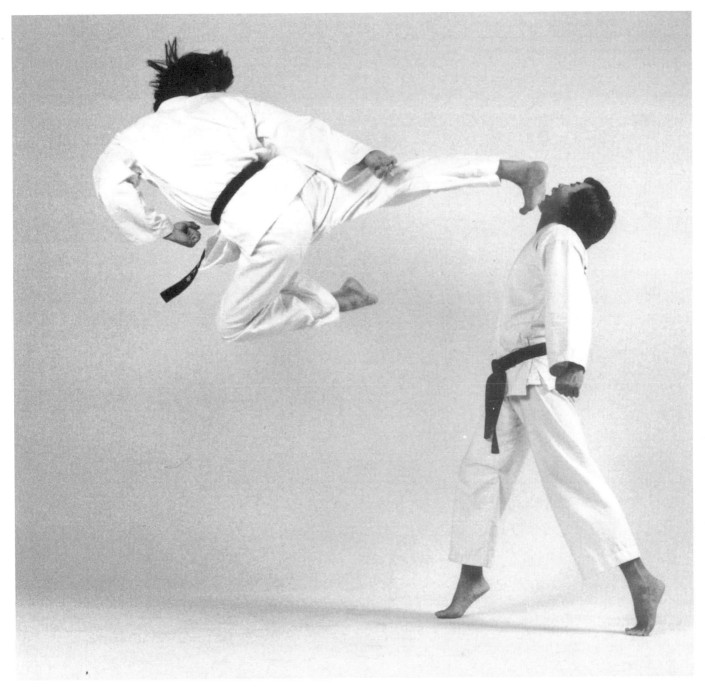

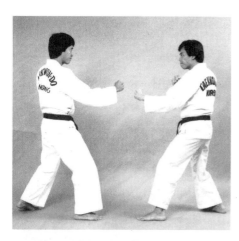

A: Face D in right natural stance with a fist guarding block.

D: Face A in left natural stance with a fist guarding block.

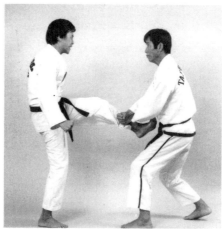

A: Execute front snap kick to D's umbilicus with the left foot.

D: Block A's leg with X-fist.

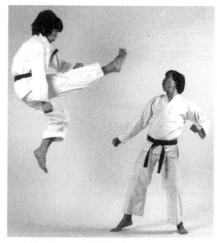

A: Execute a jumping front snap kick to D's chin with the right foot.

D: Dodge backward.

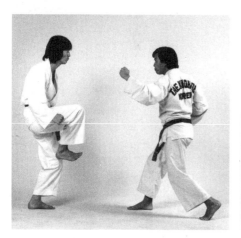

A: Land on the left foot while preparing to side kick.

D: Prepare to execute left punch.

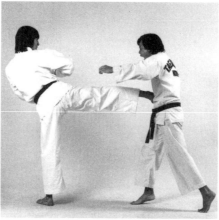

A: Execute a right side-snapping kick against D's epigastrium.

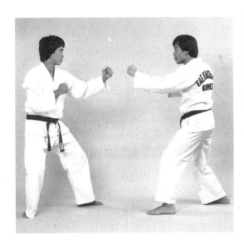

A: Face D in left L-stance with a fist guarding block.

D: Face A in left natural stance with a fist guarding block.

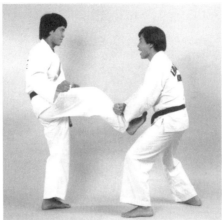

A: Execute front snap kick to D's scrotum with the left instep.

D: Block A's leg with X-fist.

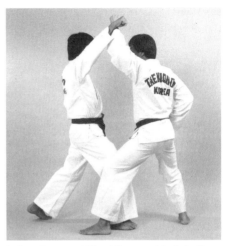

A: Punch toward D's philtrum with right fist while lowering the right foot forward.

D: Block A's arm with the left outer forearm.

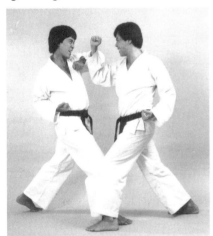

A: Strike toward D's jaw with the left side elbow.

D: Block A's arm with the right outer forearm.

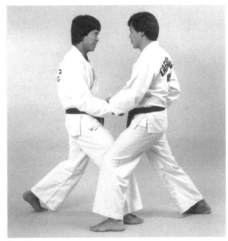

A: Execute vertical punch toward D's solar plexus with the right fist.

D: Block A's arm with the left outer forearm.

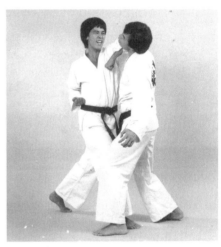

A: Execute a left side elbow strike against D's point of the jaw.

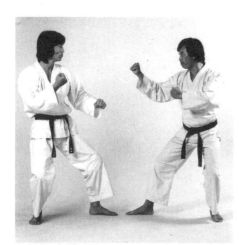

A: Face D in left L-stance with a fist guarding block.

D: Face A in right L-stance with a fist guarding block.

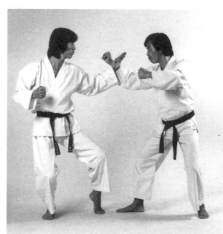

A: Fake to D's arm with the left knife-hand while pulling the right foot.

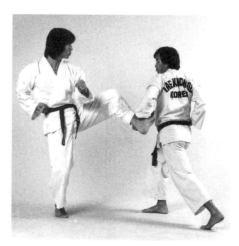

A: Execute a twisting kick to D's umbilicus with the left foot.

D: Block A's leg with the left outer forearm.

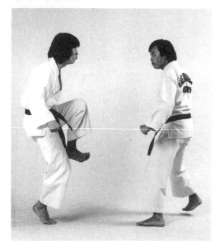

A: Prepare to execute a jumping turning kick.
D: Prepare to dodge.

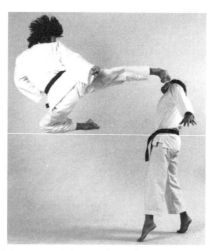

A: Execute a right jumping turning kick against D's jaw.

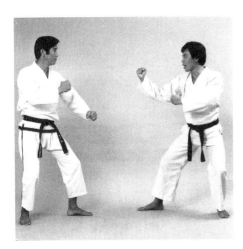

A: Face D in left L-stance with a fist guarding block.

D: Face A in right L-stance with a fist guarding block.

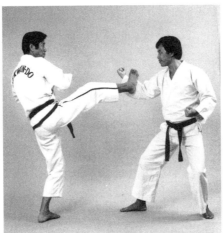

A: Crescent kick at D's arm with the right foot.

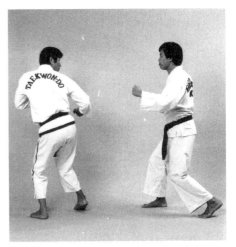

A: Lower the right foot to the right while preparing to execute back kick.

D: Prepare to execute front snap kick.

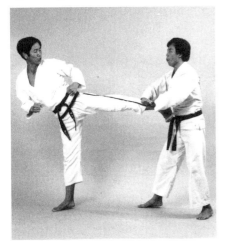

A: Execute a back side-snapping kick to D's solar plexus with the left foot.

D: Block A's leg with both palms while pulling the right foot.

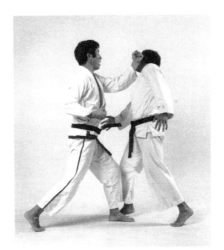

A: Execute a left back-fist strike against D's jaw while lowering the left foot forward.

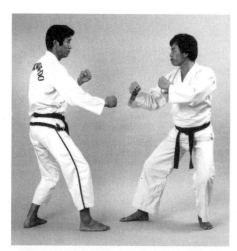

A: Face D in right natural stance with a fist guarding block.

D: Face A in right L-stance with a fist guarding block.

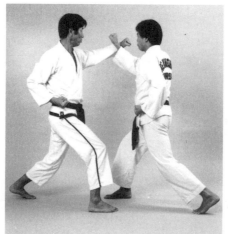

A: Punch at D's jaw with the left fist while slipping the right foot forward.

D: Block A's arm with the right outer forearm.

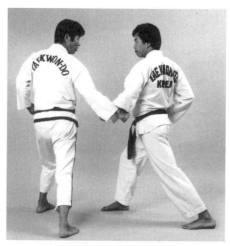

A: Punch at D's floating ribs while moving the left foot forward.

D: Block A's arm with left outer forearm while moving the right foot backward.

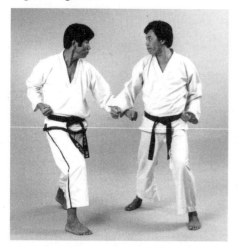

A: Punch at D's solar plexus with the left fist.

D: Block A's arm with right outer forearm.

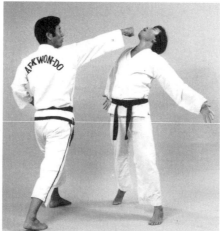

A: Execute a right punch against D's philtrum.

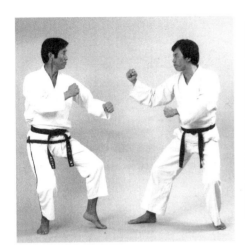

A: Face D in left vertical bending stance with a fist guarding block.

D: Face A in right L-stance with a fist guarding block.

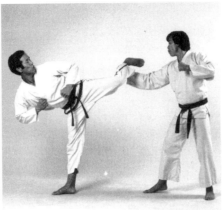

A: Execute a reverse hooking kick at D's arm with the left foot.

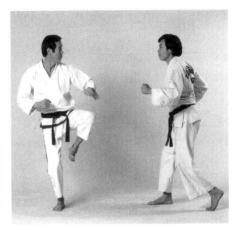

A: Prepare to side kick while pulling the left foot.

D: Prepare to execute a turning kick.

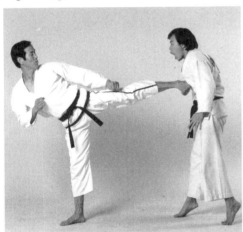

A: Execute a side checking kick at D's umbilicus with left foot.

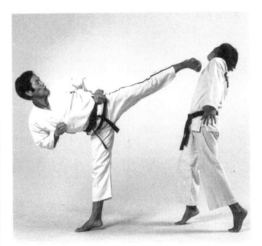

A: Execute a left side-snapping kick against D's chin.

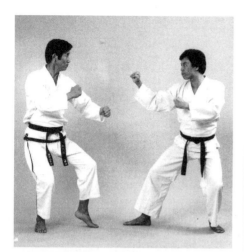

A: Face D in left vertical bending stance with a fist guarding block.

D: Face A in right L-stance with a fist guarding block.

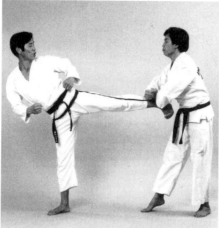

A: Execute a side-snapping kick to D's floating ribs with left foot.

D: Block A's leg with both side-fists while pulling A's right foot.

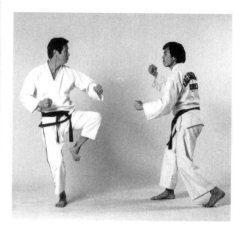

A: Prepare to execute a jumping crescent kick.

D: Prepare to left punch.

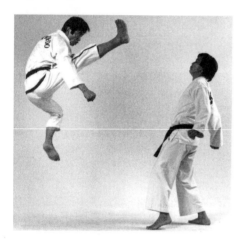

A: Execute a jumping crescent kick to D's jaw with the right foot.

D: Dodge backward.

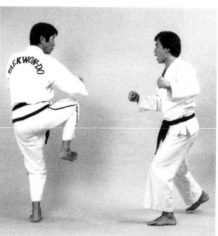

A: Land on the left foot while preparing to side kick.

D: Prepare to execute a turning kick.

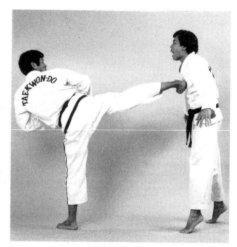

A: Execute a right side-snapping kick against D's solar plexus.

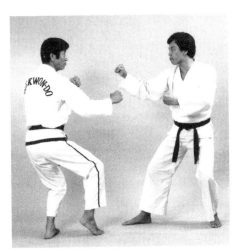

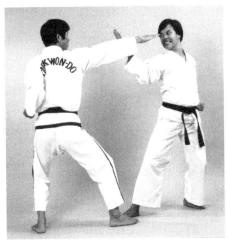

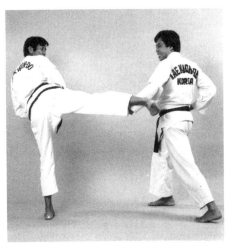

A: Face D in right vertical bending stance with a fist guarding block.

D: Face A in right L-stance with a fist guarding block.

A: Fake thrust to D's eyeball with right flat fingertip.

D: Block A's arm with the right knife-hand.

A: Execute a turning kick to D's lower abdomen with right foot.

D: Block A's leg with the left outer forearm while moving the right foot to the right.

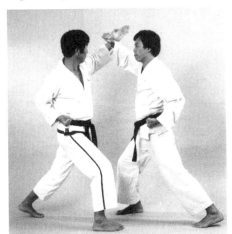

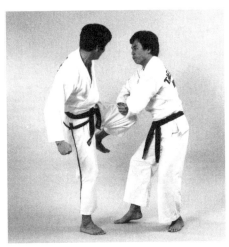

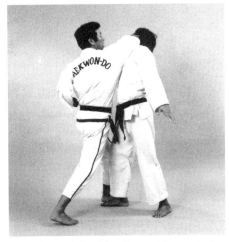

A: Strike inward to D's neck with the left knife-hand while lowering the right foot forward.

D: Block A's arm with right outer forearm.

A: Execute a turning kick to D's floating ribs with the left knee.

D: Block A's leg with both side-fists.

A: Execute a right side-elbow strike against D's jaw while lowering the left foot forward.

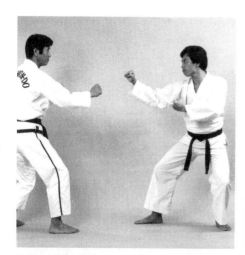

A: Face D in right natural stance with a fist guarding block.
D: Face A in right L-stance with a fist guarding block.

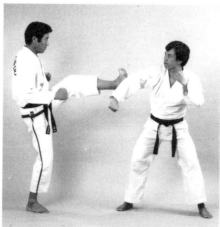

A: Execute a crescent kick to D's elbow with left foot.

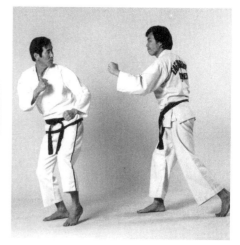

A: Prepare to execute reverse hooking kick.
D: Prepare to execute turning kick.

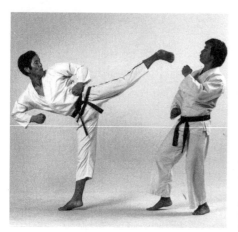

A: Execute a reverse hooking kick to D's neck with the left foot.
D: Dodge backward while pulling the right foot.

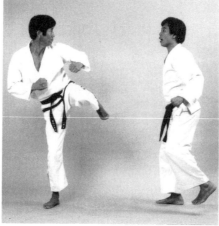

A: Prepare to side kick.
D: Prepare to execute turning kick.

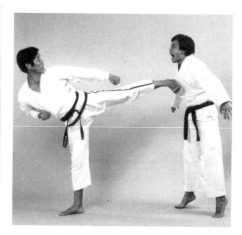

A: Execute a left side-snapping kick against D's solar plexus.

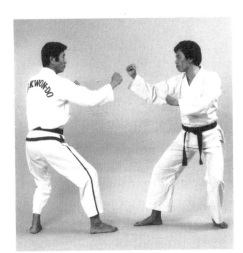

A: Face D in right L-stance with a fist guarding block.

D: Face A in right L-stance with a fist guarding block.

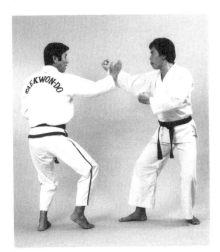

A: Fake strike to D's arm with right palm while pulling right leg.

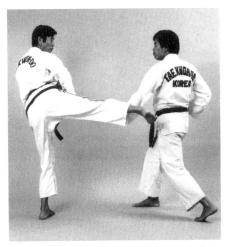

A: Execute a turning kick to D's lower abdomen with the right foot.

D: Block A's leg with the left forearm.

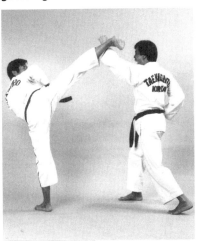

A: Execute a turning kick to D's jaw with the right foot.

D: Block A's leg with the left outer forearm while moving the right foot to the right.

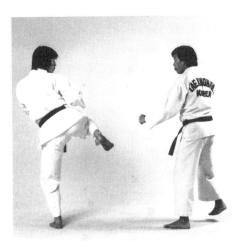

A: Prepare to execute a jumping reverse turning kick.

D: Prepare to dodge.

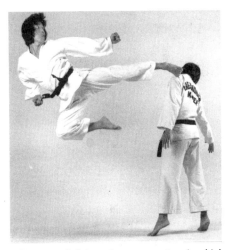

A: Execute a left jumping reverse turning kick against D's upper neck.

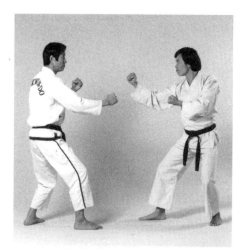

A: Face D in right natural stance with a fist guarding block.

D: Face A in right L-stance with a fist guarding block.

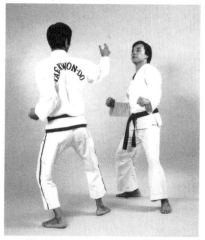

A: Fake strike to D's face with the right back-hand while moving the left foot and turning body counterclockwise.

D: Move the right foot to the right while dodging.

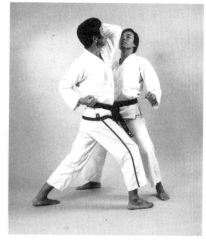

A: Execute an upward strike at D's chin with the left elbow while slipping the right foot.

D: Dodge A's elbow to the left side.

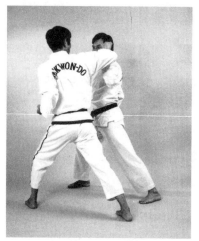

A: Strike to D's jaw with the right side-elbow.

D: Block A's arm with the left outer forearm.

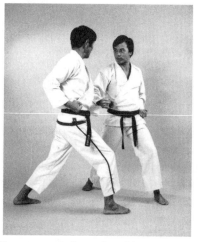

A: Execute vertical punch to D's epigastrium with left fist.

D: Block A's arm with the right outer forearm.

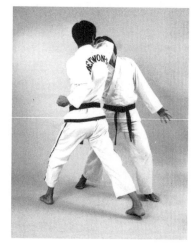

A: Execute a right elbow strike against D's jaw.

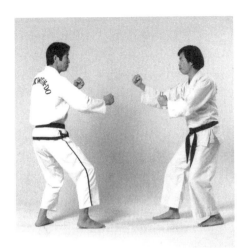

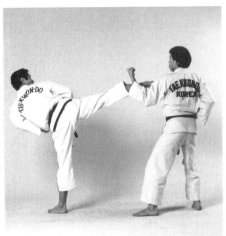

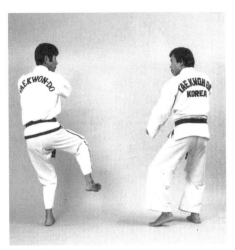

A: Face D in right natural stance with a fist guarding block.

D: Face A in right natural stance with a fist guarding block.

A: Execute a side-snapping kick to D's Adam's apple with right foot.

D: Block A's leg with the left outer forearm while moving the right foot backward.

A: Prepare to execute knife-hand strike.

D: Prepare to execute turning kick while moving left foot to the left.

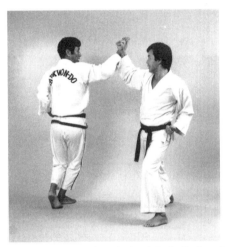

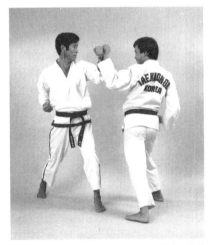

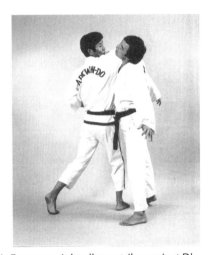

A: Strike to D's neck with the right knife-hand while forming a right X-stance.

D: Block A's arm with the right outer forearm.

A: Side strike to D's jaw with the left back-fist while turning counterclockwise and moving left foot to the left.

D: Block A's arm with left outer forearm.

A: Execute a right elbow strike against D's jaw while turning body clockwise, pivoting on left foot.

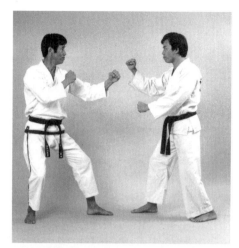

A: Face D in left L-stance with a fist guard-ing block.

D: Face A in right natural stance with a fist guarding block.

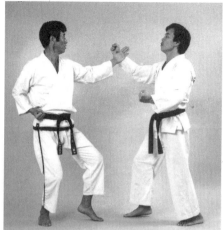

A: Fake strike to D's arm with the left back-hand while pulling the right foot.

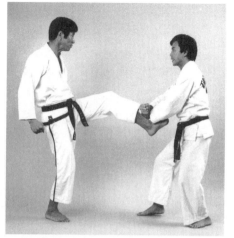

A: Execute a front snap kick to D's epigas-trium with the left foot.

D: Block A's leg with X-fist while pulling the right foot.

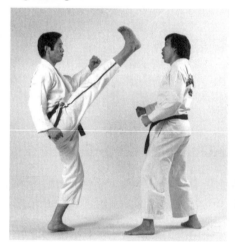

A: Execute a diagonally downward kick to D's neck with the right back heel.

D: Dodge backward while moving the right foot.

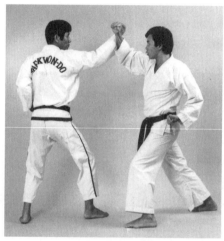

A: Execute a right back-fist strike to D's jaw while lowering the right foot to the right.

D: Block A's arm with right outer forearm.

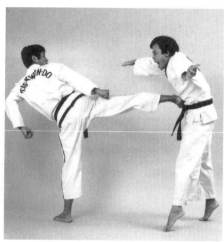

A: Execute a right side thrusting kick against D's epigastrium.

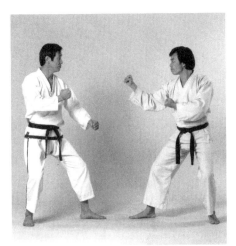

A: Face D in left L-stance with a fist guarding block.

D: Face A in right L-stance with a fist guarding block.

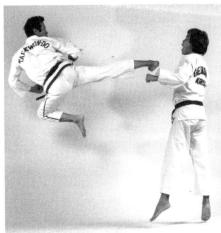

A: Execute a jumping turning kick to D's jaw with the right foot.

D: Jump to dodge while moving right foot backward.

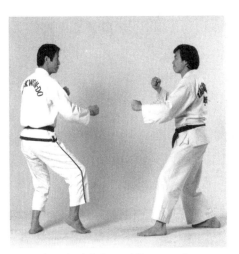

A: Land on the left foot while preparing to flying mid-air side kick.

D: Prepare to turning kick.

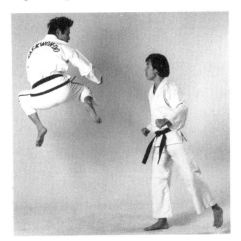

A: Fly by spinning 180 degrees.

D: Move left foot backward while dodging.

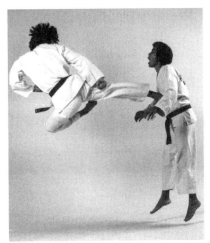

A: Execute a right side thrusting kick against D's sternum.

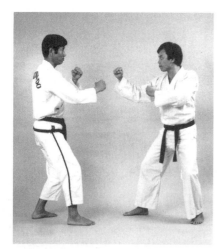

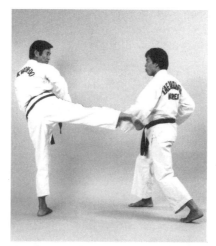

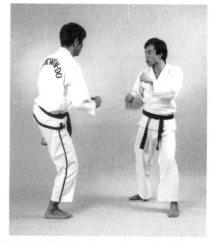

A: Face D in right natural stance with a fist guarding block.

D: Face A in right L-stance with a fist guarding block.

A: Execute a turning kick to D's epigastrium with the right foot.

D: Block A's leg with the left outer forearm while moving right foot to the right.

A: Lower the right foot to the right while preparing to execute a turning kick.

D: Prepare to block.

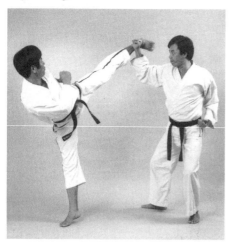

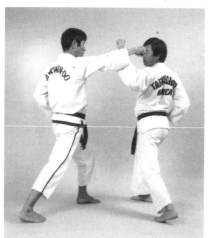

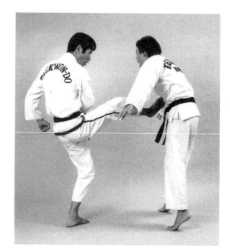

A: Execute a turning kick to D's face with the left foot.

D: Block A's leg with the right outer forearm.

A: Punch toward D's jaw with the right fist, and at the same time lower the left foot to the left.

D: Block A's arm with the left outer forearm.

A: Execute a right twisting kick against D's abdomen.

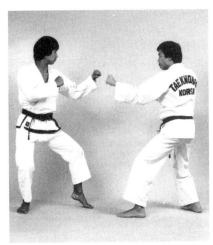

A: Face D in left natural bending stance with a fist guarding block.

D: Face A in left natural stance with a fist guarding block.

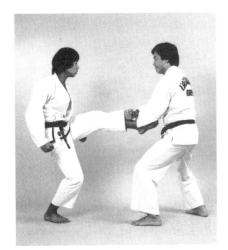

A: Execute a front snap kick to D's lower abdomen with the left foot.

D: Block A's leg with X-fist.

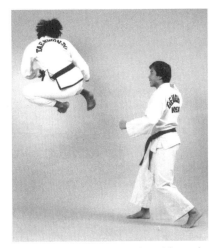

A: Prepare to execute a jumping side pushing kick.

D: Prepare to dodge backward.

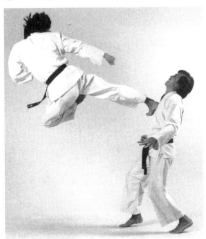

A: Execute a right side pushing kick against D's sternum.

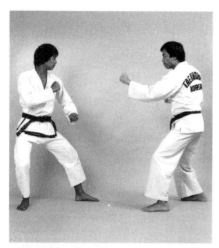

A: Face D in left L-stance with a fist guarding block.

D: Face A in left natural stance with a fist guarding block.

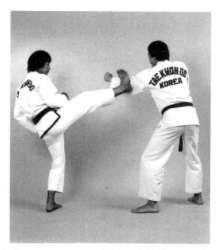

A: Execute a crescent kick at D's elbow with the right foot.

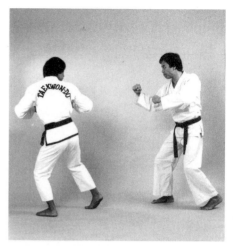

A: Lower the right foot to the right while preparing to execute a reverse turning kick.

D: Move left foot backward while dodging.

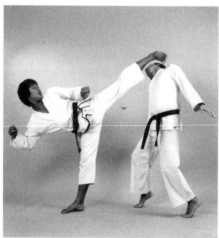

A: Execute a left reverse turning kick against D's neck.

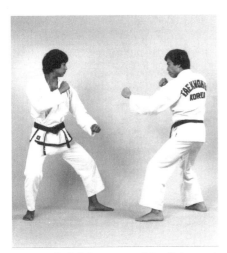

A: Face D in left L-stance with a fist guarding block.

D: Face A in left natural stance with a fist guarding block.

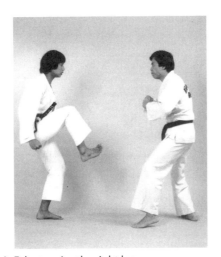

A: Fake to raise the right leg.

D: Prepare to block while pulling the left foot.

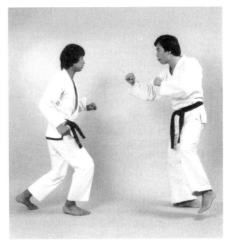

A: Lower the right foot in front of the left foot while preparing to jump.

D: Move the left foot backward while preparing to block.

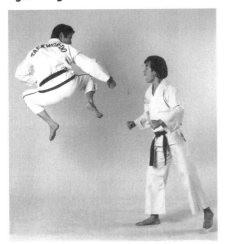

A: Prepare to execute a flying kick by jumping and spinning clockwise 180 degrees.

D: Dodge backward.

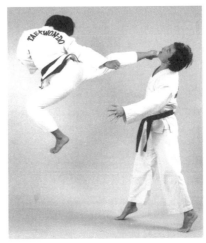

A: Execute a right reverse turning kick against D's neck while spinning clockwise.

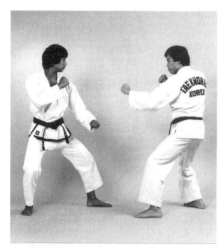

A: Face D in left L-stance with a fist guarding block.

D: Face A in left natural stance with a fist guarding block.

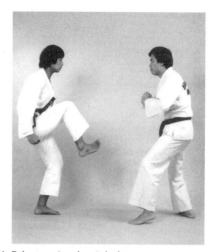

A: Fake to raise the right leg.

D: Prepare to block while pulling the left foot.

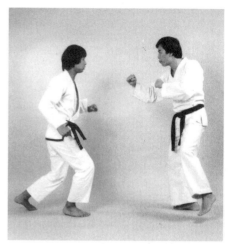

A: Lower the right foot in front of the left foot while preparing to jump.

D: Move the left foot backward while preparing to block.

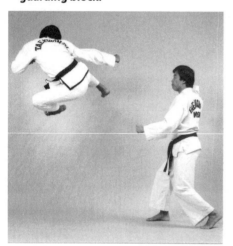

A: Prepare to execute a flying kick by jumping and spinning clockwise 180 degrees.

D: Dodge backward.

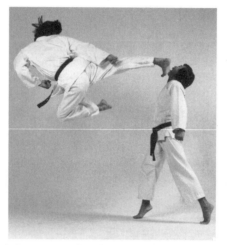

A: Execute a right side thrusting kick against D's face while spinning clockwise.

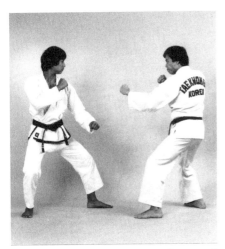

A: Face D in left L-stance with a fist guarding block.

D: Face A in left natural stance with a fist guarding block.

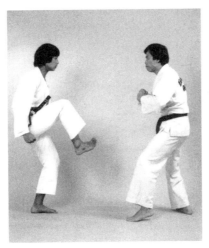

A: Fake to raise the right leg.

D: Prepare to block while pulling the left foot.

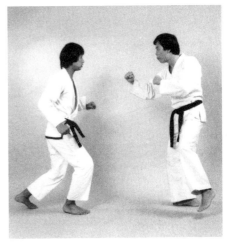

A: Lower the right foot in front of the left foot while preparing to jump.

D: Move the left foot backward while preparing to block.

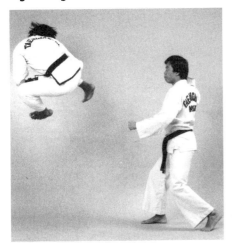

A: Fly by spinning clockwise 180 degrees.

D: Dodge backward.

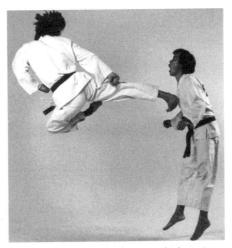

A: Execute a right side thrusting kick against D's sternum while spinning clockwise.

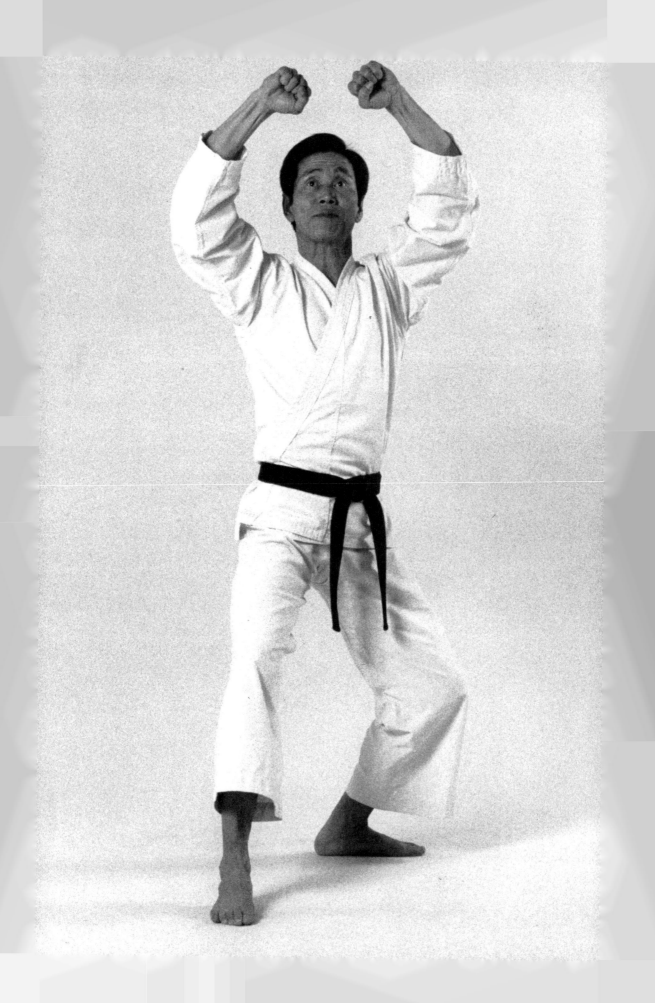

CHAPTER 4
PATTERNS

The patterns usually involve a rapid series of defense and/or attack techniques requiring proper, logical movements. Thus while performing patterns, correct posture and facing must be maintained at all times, distributing attacking and defensive techniques equally among right and left hands and feet.

By exercising the pole and knife patterns in this book, you will be able to acquire certain special techniques that cannot be obtained from either fundamental exercises or sparring.

The pattern practice can help to improve your flexibility of movements, control breathing, and develop smooth and rhythmical motions as well as building a muscular physique.

DIRECTION OF DIAGRAM

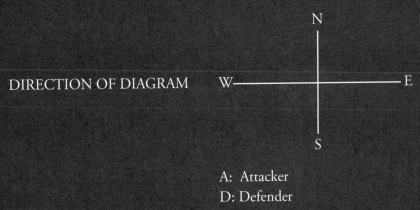

A: Attacker
D: Defender

This diagram shows the four directions the student will follow during the performance of patterns, under the assumption that the student is facing N.

Silla Patterns

The Silla Pattern as the name implies has its origin in the Silla dynasty about 1,350 years ago during the reign of Pak Hyokkose. The pattern, which is also known as Hwa Rang Pattern, was practiced by a group of young noblemen warriors who trained themselves in martial arts and refined their souls to provide the fountainhead for the defense of their country and to eventually become the actual driving force for the unification of the three kingdoms—Koryo, Silla, and Baek-je.

Silla Pattern I

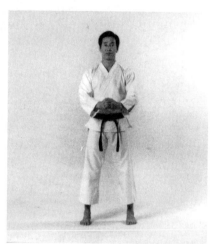

Parallel ready stance. Student facing N

Diagram:

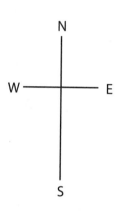

72 Movements

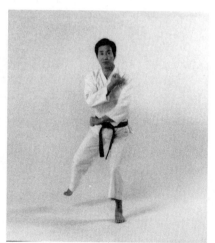

Preparing to execute a right 9-shape block.

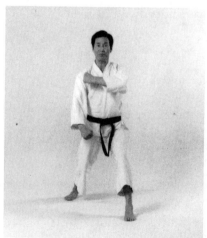

1. Move the right foot to S, forming a left long walking stance while executing a right 9-shape block.

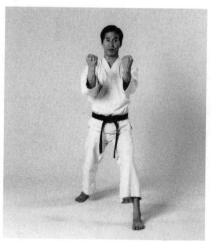

2. Execute a middle wedging block with inner forearm.

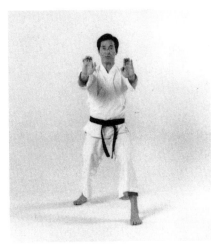

3. Execute a middle pushing block to N with both palms.

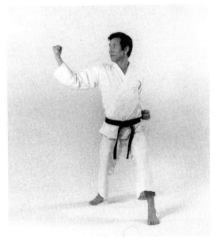

4. Execute a high side block to E with right inner forearm.

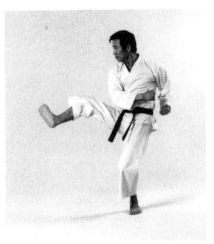

5. Execute a low twisting kick to E with right foot.

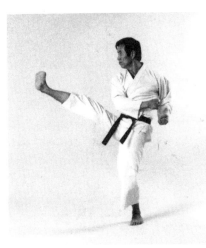

6. Execute a middle twisting kick to E with right foot.

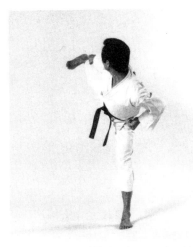

7. Execute a middle back snapping kick to S with right foot.

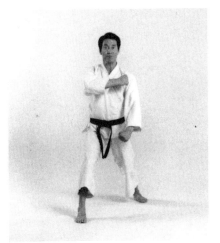

8. Bring the right foot close beside left foot and then move the left foot to S, forming a right long walking stance while executing a left 9-shape block.

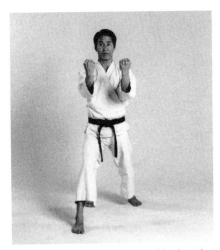

9. Execute a middle wedging block with the inner forearm.

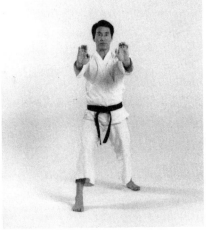

10. Execute a middle pushing block to N with both palms.

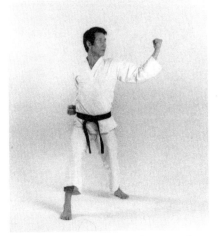

11. Execute a high side block to W with left inner forearm.

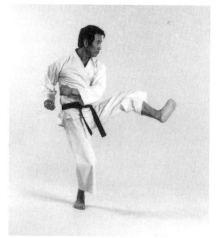

12. Execute a low twisting kick to W with the left foot.

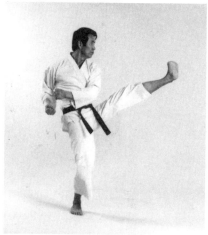

13. Execute a middle twisting kick to W with the left foot.

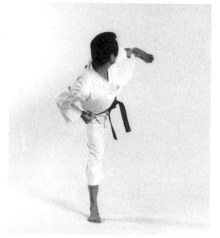

14. Execute a middle back snapping kick to S with the left foot.

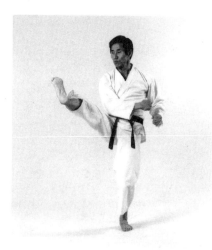

15. Bring the left foot close beside right foot and then execute a middle twisting kick to NE with the right foot.

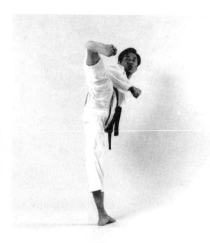

16. Execute a middle turning kick to N with the right foot.

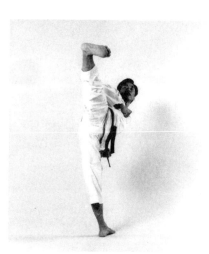

17. Execute a high turning kick to N with the right foot.

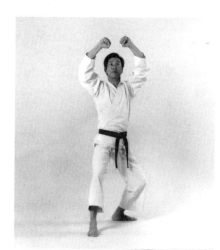

18. Lower the right foot to N, forming a right L-stance, and execute a rising block with both outer forearms.

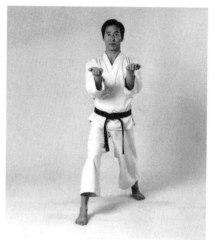

19. Execute a middle scooping block with both palms while forming a right long walking stance, slipping the right foot.

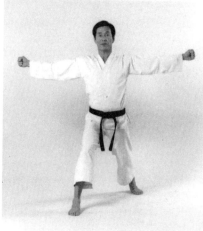

20. Execute a middle strike to W and E with the back fists.

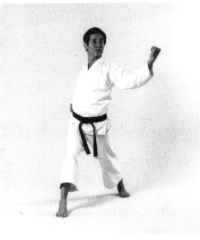

21. Execute a high circular block to NW with left inner forearm.

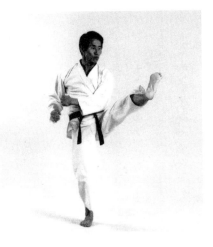

22. Execute a middle twisting kick to NW with the left foot.

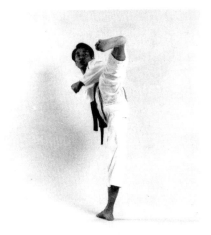

23. Execute a middle turning kick to N with the left foot.

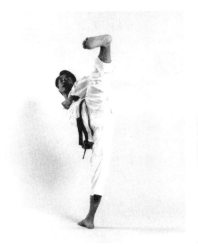

24. Execute a high turning kick to N with the left foot.

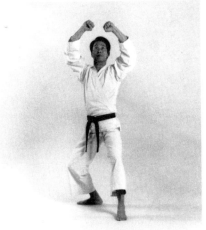

25. Lower the left foot to N, forming a left L-stance, and execute a rising block with both outer forearms.

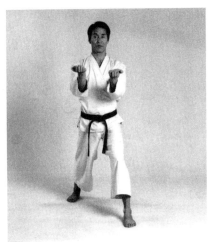

26. Execute a middle scooping block to N with both palms while forming a left long walking stance, slipping the left foot.

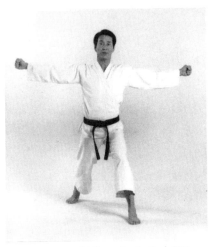

27. Execute a middle strike to E and W with the back fists.

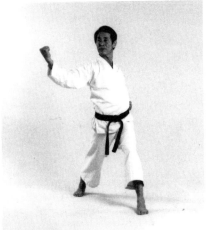

28. Execute a high circular block to NE with right inner forearm.

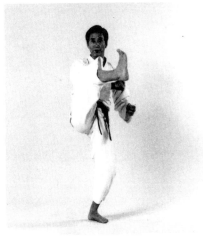

29. Execute a middle crescent kick to N with the right foot.

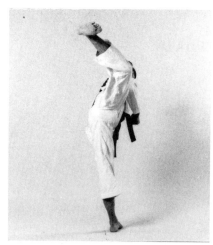

30. Execute a high reverse hooking kick to N with the right foot.

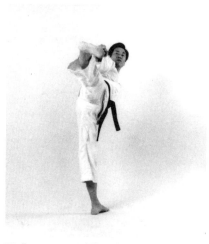

31. Execute a middle side-snapping kick to N with the right foot.

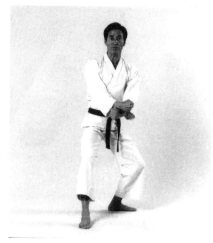

32. Lower the right foot to N, forming a right L-stance, and execute pressing block to N with an X-fist.

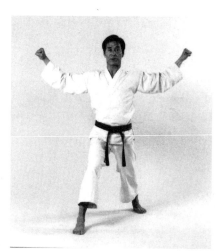

33. Execute a high W-shape block with outer forearms while forming a right long walking stance, slipping the right foot.

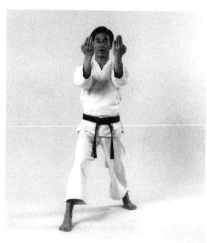

34. Execute a high inward strike to N with both knife-hands.

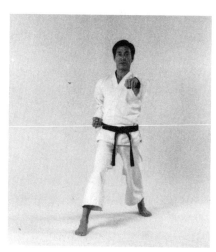

35. Execute a middle punch with the left fist.

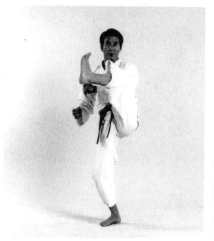

36. Execute a middle crescent kick to N with the left foot.

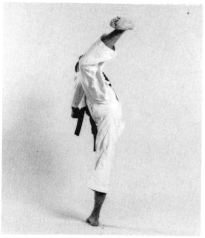

37. Execute a high reverse hooking kick to N with the left foot.

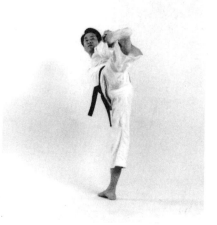

38. Execute a middle side-snapping kick to N with the left foot.

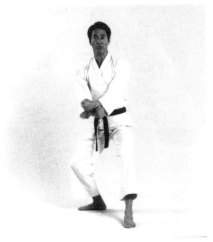

39. Lower the left foot to N, forming a left L-stance, and execute a pressing block to N with an X-fist.

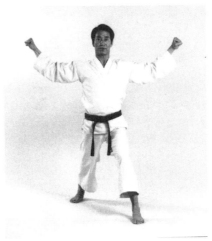

40. Execute a high W-shape block with outer forearms while forming a left long walking stance, slipping the left foot.

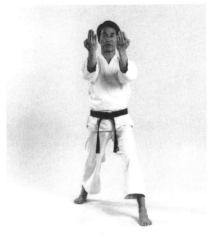

41. Execute a high inward strike to N with both knife-hands.

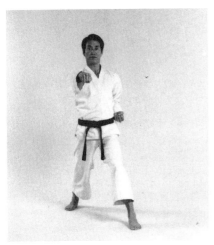

42. Execute a middle punch with the right fist.

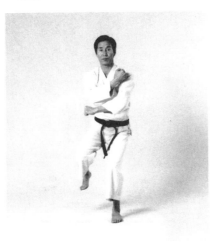

43a. Preparing to execute a low block with the right outer forearm.

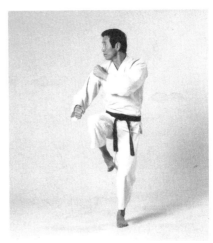

43b. Bring the right foot to the left knee joint forming a left one-leg bending stance toward N while executing a low block with the right outer forearm, bringing the left semi-prone fist horizontally in front of the right chest and turning face toward E.

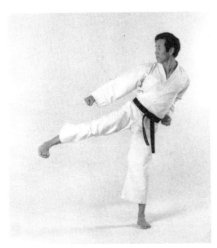

44. Execute a low side pressing kick to E with the right foot.

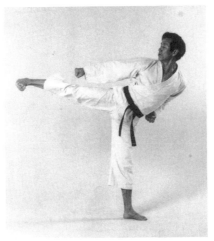

45. Execute a middle side-snapping kick to E with the right foot.

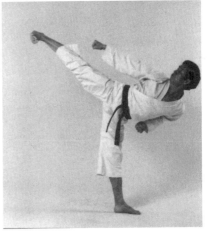

46. Execute a high side-snapping kick to E with the right foot.

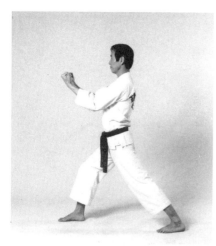

47. Lower the right foot to E, forming a right long walking stance toward E, and execute a middle wedging block with inner forearms.

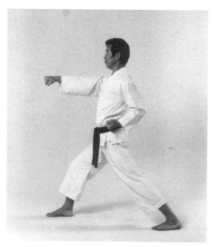

48. Execute a middle punch with the right fist.

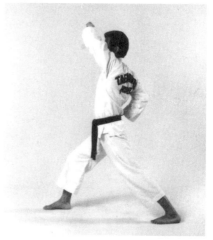

49. Execute a rising block with the left outer forearm.

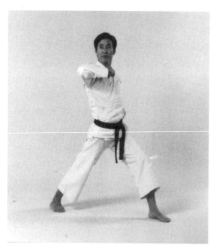

50. Execute a middle strike to N with the right side elbow while forming a left long walking stance toward N pivoting on both feet.

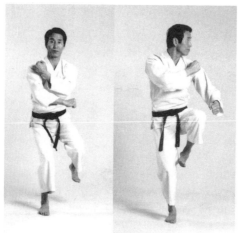

51. Bring the left foot to the right knee joint, forming a right one-leg bending stance toward N while executing a low block with a left outer forearm, bringing the right semi-prone fist horizontally in front of the left chest and turning face toward W.

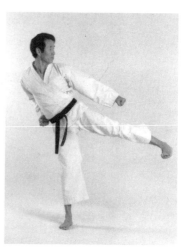

52. Execute a low side pressing kick to W with the left foot.

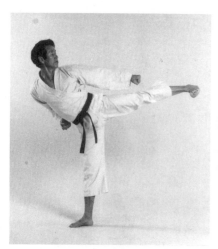

53. Execute a middle side-snapping kick to W with the left foot.

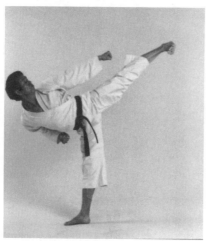

54. Execute a high side-snapping kick to W with the left foot.

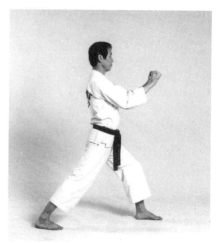

55. Lower the left foot to W, forming a left long walking stance toward W, and execute a middle wedging block with the inner forearms.

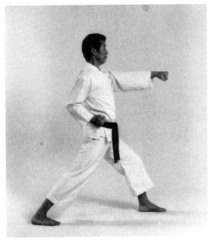

56. Execute a middle punch with the left fist.

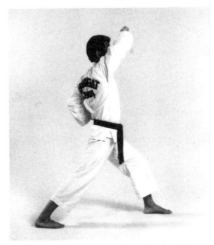

57. Execute a rising block with the right outer forearm.

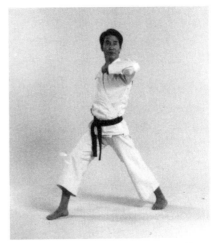

58. Execute a middle strike to N with the left side elbow while forming a right long walking stance toward N, pivoting on both feet.

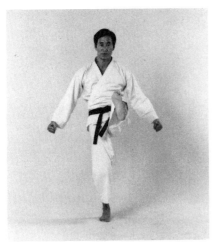

59. Execute a middle front snap kick to N with the left foot.

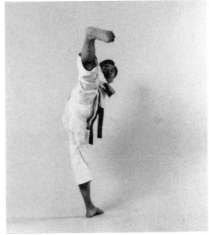

60. Lower the left foot to the right foot and then execute a high turning kick to N with the right foot.

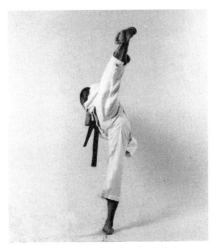

61. Lower the right foot to the left foot and then execute a high reverse turning kick to N with the left foot.

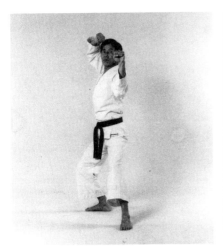

62. Lower the left foot to N, forming a left L-stance, and execute a square outer forearm block.

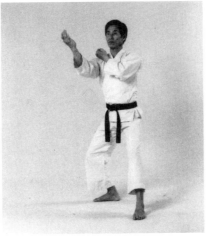

63. Execute a high inward strike to NE with the right knife-hand and bring the left side fist in front of the right shoulder.

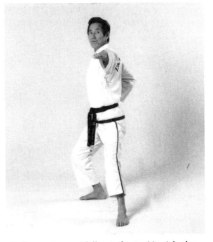

64. Execute a middle strike to N with the left knife-hand.

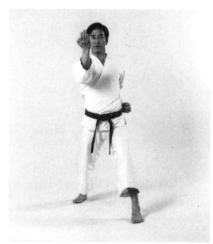

65. Execute a high inward strike to N with the right knife-hand while forming a left long walking stance, slipping left foot.

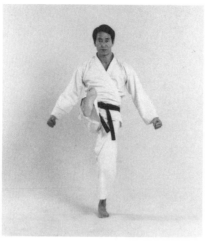

66. Execute a middle front snap kick to N with the right foot.

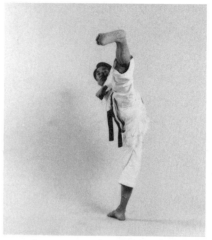

67. Lower the right foot to the left foot and then execute a high turning kick to N with the left foot.

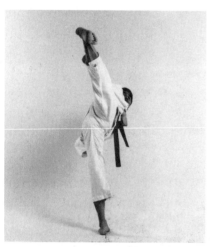

68. Lower the left foot to the right foot and then execute a high reverse turning kick to N with the right foot.

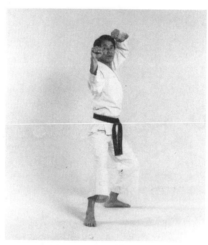

69. Lower the right foot to N, forming a right L-stance and execute a square outer forearm block.

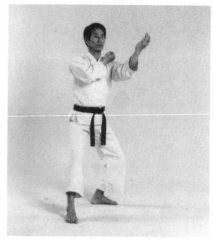

70. Execute a high inward strike to NW with the left knife-hand while bringing the right side fist in front of the left shoulder.

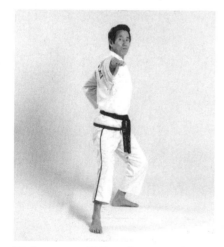

71. Execute a middle strike to N with the right knife-hand.

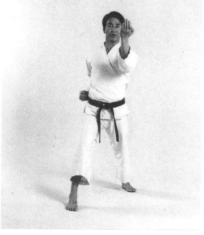

72. Execute a high inward strike to N with the left knife-hand while forming a right long walking stance, slipping the right foot.

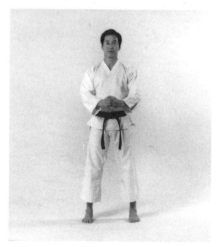

End. Bring the left foot forward to form a ready stance.

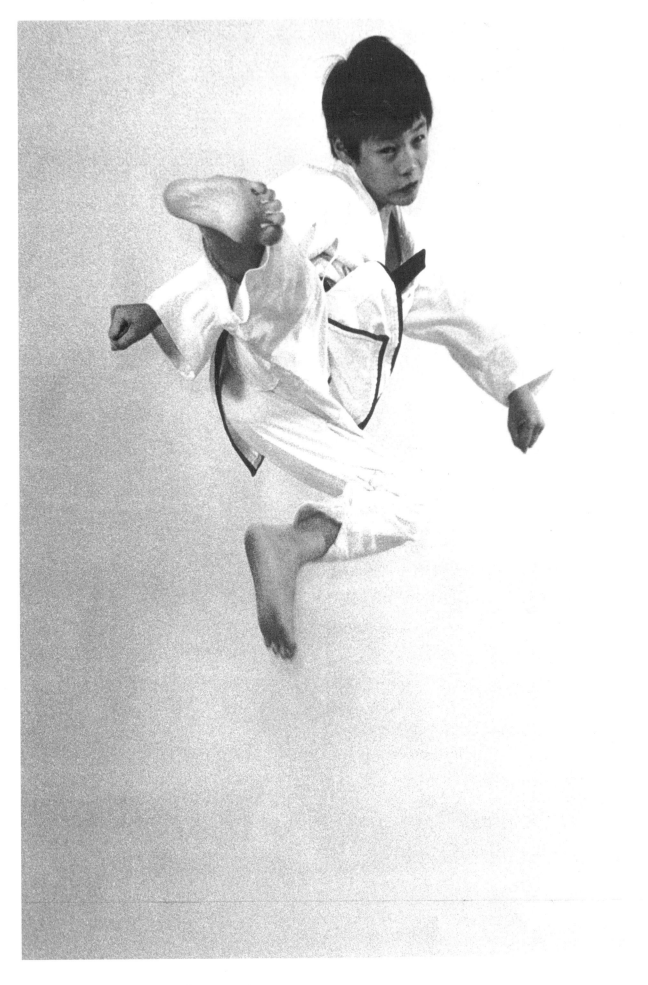

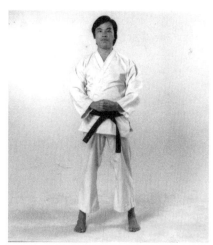

Diagram:

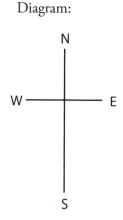

58 Movements

Parallel ready stance. Student facing N.

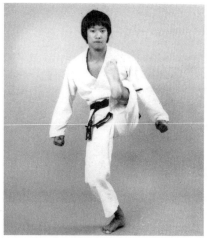

1. Execute a middle crescent kick to N with the left foot.

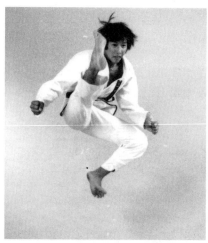

2. Execute a jumping crescent kick to N with the right foot without lowering the left foot.

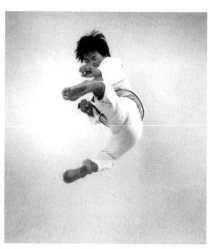

3. Execute a jumping side-snapping kick to N with the left foot without lowering the right foot.

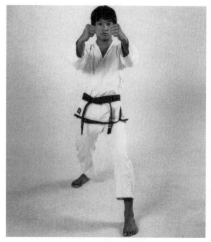

4. Lower the left foot to N forming a left long walking stance while executing a high vertical punch to N with the twin fist.

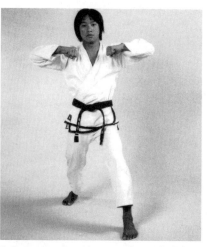

5. Execute a thrusting to sides with the double side elbow.

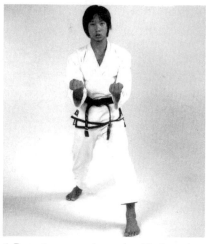

6. Execute an upset punch with the twin fist.

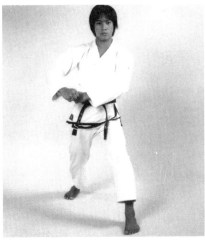

7. Execute a middle pressing block to NE with both side fists.

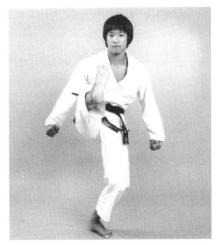

8. Execute a middle crescent kick to N with the right foot.

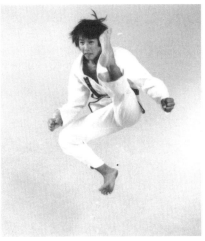

9. Execute a jumping crescent kick to N with the left foot without lowering the right foot.

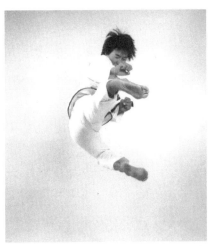

10. Execute a jumping side-snapping kick to N with the right foot without lowering the left foot.

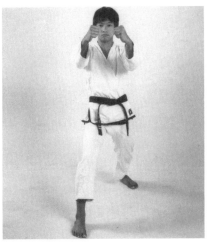

11. Lower the right foot to N forming a right long walking stance while executing a high vertical punch to N with the twin fists.

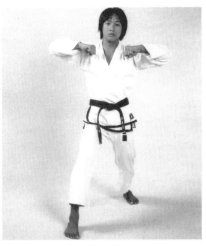

12. Execute a thrust to sides with the double side elbow.

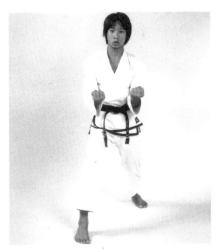

13. Execute an upset punch with the twin fists.

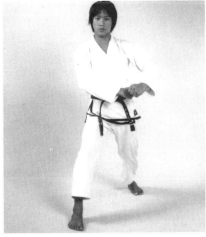

14. Execute a middle pressing block to NW with both side fists.

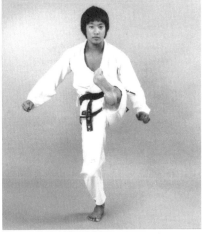

15. Execute a middle front snap kick to N with the left foot.

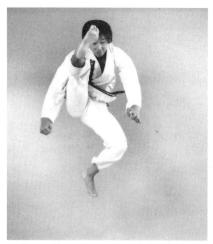

16. Execute a jumping front snap kick to N with the right foot without lowering the left foot.

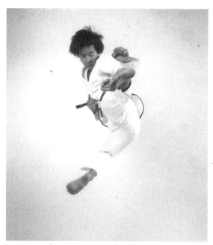

17. Execute a jumping turning kick to N with the left foot without lowering the right foot.

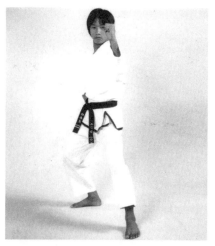

18. Lower the left foot to N, forming a left L-stance while executing a high strike to N with the left back fist.

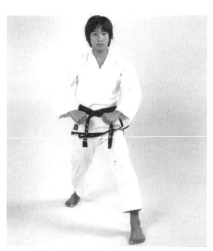

19. Execute a low block with both outer forearms while forming a left long walking stance, slipping the left foot.

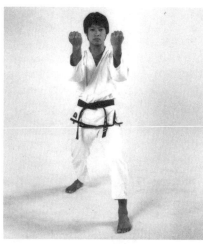

20. Execute a high wedging block with the inner forearms.

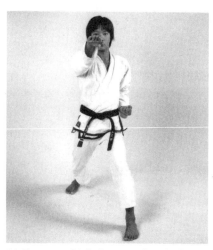

21. Execute a high thrust with right flat fingertip.

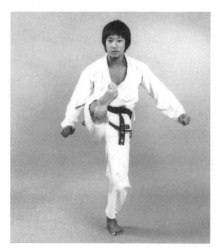

22. Execute a middle front snap kick to N with the right foot.

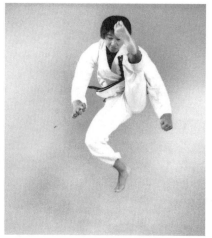

23. Execute a jumping front snap kick to N with the left foot without lowering the right foot.

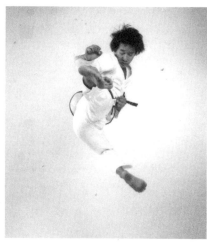

24. Execute a jumping turning kick to N with the right foot without lowering the left foot.

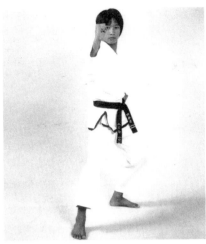

25. Lower the right foot to N, forming a right L-stance while executing a high strike to N with the right back fist.

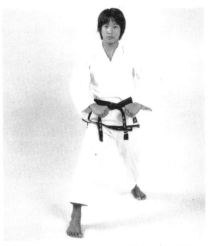

26. Execute a low block with both outer forearms while forming a right long walking stance, slipping the right foot.

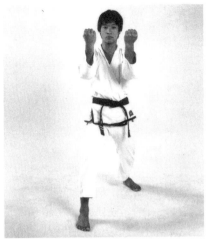

27. Execute a high wedging block with the inner forearms.

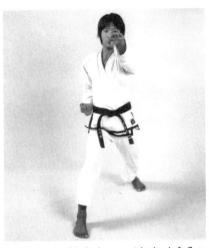

28. Execute a high thrust with the left flat fingertip.

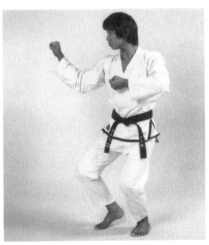

29. Bring the left foot to close beside the right foot, forming a right natural bending stance toward E while executing a high guarding block with a right outer forearm.

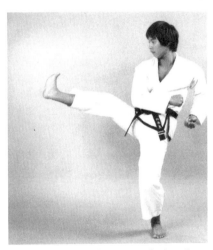

30. Execute a middle twisting kick to E with the right foot.

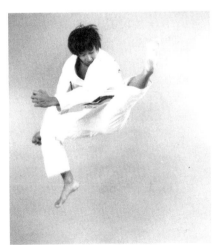

31. Execute a jumping twisting kick to N with the left foot without lowering the right foot.

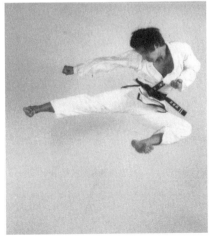

32. Execute a jumping side-snapping kick to E with the right foot without lowering the left foot.

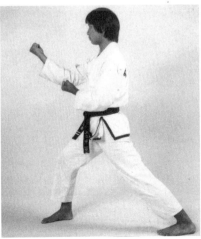

33. Lower the right foot to E, forming a right long walking stance while executing a middle block to E with right double forearm.

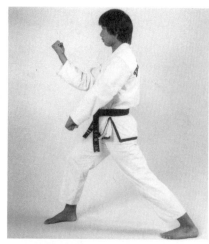

34. Execute a low block with a left fore-arm, keeping the right forearm as it was in 33.

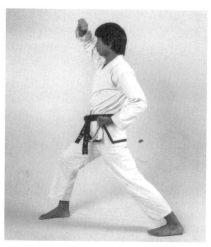

35. Execute a rising block with the right forearm.

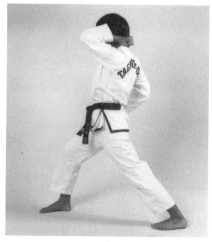

36. Execute a high strike to E with the left upper elbow.

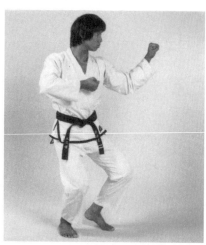

37. Bring the right foot to close beside left foot, forming a left natural bending stance toward W while executing a high guarding block with left outer forearm.

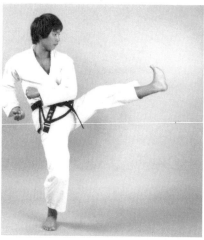

38. Execute a middle twisting kick to W with the left foot.

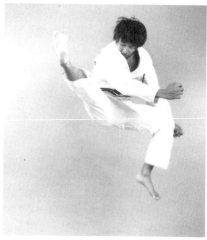

39. Execute a jumping twisting kick to N with the right foot without lowering the left foot.

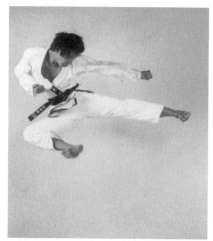

40. Execute a jumping side-snapping kick to W with the left foot without lower-ing the right foot.

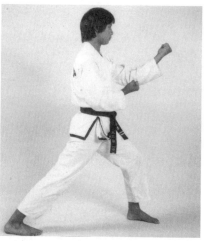

41. Lower the left foot to W, forming a left long walking stance while executing a middle block to E with a left double forearm.

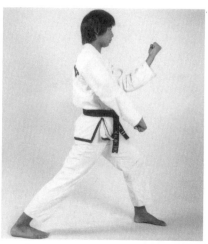

42. Execute a low block with a right forearm, keeping the left forearm as it was in 41.

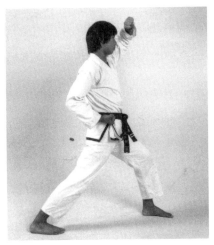

43. Execute a rising block with a left forearm.

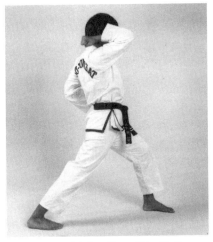

44. Execute a high strike to W with the right upper elbow.

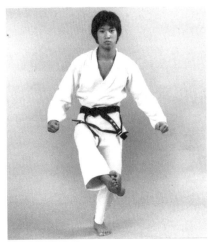

45. Bring the left foot to close beside right foot while executing a low sweeping kick to N with the right foot.

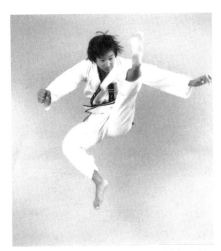

46. Execute a jumping crescent kick to N with the left foot without lowering the right foot.

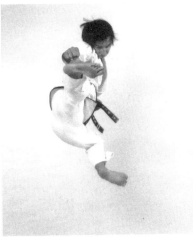

47. Execute a jumping side-snapping kick to N with the right foot while spinning clockwise 180 degrees.

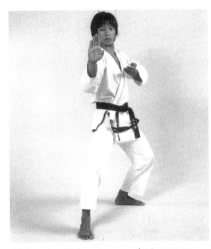

48. Land at N, forming a right L-stance while executing a middle guarding block with a right knife-hand.

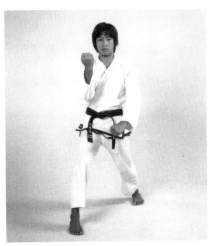

49. Execute a low block with a left outer forearm and then middle block with a right inner forearm while forming a right long walking stance, slipping the right foot.

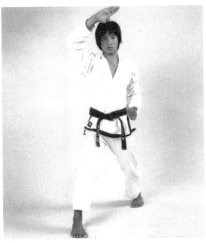

50. Execute a rising block with a right knife-hand.

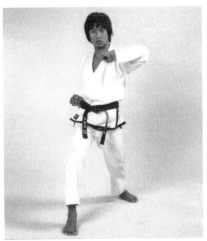

51. Execute a middle strike with the left side elbow.

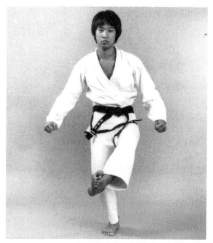

52. Execute a sweeping kick to N with the left foot.

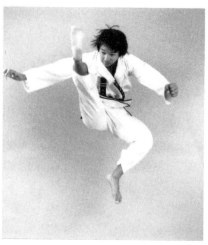

53. Execute a jumping crescent kick to N with the right foot.

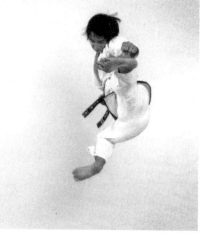

54. Execute a jumping side-snapping kick to N with the left foot while spinning counterclockwise 180 degrees.

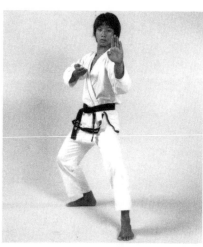

55. Landing at N, forming a left L-stance while executing a middle guarding block with the left knife-hand.

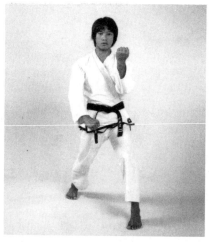

56. Execute a low block with a right outer forearm and then middle block with a left inner forearm while forming a left long walking stance, slipping the left foot.

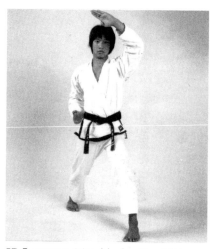

57. Execute a rising block with a left knife-hand.

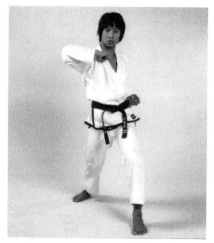

58. Execute a middle strike with the right side elbow.

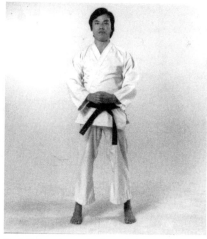

End: Bring the right foot forward to form a ready stance.

Silla Knife Pattern

Silla Knife Pattern, which is also known as Hwa Rang Knife Pattern, has its origin in the Silla dynasty about 1,350 years ago. The knife pattern, equivalent to the release from a knife attack, emphasizes accuracy and speed of movement and proper judgment of the attacker's direction of movement. Above all, the truncal twist technique forms a very essential part in the counterattack if the counterattack is to be a decisive and powerful one.

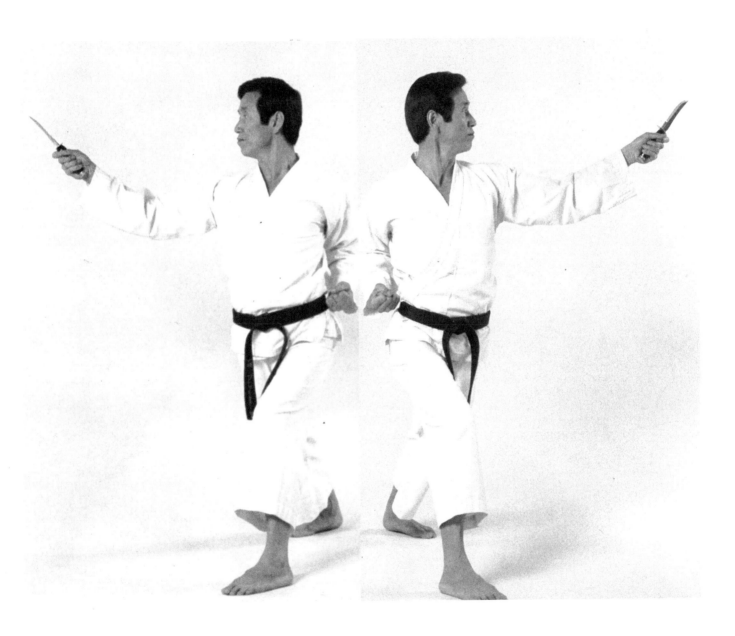

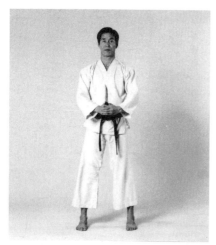

Parallel ready stance. Student facing N.

Diagram:

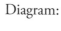
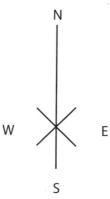

46 Movements

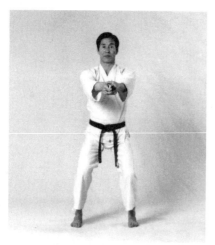

1. Execute a middle stab to N with both hands holding knife in right hand while forming a sitting stance.

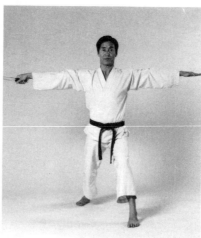

2. Move the right foot to S, forming a left long walking stance while executing a middle horizontal slash to E with the right knife-hand, and at the same time middle strike to W with the left knife-hand.

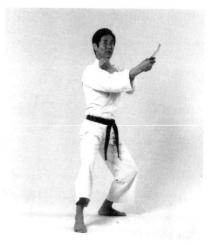

3. Move right foot to N, forming a right L-stance while executing a high inward slash to NW with the right knife; simultaneously bring the left side-fist in front of the right shoulder.

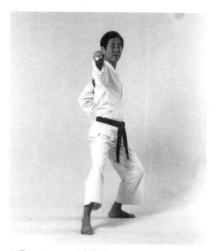

4. Execute a middle horizontal outward slash to N with the right knife-hand while shifting to N, maintaining a right L-stance.

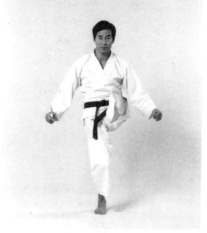

5. Execute a middle front snap kick to N with the left foot.

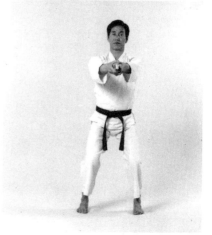

6. Lower the left foot beside the right foot, forming a sitting stance, and pass the knife to the left hand while executing a middle stab to N with both hands.

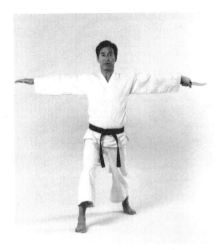

7. Move left foot to S, forming a right long walking stance while executing a middle horizontal slash to W with the left knife, and simultaneously middle strike to E with the right knife-hand.

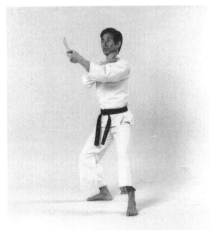

8. Move left foot to N, forming a left L-stance while executing a high inward slash to NE with the left knife, and simultaneously bring the right side-fist in front of the left shoulder.

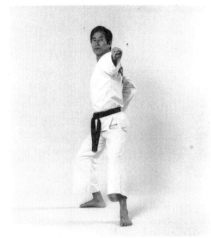

9. Execute a middle horizontal outward slash to N with the left knife while shifting to N maintaining a left L-stance.

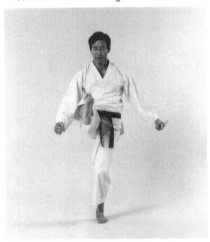

10. Execute a middle front snap kick to N with the right foot.

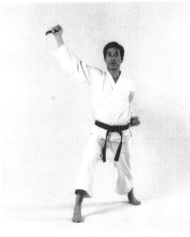

11. Lower the right foot to N, forming a right long walking stance, and pass the knife to the right hand while executing a high diagonal outward slash to N with the right knife-hand.

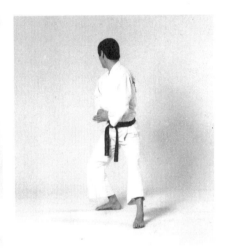

12. Move right foot to S, forming a left L-stance while executing a middle stab to S with the right knife, simultaneously support the right butt end of the knife with the left palm and turn face toward S.

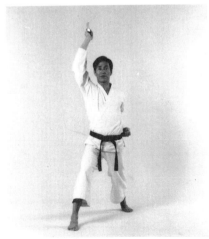

13. Move right foot to N, forming a right long walking stance while executing a vertical upward slash to N with the right knife-hand.

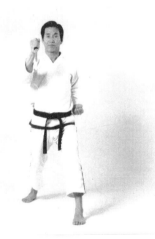

14. Move left foot to N, forming a left long walking stance, while executing a middle vertical downward stab to N with the right knife-hand.

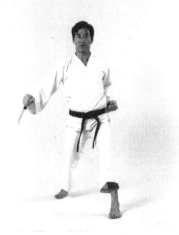

15. Execute a middle diagonal downward stab to NE with the right knife-hand.

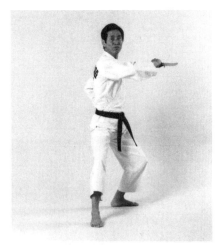

16. Move right foot to N, forming a right L-stance while executing a middle horizontal inward slash to N with the right knife.

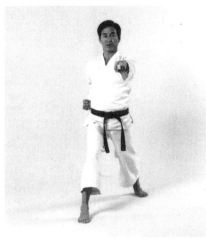

17. Pass the knife to the left hand, simultaneously middle stab to N with the left knife while slipping the right foot to form a right long walking stance.

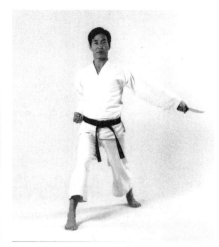

18. Execute a low slash to W with the left knife.

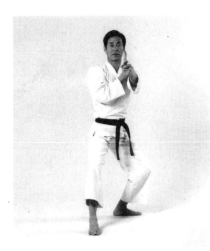

19. Execute a high vertical upward stab to N with the left knife, and simultaneously bring the right side-fist in front of the left shoulder while pulling the left foot to form a right L-stance.

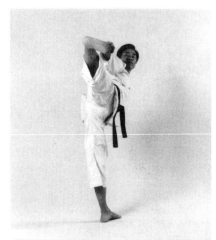

20. Execute a middle side-snapping kick to N with the right foot while pulling the left knife backward along the left hip.

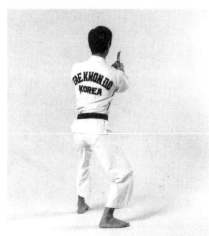

21. Lower the right foot to N, forming a left L-stance toward S, and pass the knife to the right hand while executing a high vertical upward stab to S with the right knife, simultaneously bring the left side fist in front of the right shoulder.

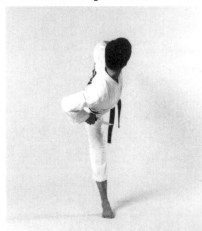

22. Execute a middle side-snapping kick to S with the left foot while pulling the right knife backward along the right hip.

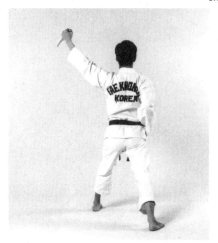

23. Lower the left foot to S, forming a left long walking stance, and pass the knife to the left hand while executing a high diagonal outward slash to S with the left knife.

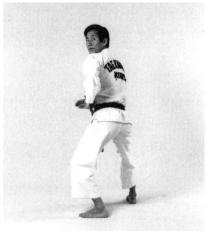

24. Move left foot to N, forming a right L-stance while executing a middle stab to N with the left knife, and simultaneously support the left butt end of the knife with the right palm and turn face toward N.

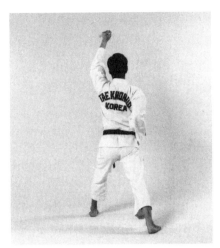

25. Move left foot to S, forming a left long walking stance while executing a vertical upward slash to S with the left knife.

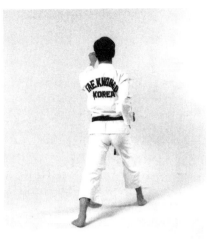

26. Move right foot to S, forming a right long walking stance while executing a middle vertical downward stab to S with the left knife.

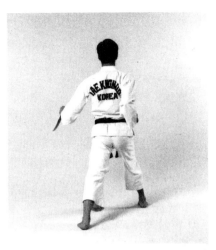

27. Execute a middle diagonal downward stab to SW with the left knife.

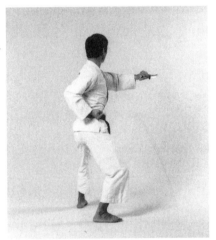

28. Move the left foot to S, forming a left L-stance while executing a middle horizontal inward slash to S with the left knife.

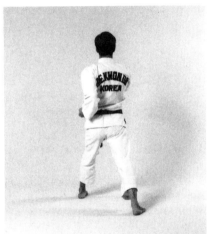

29. Pass the knife to the right hand, and simultaneously middle stab to S with the right knife while slipping the left foot to form a left long walking stance.

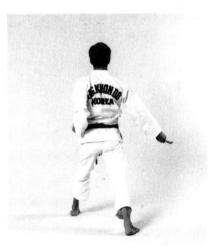

30. Execute a low slash to E with the right knife.

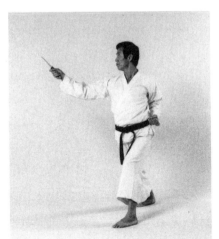

31. Move right foot to S, forming a left long walking stance toward W while executing a high diagonal inward slash to SW with the right knife.

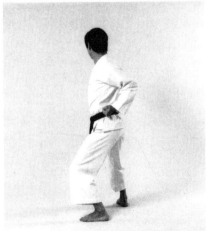

32. Execute a middle horizontal outward slash to S with the right knife while pulling the right foot to form a right L-stance.

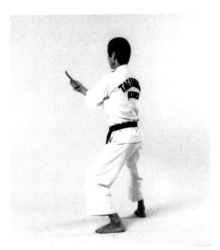

33. Execute a high inward chop to SW with the right knife, and simultaneously bring the left knife-hand in front of the right shoulder.

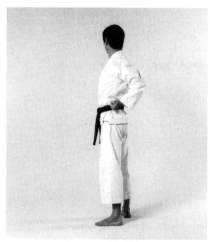

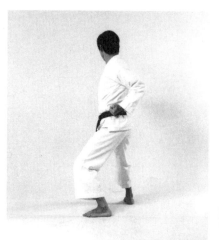

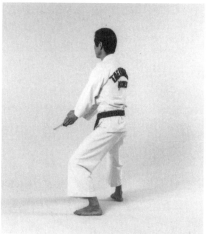

34. Execute a middle downward chop to S with the right knife while pulling the right foot to form a right vertical stance.

35. Execute a middle stab to S with the right knife while sliding the right foot to form a right L-stance.

36. Execute a low inward chop to SW with the right knife while bringing the left finger-belly onto the right under forearm.

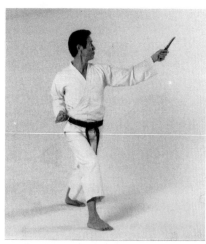

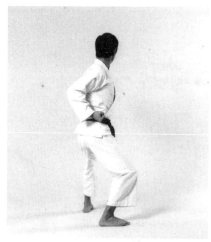

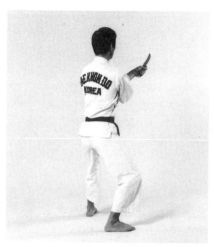

37. Move left foot to S, forming a right long walking stance toward W, and pass the knife to the left hand while executing a high diagonal inward slash to SW with the left knife.

38. Execute a middle horizontal outward slash to S with the left knife while pulling the left foot to form a left L-stance.

39. Execute a high inward chop to SW with the left knife, and simultaneously bring the right knife-hand in front of the left shoulder.

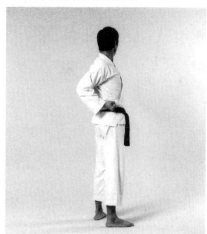

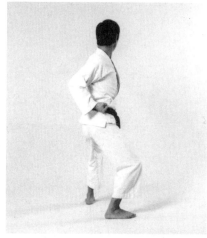

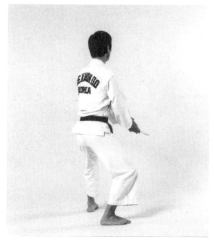

40. Execute a middle downward chop to S with the left knife while pulling the left foot to form a left vertical stance.

41. Execute a middle stab to S with the left knife, while sliding the left foot to form a left L-stance.

42. Execute a low inward chop to SW with the left knife, while bringing the right finger-belly onto the left under forearm.

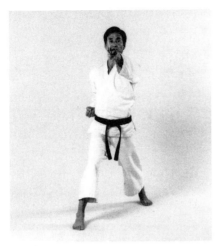

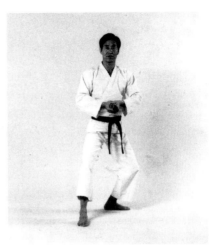

43. Move left foot on line NS forming a right long walking stance toward S while executing a high stab to N with the left knife.

44. Pull the right foot to form a right L-stance, and simultaneously bring the right hand onto the left fist while pulling the knife.

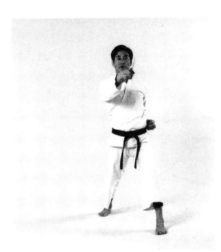

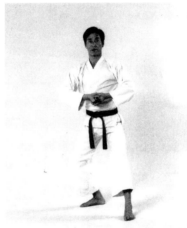

45. Move left foot to N, forming a left long walking stance, and pass the knife to the right hand while executing a high stab to N with the right knife.

46. Pull the left foot to form a left L-stance, and simultaneously bring the left hand onto the right fist while pulling the knife.

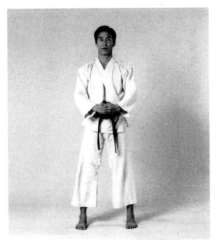

End: Bring the left foot back to ready stance.

Silla Pole Pattern

Like Silla Knife Pattern, Silla Pole Pattern is named after the Hwa Rang youth group, which originated in the Silla dynasty about 1,350 years ago. Similar to the defense against a pole attack, the pole pattern requires dodging from the direction the weapon is striking and lengthening your strike. Your palm may be used as a blocking tool, but never when the attacker thrashes at full range.

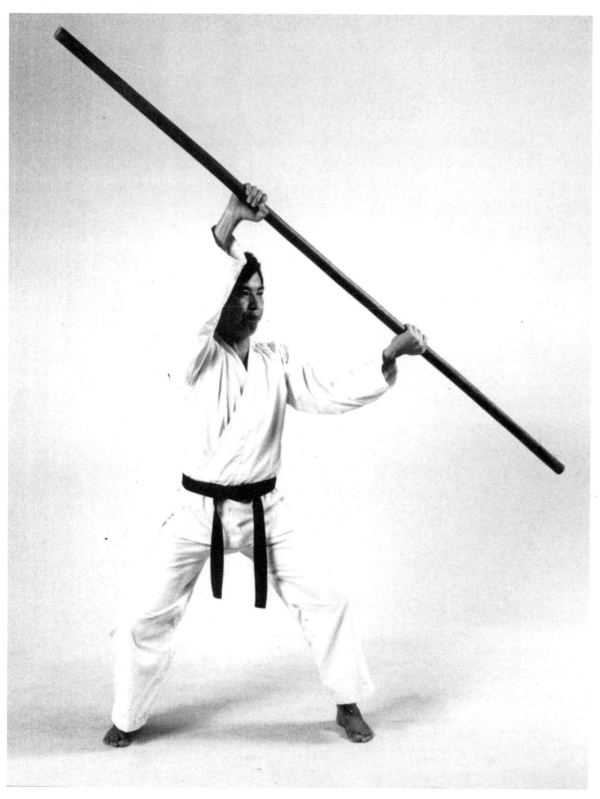

Silla Pole Pattern

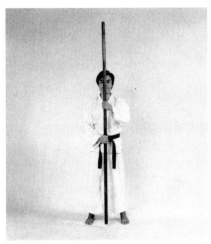

Hold the pole vertically in front of the chest and parallel ready stance. Student is facing N.

Diagram

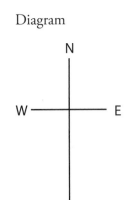

57 Movements

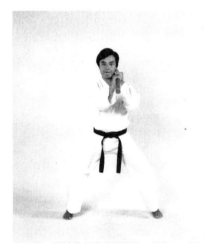

1. Move the right foot to E, forming a riding stance, while executing a middle vertically upward striking toward N with the right end of the pole.

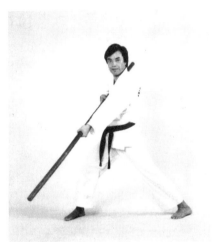

2. Execute a low diagonally upward block toward NE with the left end of the pole while forming a right long walking stance, turning body clockwise and pivoting on both feet.

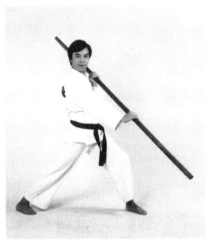

3. Execute a low diagonally upward block toward NW with the right end of the pole while forming a left long walking stance; turn body counterclockwise and pivot on both feet.

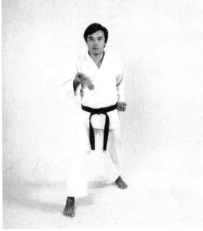

4. Move right foot to N, forming a right long walking stance, and hold the pole in right hand while executing a middle horizontally outward strike toward N with the right end of the pole.

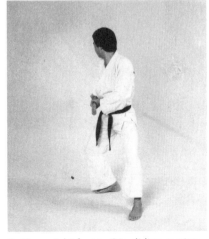

5. Move right foot to S in sliding motion, forming a left L-stance while executing a middle thrust toward S with right end of the pole and facing toward S.

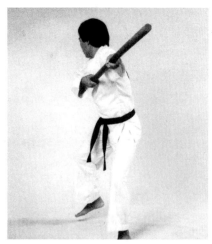

6a. Prepare to execute a middle thrust.

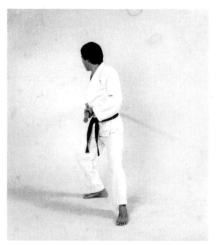

6b. Execute a middle thrust toward S with the right end of the pole, while shifting to S and maintaining a left L-stance.

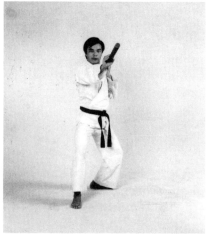

7. Move the right foot to N, forming a right L-stance while executing a high vertically upward strike toward N with the right end of the pole.

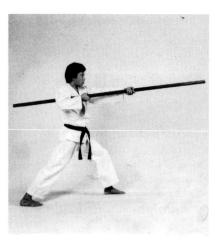

8. Move left foot to W, forming a left long walking stance while executing a middle horizontally inward strike toward W with the left end of the pole.

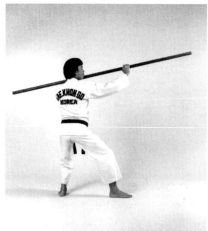

9. Move right foot to W, forming a right L-stance while executing a high vertically upward strike toward W with the right end of the pole.

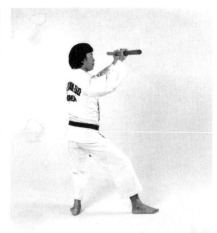

10. Execute a high horizontally inward and outward strike toward NS with both ends of the pole.

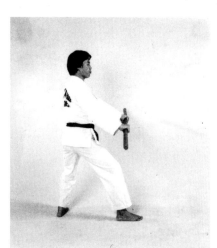

11. Execute a low block toward W with the pole.

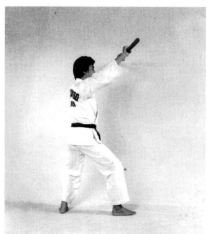

12. Execute an upward block toward W with the pole.

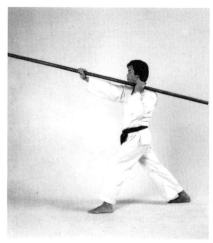

13. Move right foot on line EW, forming a left long walking stance toward E while executing a high diagonally upward strike toward E with the right end of the pole.

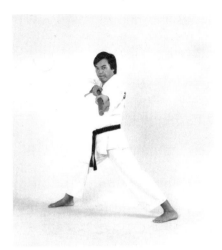

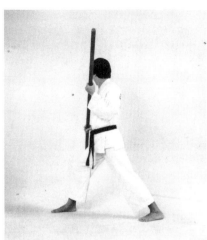

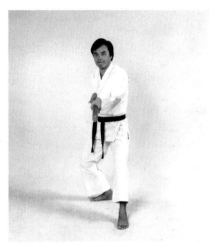

14. Move right foot to E, forming a right long walking stance while executing a middle horizontally inward strike toward N with the left end of the pole and facing toward N.

15. Execute a low diagonally downward thrust toward S with the right end of the pole, and face toward S.

16. Move left foot to N, forming a left L-stance while executing a middle vertically downward strike toward N with the left end of the pole.

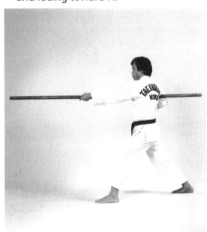

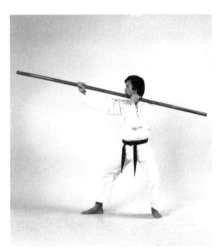

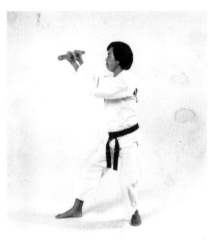

17. Move left foot to E, forming a left long walking stance while executing a middle horizontally upward strike toward E with the left end of the pole.

18. Move right foot to E, forming a right L-stance while executing a high vertically upward strike toward E with the right end of the pole.

19. Execute a high horizontally inward and outward strike toward NS with both ends of the pole.

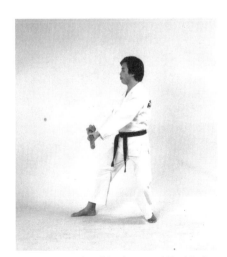

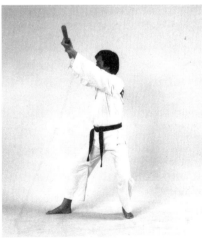

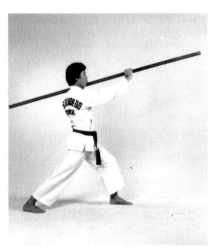

20. Execute a low block toward E with the pole.

21. Execute an upward block toward E with the pole.

22. Move right foot on line EW, forming a left long walking stance toward W while executing a high diagonally upward strike toward W with the right end of the pole.

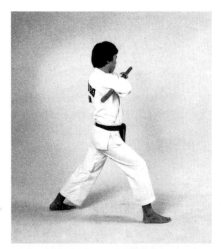

23. Move right foot to W, forming a right long walking stance while executing a middle horizontally inward strike toward S with left end of the pole and facing toward S.

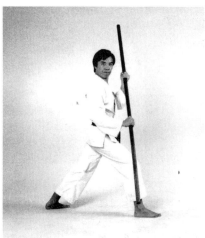

24. Execute a low diagonally downward thrust toward N with the right end of the pole and face toward N.

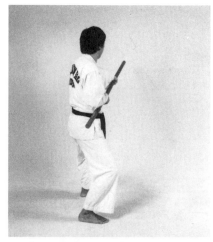

25. Move left foot to S, forming a left L-stance while executing a middle vertically downward strike toward S with the left end of the pole.

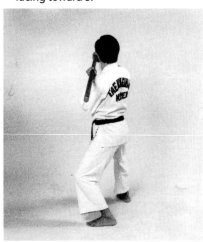

26. Move right foot to S, forming a right L-stance while executing a high vertically upward strike toward S with the right end of the pole.

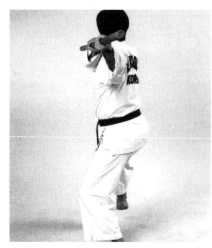

27a. Prepare to execute a high thrust

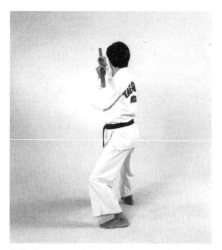

27b. Execute a high thrust toward S with the right end of the pole while shifting to S maintaining a right L-stance. Perform 26 and 27 in fast motion.

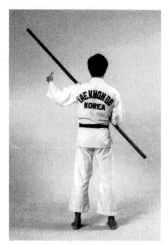

28a. Bring the left foot beside right foot to form a parallel stance toward S while preparing to swing the pole diagonally downward.

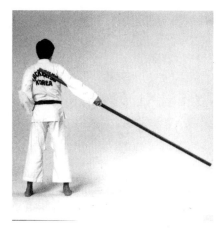

28b. Swing the pole diagonally downward toward E with the right hand.

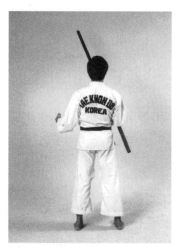

29a. Rotate the pole upward clockwise

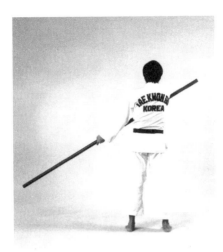

29b. Swing the pole diagonally downward toward W to hold the pole with the left hand.

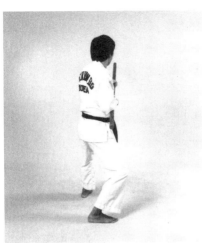

30. Move the right foot to N, forming a left L-stance toward S while executing a middle vertically downward strike toward S with the left end of the pole. Perform 28, 29, and 30 in continuous motion.

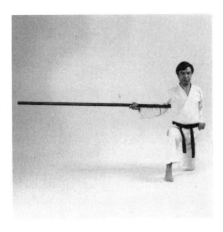

31. Move left foot on line NS to form a right kneeling stance toward N while executing a horizontally outward strike from W to E; hold the pole in right hand.

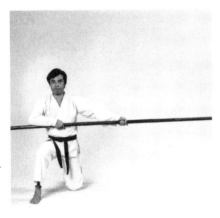

32. Execute a horizontally inward strike from E to W and hold the pole in left hand.

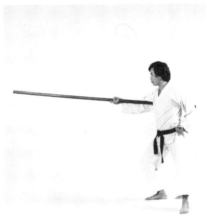

33. Move left foot to N, forming a left L-stance while executing a high horizontally outward strike from W to E, and hold the pole in right hand.

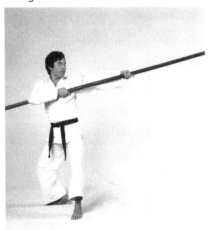

34. Execute a high horizontally inward strike from E to W and hold the pole in left hand.

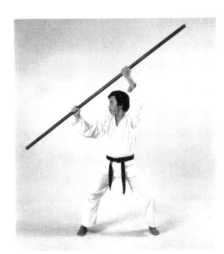

35. Move the right foot on line EW, forming a riding stance toward N while executing a high side block to NE with the pole.

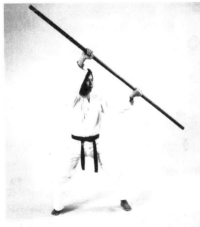

36. Execute a high side block to NW with the pole.

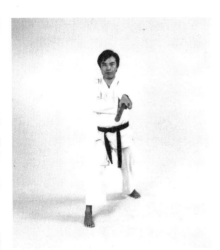

37. Move right foot to N, forming a right long walking stance while executing a middle vertically downward strike toward N with the left end of the pole; bring the right hand under the left armpit.

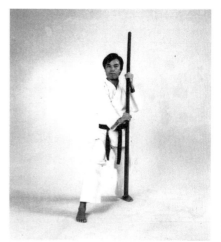

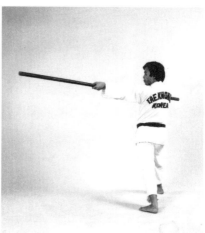

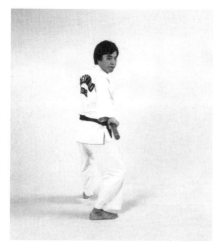

38. Execute a low vertically upward block toward N with the right end of the pole.

39. Move left foot to N, forming a right long walking stance toward NW and turning body clockwise, pivoting on both feet while executing a high diagonally upward strike toward NE with the left end of the pole; face toward NE.

40. Move right foot to N, forming a left L-stance and turning body clockwise, pivoting on left foot while executing a middle thrust toward N with right end of the pole; face toward N.

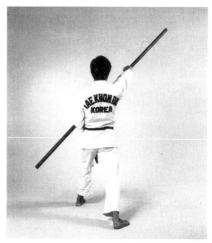

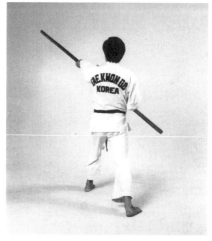

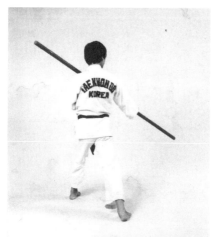

41. Execute a high diagonally downward strike toward SE with the right end of the pole while slipping the left foot to form a left long walking stance.

42. Execute a high diagonally downward strike toward SW with the left end of the pole.

43. Execute a low diagonally upward block toward SE with the right end of the pole.

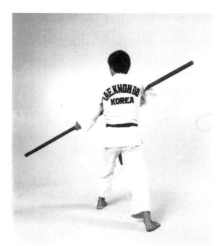

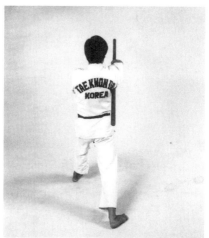

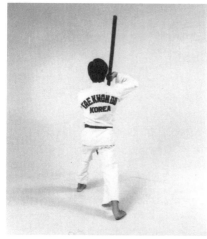

44. Execute a low diagonally upward block toward SW with the left end of the pole.

45. Execute a middle vertically downward strike toward S with the right end of the pole and bring the left hand under the right armpit.

46. Execute a low vertically upward block toward S with the left end of the pole.

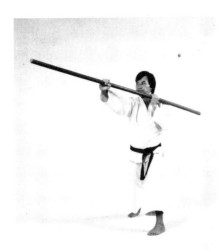

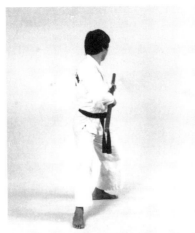

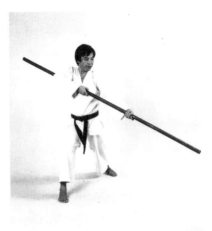

47. Move right foot to S, forming a left long walking stance toward NE and turning body counterclockwise pivoting on both feet while executing a high diagonally upward strike toward SW with the right end of the pole; face toward SW.

48. Move left foot to S, forming a right L-stance and turning body counterclockwise, pivoting on right foot while executing a middle thrust toward S with the left end of the pole; face toward S.

49. Execute a low diagonally upward block toward NW with the left end of the pole while slipping the right foot to form a right long walking stance.

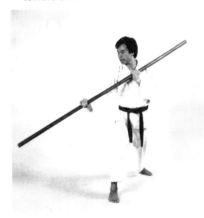

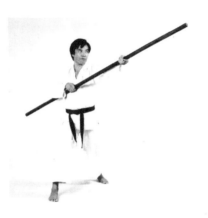

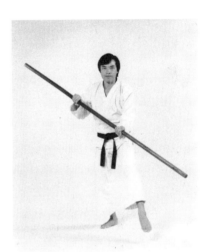

50. Execute a low diagonally upward block toward NE with the right end of the pole.

51. Execute a high diagonally downward strike toward NW with the left end of the pole.

52. Execute a high diagonally downward strike toward NE with the right end of the pole.

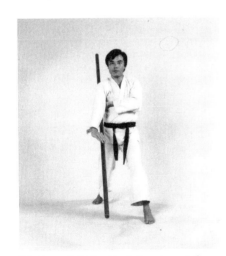

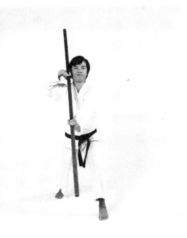

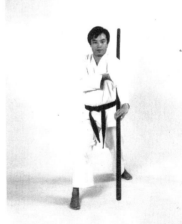

53. Move right foot to S, forming a left walking stance while executing a downward strike to N, rotating once from the right armpit with the right end of the pole and bringing the left hand under the right armpit.

54. Execute a low vertically upward block toward N with the left end of the pole.

55. Move the left foot to S, forming a right walking stance while executing a downward strike to N, rotating once from the left armpit with the left end of the pole and bringing the right hand under the left armpit.

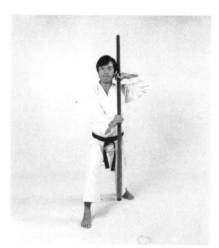 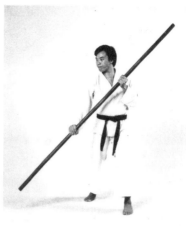

56. Execute a low vertically upward block toward N with the right end of the pole.

57. Move left foot to N, forming a left walking stance while executing a low diagonally downward thrust toward E with the right end of the pole; face toward E.

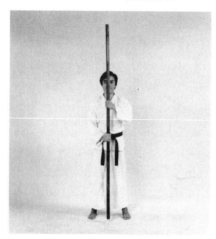

End: Bring the right foot forward to form a ready stance.

CHAPTER 5
TRAINING

Proper training in taekwondo gives the student solid groundwork for advancement toward expertise in skill and technique. The training part in this book is mainly for advanced students who are already familiar with basic hand and foot movements, as well as the truncal twist. Students need continuous training that will enable them to do fast, accurate kicks, jumps, and hand movements. When under training, they should concentrate on those important factors which contribute to the scientific use of force. These factors are speed, agility, balance, accurate timing, and target focus.

The whole body is mobilized as the source of energy for various actions; therefore, recognition of and through training in the above important factors will make it possible to concentrate potential energy and enormously magnified power and force, once it is unleashed.

An important point, which is worth mentioning, is that only restricted, trained, and coordinated movements and actions can enable you to attain the desired energy output. Excessive, uncontrolled, and disorganized movements not only deplete your energy rather quickly, but would also induce the attacker to exploit the situation and thus gain the upper hand.

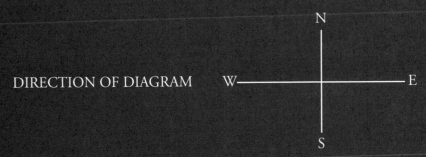

DIRECTION OF DIAGRAM

The diagram shows the four directions you will follow during the performance of patterns, under the assumption that you are beginning with facing N.

Preparatory Exercises

It is essential to do basic preparatory exercises to make the joints and muscles limber and increase blood circulation prior to commencing daily training. A student who immediately begins strenuous jumping, kicking, or punching exercises risks pulling muscles and straining ligaments or other injury.

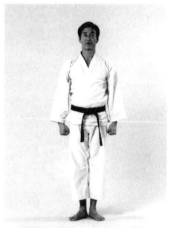 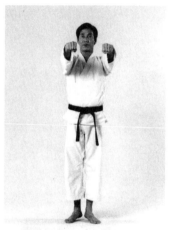 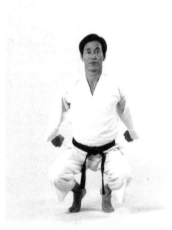 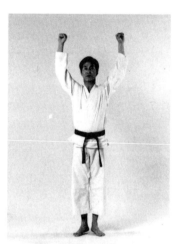

1. Knee and arm exercise.

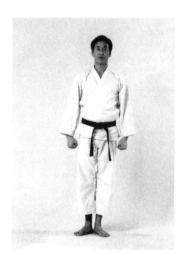

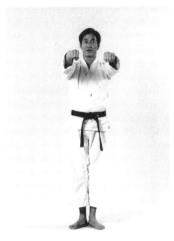 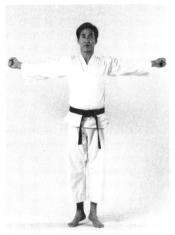 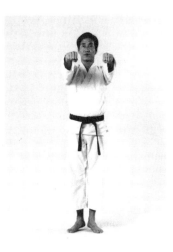 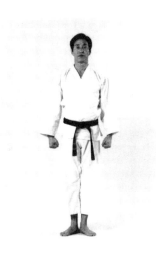

2. Arm exercise.

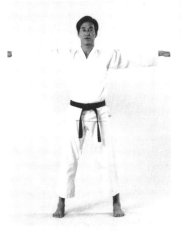 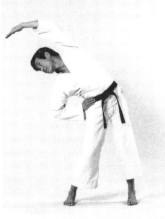 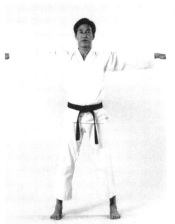 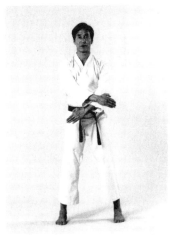

3. Side-hip exercise.

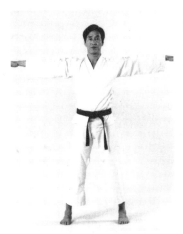 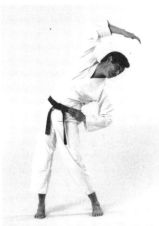 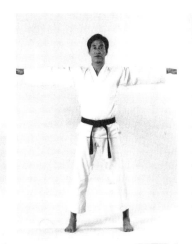 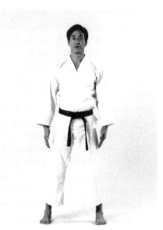

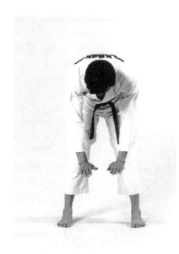 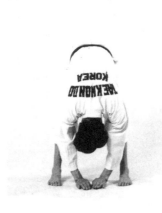 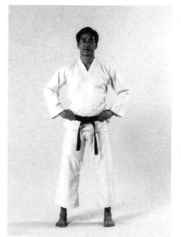 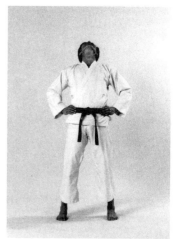

4. Back and forth exercise.

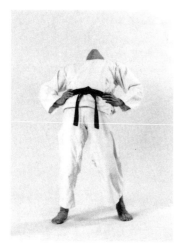 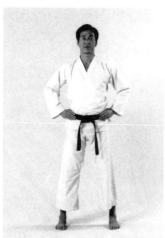

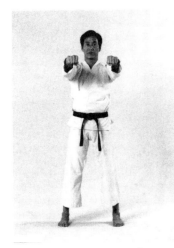 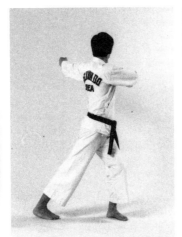 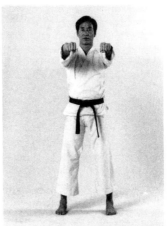 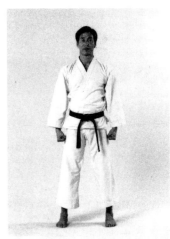

5. Side-hip twisting exercise.

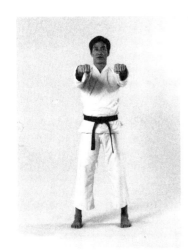 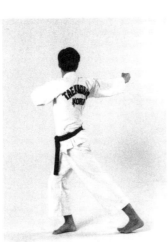 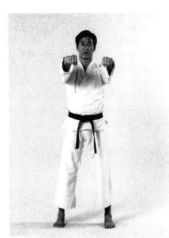 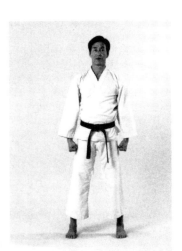

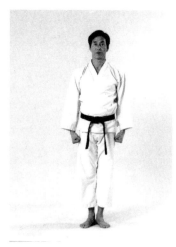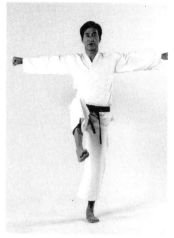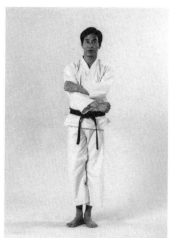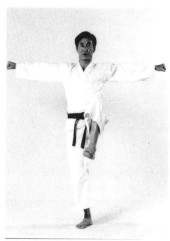

6. Arm and leg exercise.

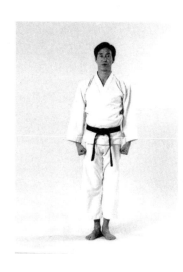

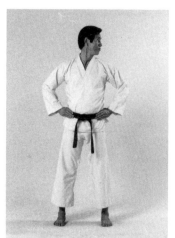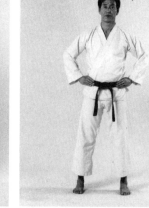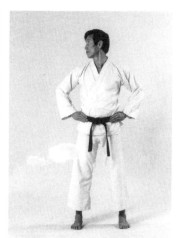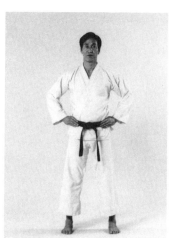

7. Neck side-turning exercise.

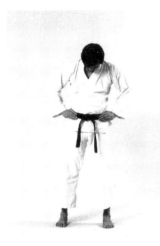 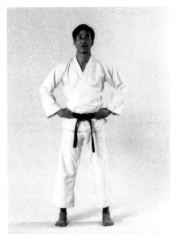 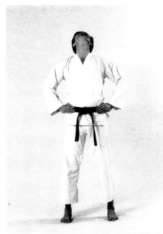 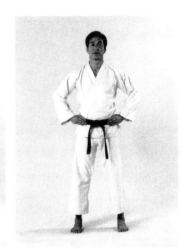

8. Neck forward and backward bending exercise.

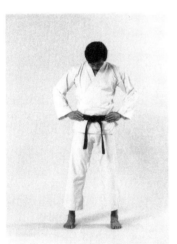 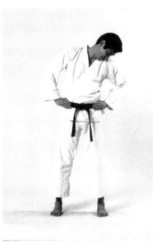 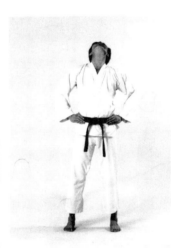 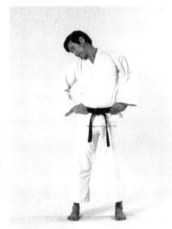

9. Neck turning exercise.

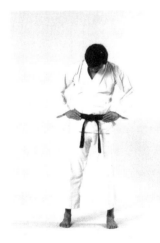 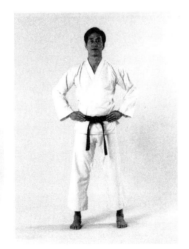

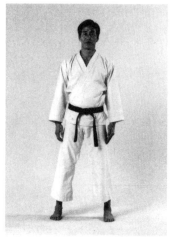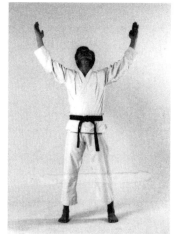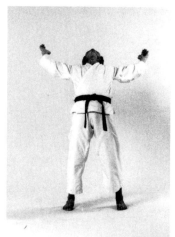

10. Breathing exercise.

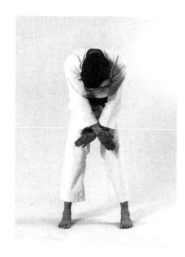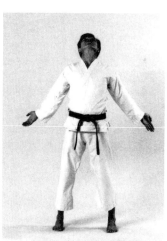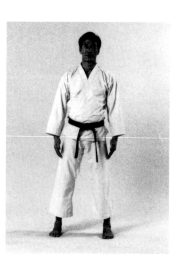

Calisthenics

As these are body-conditioning exercises, they require the maneuvering of almost all parts of the body. Before and after performing the strenuous movements in taekwondo, the student is advised to do calisthenics in order to loosen up muscles and joints.

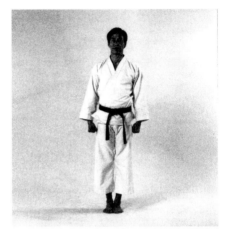 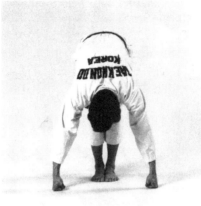 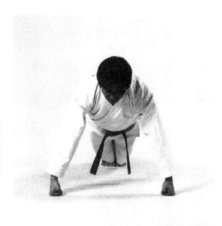

1. Close-leg pushups.

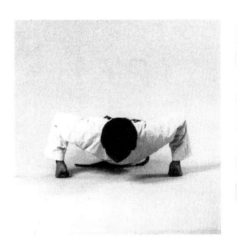 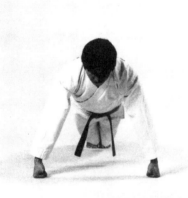

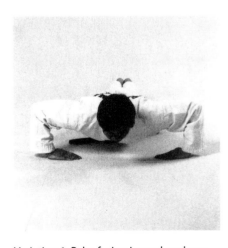 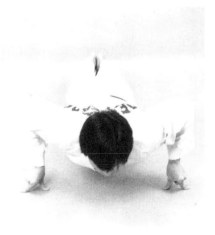

Variation 1: Palm facing inward pushups.   Variation 2: Two-finger pushups.

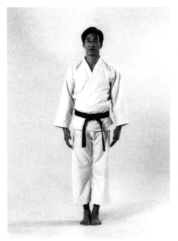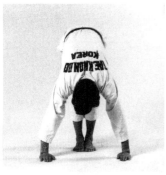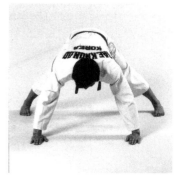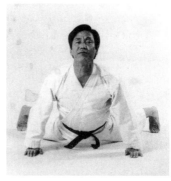

2. Open-leg pushups.

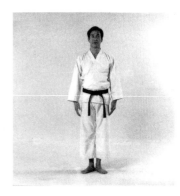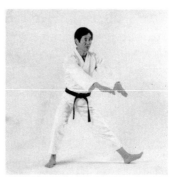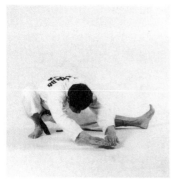

3. Squatting position stretch.

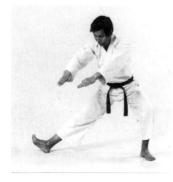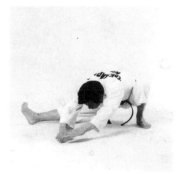

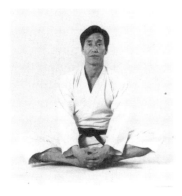 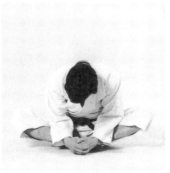 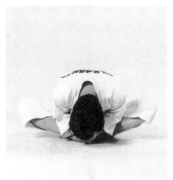 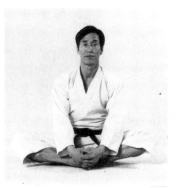

4. Close-soles flexed position
   forward bend stretch.

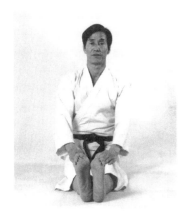 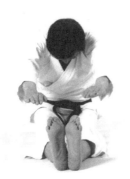 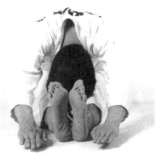 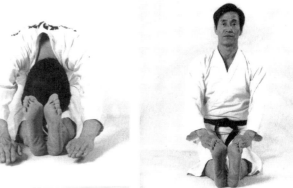

5. Straight close-leg position
   forward bend stretch.

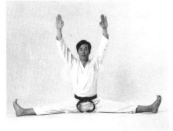 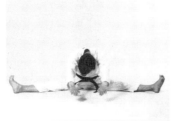 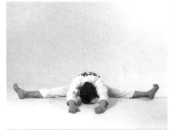 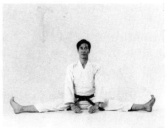

6. Straight open-leg position
   foward bend stretch.

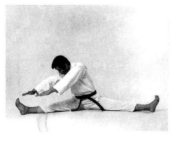 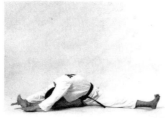 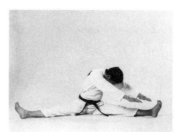 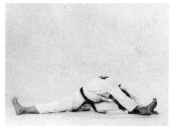

7. Straight open-leg position
   twisting side-bend stretch.

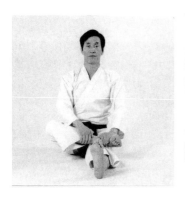 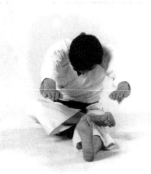 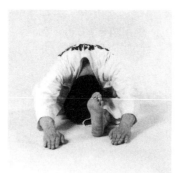 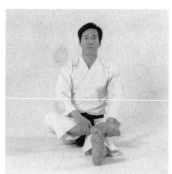

8. Flexed astride knee position
   forward bend stretch.

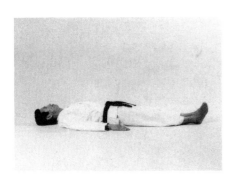 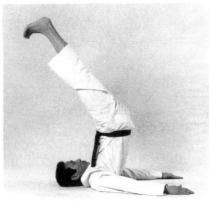 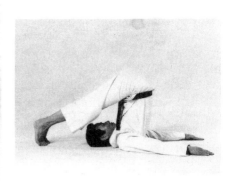

9. Lie down position backstretch.

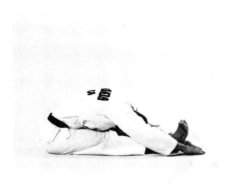 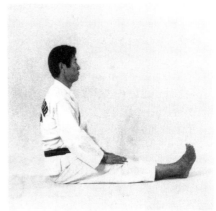

Basic Principles of Taekwondo Action

The physical power of taekwondo is produced by a central trunk twist, delivering peripheral limb parts at a powerful speed onto a target with practiced precision, concentration, and balance. While by practice, you can manifest the latter qualities, the truncal twist is perhaps the most elusive for a beginner to acquire and the teacher to explain. However, it is the most important element in the whole process of power generation and is a built-in action-reaction equalizer, allowing, for example, a practitioner to effect powerful strikes while both feet are off the ground.

Take the right hand punch on a forward stance as an example. During training, you are taught to punch with the right fist while pulling the left arm back at the same time. The latter movement produces the reactionary force to add to the former. Yet, if you should do so without truncal movements, maximum power is not attained. In fact, the very first body movement should arise from the trunk, twisting on a vertical axis, swinging the shoulders in turn to bring the arms into their final paths. All muscles involved are summoned into action in a split second, together but in sequence—trunk, shoulder, arms, hands. Relaxation of the intervening parts during motion is essential so as not to impede the smoothness of operation and therefore speed. If there is no preparatory trunk movements (see below), the end position will find the right shoulder slightly in front of the left and slightly behind the frontal plane. (There is of course another twisting motion of supination to pronation of the right forearm and vice versa of the left.) In time, the truncal twist will be spontaneous in all actions, will become shortened in execution time, and will be almost imperceptible to an observer. This is the reason why it is so difficult for students to learn the movement from their instructors unless it is purposely exaggerated to allow observation. Certain points need elaboration.

Preparatory Trunk Movement (PTM)

In the execution of the truncal countertwist, there are occasions that will allow movement of the shoulders and pelvis, in preparation, in directions opposite to that used during the countertwist itself—such as during long stride attacks and breaking sessions. The PTM does two things: (1) It gives an opportunity for the muscle tone to wind up before the all-out contractions at the countertwist; (2) It permits alignment of the shoulders and pelvis at the end of an action.

The adjective "preparatory" is used instead of "preceding" because there are occasions that will not allow PTM, such as during sudden strike attacks and abrupt defensive blocking movements. In these latter incidences, you will find an end position misalignment. In the case of a right arm punch, for example, the right shoulder will be slightly forward and the left slightly backward in relation to the frontal plane at the termination of action. If balance is disturbed in these cases, it may be restored by either doing a slight spring-like knee bend for shock absorption or by taking one step forward with the right foot.

End Position

At the termination of an action, the shoulders and pelvis may be aligned or misaligned depending on the presence or absence of PTM, respectively, as explained above. The end position of leg actions is more complicated. In a side kick, the pelvis, besides rotating on the vertical axis of the body to effect truncal countertwist, is also tilted outward and upward in the direction of the kick—the pelvis now rotating in the opposite direction of the body. Examples of their final alignment are shown in the diagrams.

Truncal Twist In Three Axes

In a side kick, it is seen from the diagrams that the shoulders and pelvis swing in opposite directions on two axes. In a front kick, they will do the same but on a vertical axis passing through the center of the body, as before, and a horizontal axis passing through the loins.

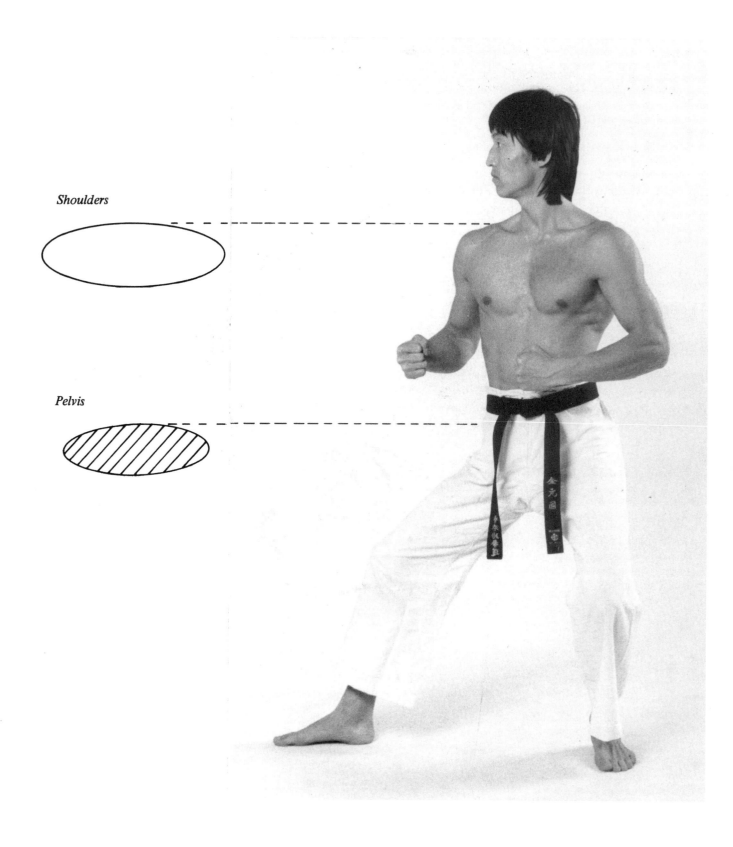

Shoulders

Pelvis

Short Action (e.g., right arm punch)

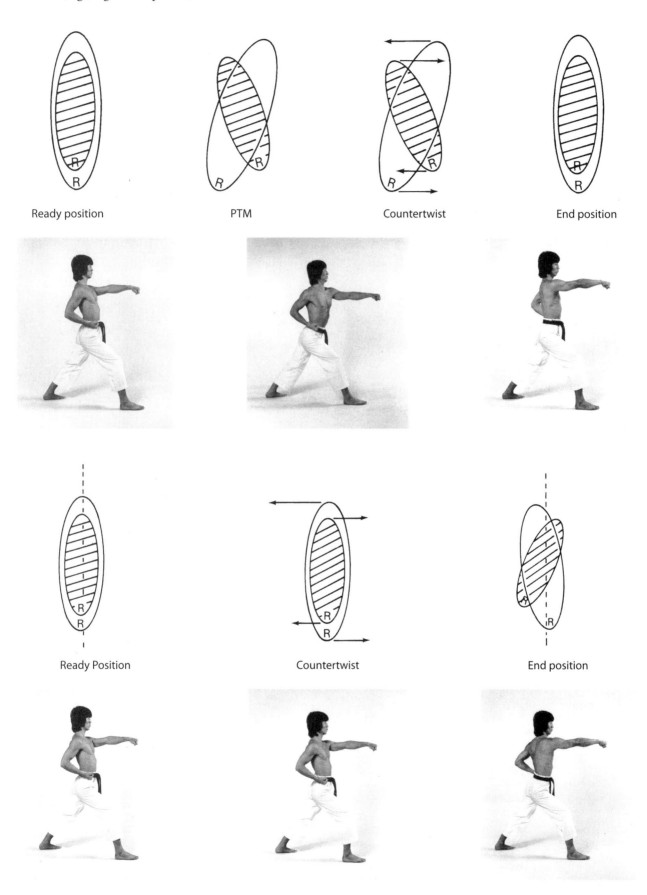

Ready position   PTM   Countertwist   End position

Ready Position   Countertwist   End position

Long Action (e.g., right arm punch)

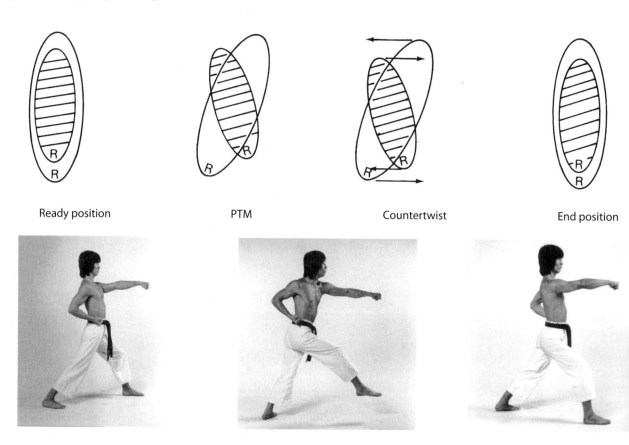

Ready position   PTM   Countertwist   End position

End Kick (e.g., right foot—Short Action)

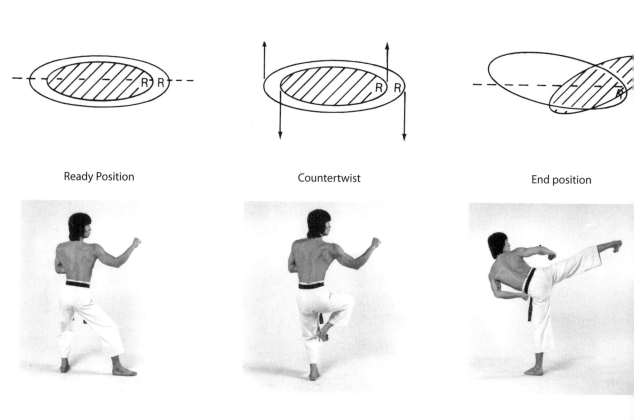

Ready Position   Countertwist   End position

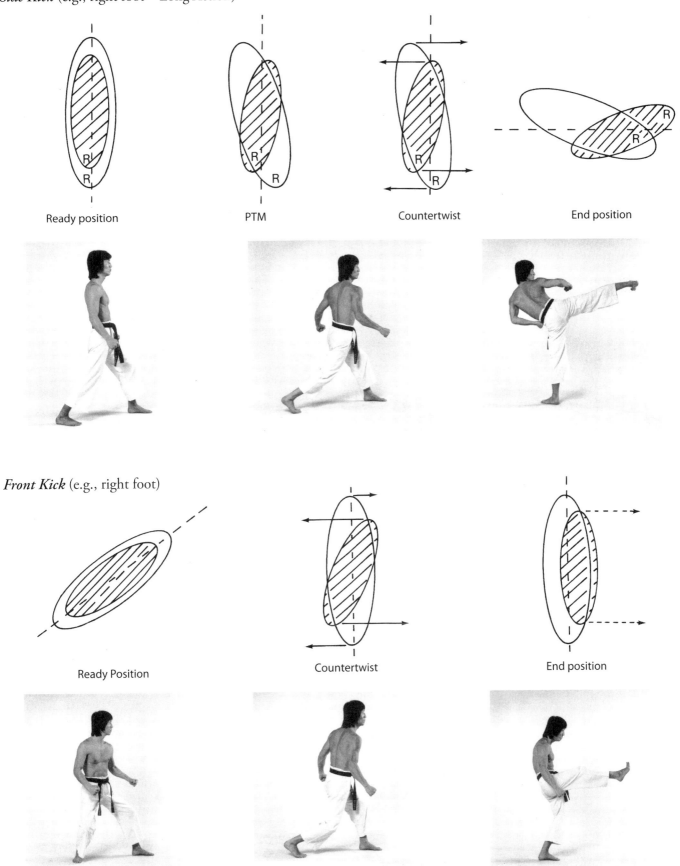

Side Kick (e.g., right foot—Long Action)

Ready position

PTM

Countertwist

End position

Front Kick (e.g., right foot)

Ready Position

Countertwist

End position

Elbow Breaking of Boards

This breaking action is an excellent test of the maturity of the truncal countertwist on a vertical body axis. Even an untrained individual may be able to break one piece of 1" thick board with an elbow strike. But the breaking of two and especially three 1" thick boards requires proper practice and execution of the countertwist. It can be seen sometimes in taekwondo or akin demonstrations that a very muscular and well-built participant fails to deliver in an elbow breaking of two 1" thick boards, whereas a thinner one may do it with apparent ease and grace.

Elbow Breaking

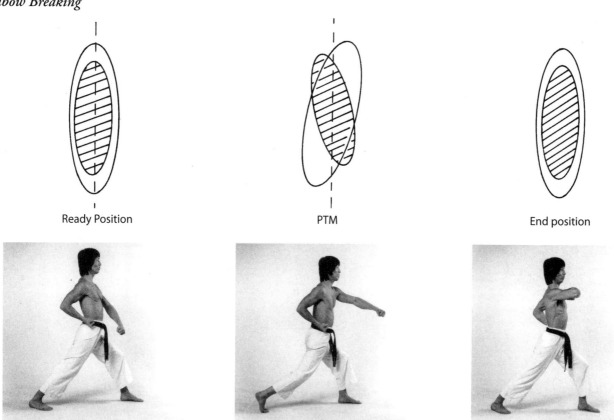

Ready Position   PTM   End position

Contribution of Truncal Twist to Speed

It is not often realized that apart from the relaxation of muscular tension between the start and end of actions, the truncal twist is the most important contributor to the speed of strikes. The trunk occupies a central position close to the axis of rotation, while the limbs, especially the arms, are attached to the body on the more peripheral part of the circle of movement. Any amount of movement of the trunk revolving on any one of the three axes mentioned in the diagrams below will produce a magnified distance of travel on the periphery.

Diagrammatically it may be represented thus:

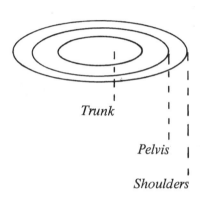

Trunk

Pelvis

Shoulders

e.g. vertical axis rotation

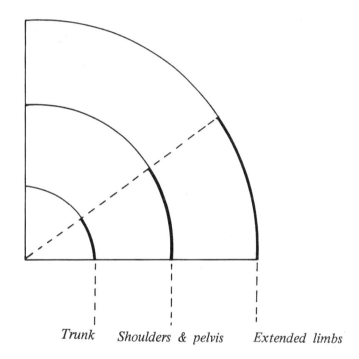

Trunk   Shoulders & pelvis   Extended limbs

Classification of Strikes

The next area of confusion in taekwondo training is the tremendous varieties of punches and kicks and their lack of a system of integration. Instructors themselves often do not agree on, for example, what is meant by a piercing kick, a thrusting kick, a pushing kick, etc., let alone students understanding them. The following classification of strikes is, therefore, proposed to try to clear up this area of contention.

In principle, different forms of strikes, whether punches, kicks, or other forms of attack with body parts, share different characteristics if viewed from their effects on the target. All strikes may be classified into First, Second, and Third degrees, and into combinations of these, according to their contact time, target displacement, tissue injury, or target damage, as explained in the table below:

Type of strike	First degree	Second degree	Third degree
1. Contact time (of body parts to target)	0 or + -	Short (small fraction of a second)	Long (up to ½ sec or more)
2. Target displacement after impact	0 or + -	+	++ to +++
3. Tissue injury or target damage	0	+++	0 to +++
4. Other characteristics: Other terminology: Use in martial art: Use in sport:	Snapping + +++ (free sparring)	Thrusting Piercing +++ +++ (breaking)	Pushing 0 to ++ 0 to ++

NB　　0 = nil

+ - = minimal or occasional

+ = mild or sometimes

++ = moderate or frequent

+++ = severe or very frequent

A First-degree strike during training sessions in free sparring is supposed to stop, say, within two centimeters short of body contact. Occasionally, of course, the attacking part touches the target. Contact time is therefore zero or minimal; displacement is also zero or minimal. No damage can occur. In Second- or Third-degree strikes, the attacking part travels into the target for a variable distance. Accordingly, the latter will be displaced to an amount depending on the force, the contact time, and the target mass. In Second-degree strikes, the total energy is dissipated within a small fraction of a second, rendering maximal shearing and damage of a target for the amount of force used. In Third-degree strikes, the attacking part pushes a target for a variable distance; the total force of the strike is applied over the whole duration of that travel. Contact time is therefore long. With control, the extent of target damage can actually by gauged.

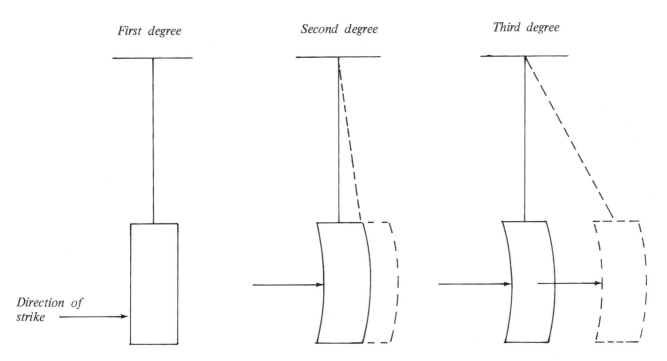

The significance of this classification can be far-reaching. Firstly, it clears up the terminology muddle. Thus, a side kick will be either First-degree, Second-degree, Third-degree, or a combination of these, viz, First plus Second, Second plus Third, First plus Third, etc. These combinations are practicable, especially in hand actions. If they were explained in "longhand," it might take half a day. Secondly, this classification gives a clear concept of the type of movements, their relationship with the target, and their consequences upon the latter, to the beginner from the start. Thirdly, only First-degree strikes should be used at free sparring, and the ability to deliver controlled attacks should be tested at intervals and at grading—by striking a Hanging Bag. First-degree strikes should produce nil or minimal displacement of the Bag. This, of course, applies to taekwondo as a sport.

I am very thankful to Dr. David C.T. Wong who has shared much time with me for the discussion of the above section. This represents one of the products of our discussions, experimentations, and thoughts on taekwondo and martial arts in general. Only through shared interests, free interchange of ideas, and a spirit of adventure can progress be made and continue to be made. Taekwondo is not an end but a means. The end is the way of life itself.

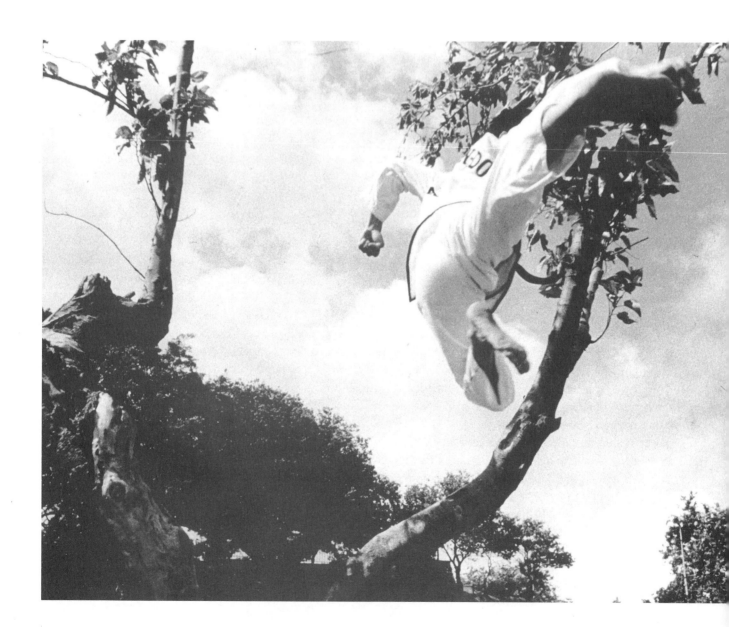

Hand Techniques

The hand is most effective when the hand, wrist, and elbow are perfectly straight at the moment of contact. The hand techniques illustrated in this chapter are designed for advanced students who are already familiar with basic hand movements, such as standard attacking and blocking techniques.

Though hand techniques are useful for attack, defense, and free sparring, they are most important in defense for blocking attacks. For example, good hand techniques are considerably more useful than foot techniques when being attacked at close range. The basic principle for all hand movements is to twist the hip and abdomen in the same direction as the hand in order to gain maximum acceleration and body power.

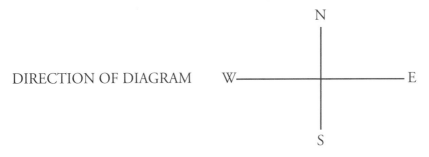

This diagram shows the four directions the student will follow during the performance of patterns, under the assumption that the student is facing N.

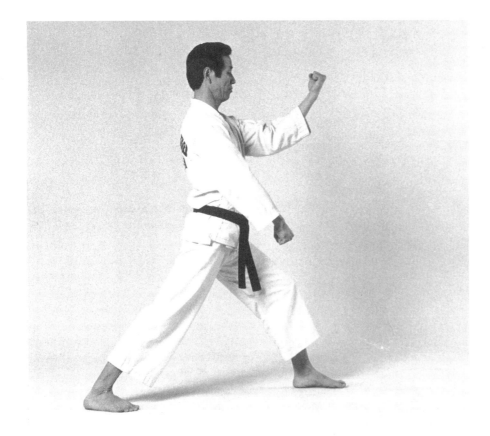

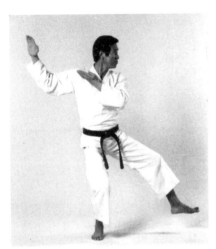

1. Move left foot to N forming a left L-stance while preparing to execute a high guarding block.

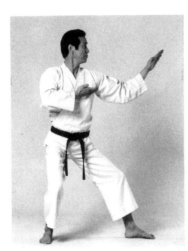

2. Execute a high guarding block with the left knife-hand.

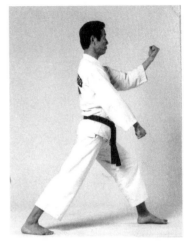

3. Execute a low block with the right forearm and high side block with the left inner forearm while slipping the left foot.

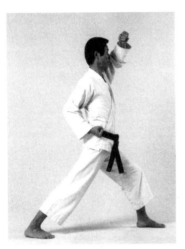

4. Execute a rising block with the left outer forearm.

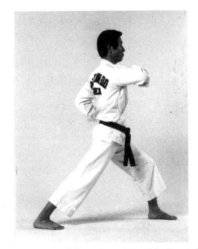

5. Execute a middle side strike with the right elbow.

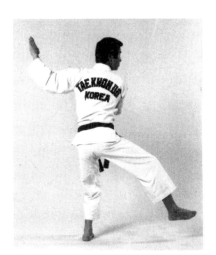

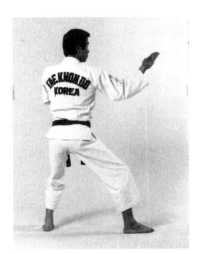

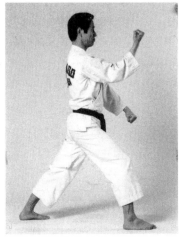

1. Move right foot to N, forming a right L-stance whole preparing to execute a high guarding block.

2. Execute a high guarding block with the right knife-hand.

3. Execute a low block with the left forearm and a high side block with the right inner forearm while slipping right foot..

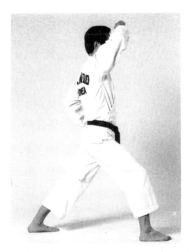

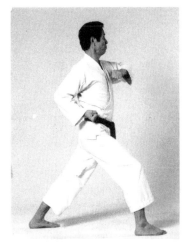

4. Execute a rising block with the right outer forearm.

5. Execute a middle side strike with the left elbow.

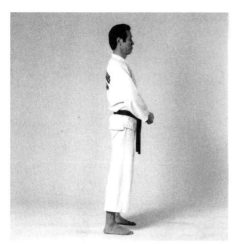

Parallel ready stance.

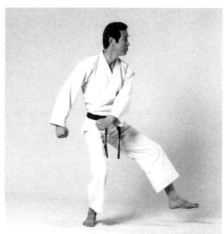

1. Prepare to twin forearm block.

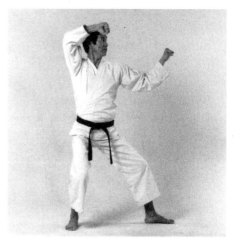

2. Move left foot to N, forming a left L-stance while executing a square outer forearm block.

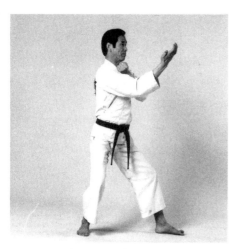

3. Execute a high inward strike to NE with the right knife-hand while bringing the left side fist in front of the right shoulder.

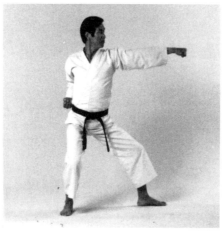

4. Execute a middle punch with the left fist.

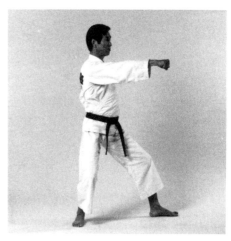

5. Execute a middle punch to NW with the right fist.

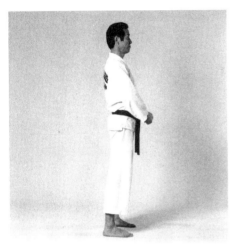

Parallel ready stance.

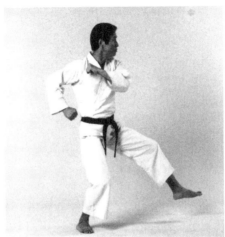

1. Prepare to double forearm block.

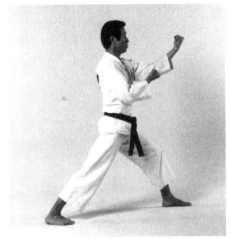

2. Move left foot to N, forming a left long walking stance while executing a high block with the left double forearm.

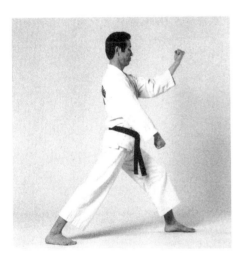

3. Execute a low block with the right outer forearm while keeping the left forearm as it is.

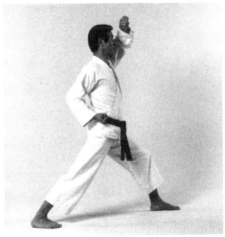

4. Execute a rising block with the left outer forearm.

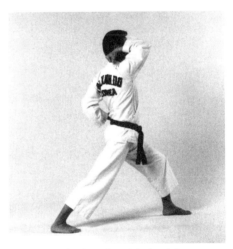

5. Execute a high strike with the right upper elbow.

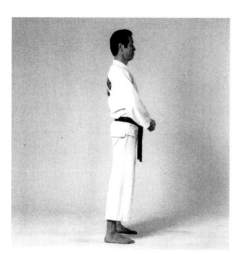

Parallel ready stance.

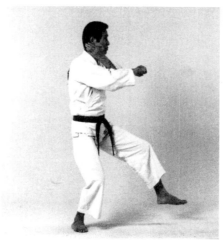

1. Prepare to execute palm hooking block.

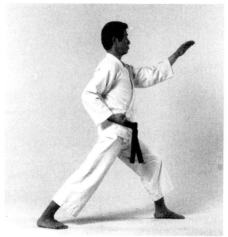

2. Move left foot to N, forming a left long walking stance while executing a high hooking block with the left palm.

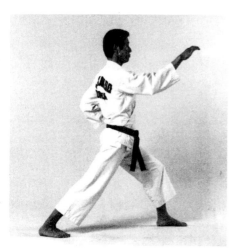

3. Execute a high hooking block with the right palm.

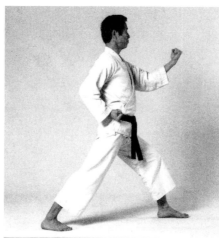

4. Execute a middle inward block with the left outer forearm.

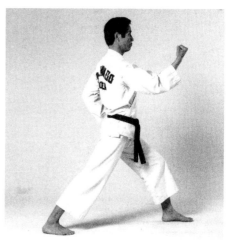

5. Execute a middle inward block with the right outer forearm.

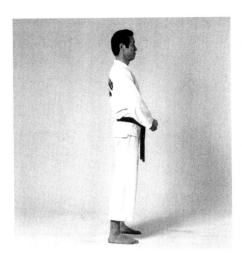

Parallel ready stance.

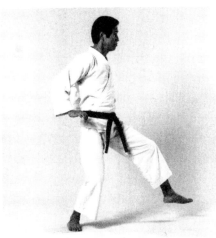

1. Prepare to twin palm upward block.

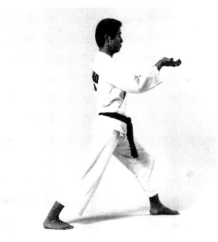

2. Move left foot to N, forming a left long walking stance while executing a middle upward block with both palms.

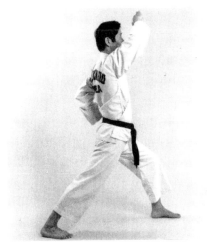

3. Execute a rising block with the right knife-hand.

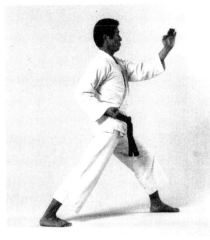

4. Execute a high inward block with the left palm.

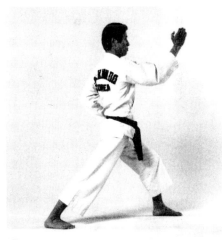

5. Execute a high inward block with the right palm.

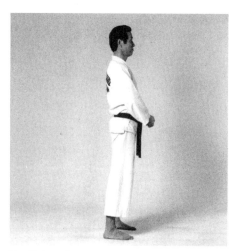

Parallel ready stance.

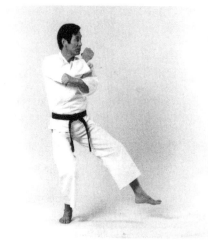

1. Prepare to inner forearm block.

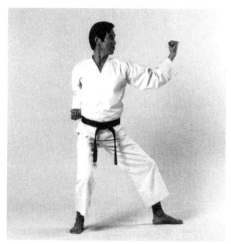

2. Move left foot to N, forming a left L-stance while executing a high block with the left inner forearm.

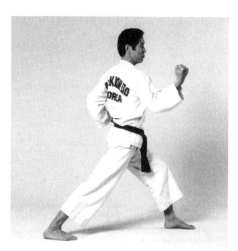

3. Execute a middle circular block to NE with the right inner forearm while slipping the left foot.

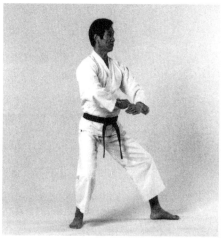

4. Execute a downward block with both palms while forming a left L-stance and pulling the left foot.

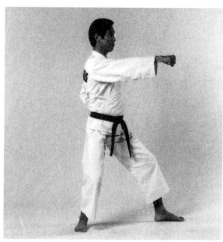

5. Execute a middle punch to NE with the right fist.

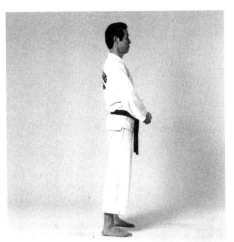

Parallel ready stance.

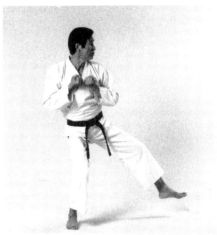

1. Prepare to execute a twin fist vertical punch.

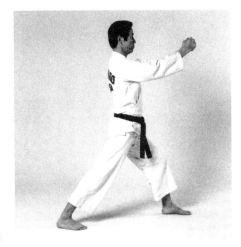

2. Move left foot to N forming a left long walking stance while executing a high vertical punch with twin fists.

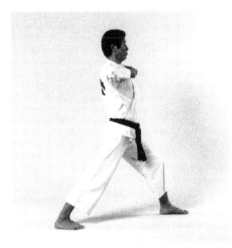

3. Thrust to sides with double side elbow.

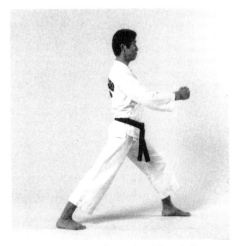

4. Execute a vertical punch with twin fists.

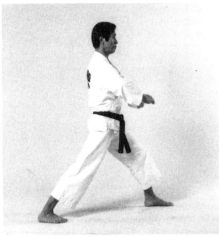

5. Execute a middle side block with both palms.

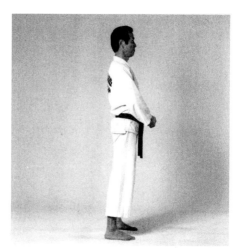

Parallel ready stance.

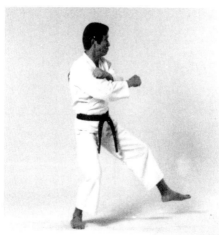

1. Prepare to execute inner forearm wedging block.

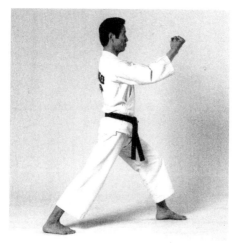

2. Move left foot to N, forming a left long walking stance while executing a high wedging block with the inner forearm.

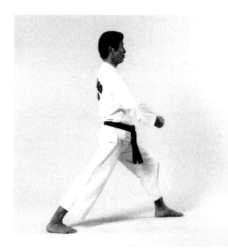

3. Execute a low block with both outer forearms.

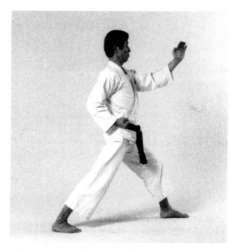

4. Execute a high inward block with the left palm.

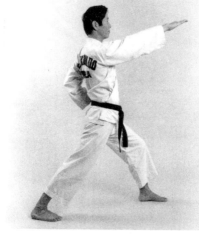

5. Execute a high thrust with the right flat fingertip.

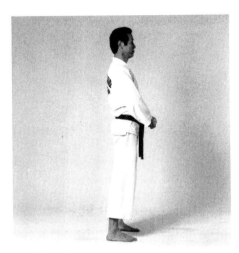

Parallel ready stance.

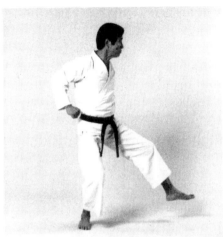

1. Prepare to execute twin upset punch.

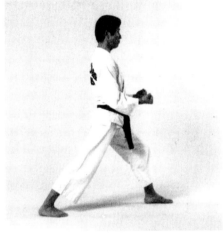

2. Move left foot to N forming a left long walking stance while executing an upset punch with twin fists.

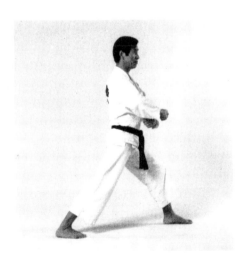

3. Execute a downward side block with the twin side fists.

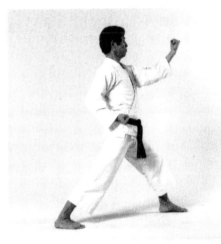

4. Execute a high block with the left inner forearm.

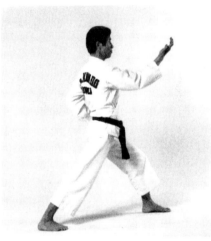

5. Execute a high inward strike with the right knife-hand.

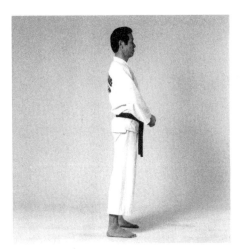

Parallel ready stance.

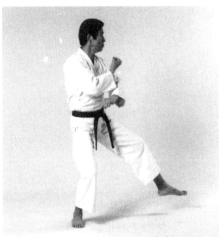

1. Prepare to execute a low block with the right forearm and middle side block with the left forearm.

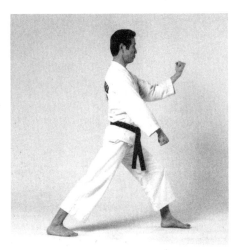

2. Move left foot to N, forming a left long walking stance while executing a low block with the right forearm and a middle side block with the left inner forearm.

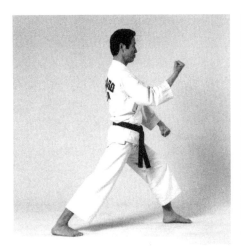

3. Execute a low block with the left forearm and a middle side block with the right inner forearm.

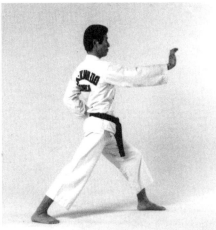

4. Execute a middle pushing block with the right palm.

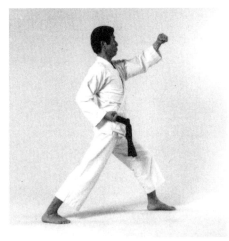

5. Execute a high crescent punch with the left fist.

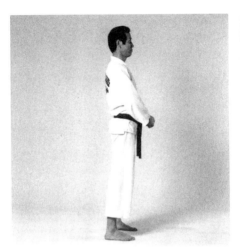

Parallel ready stance.

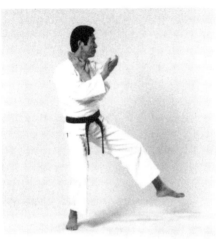

1. Prepare to execute knife-hand wedging block.

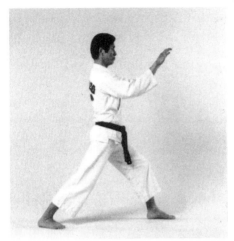

2. Move left foot to N, forming a left long walking stance while executing a high wedging block with the knife-hand.

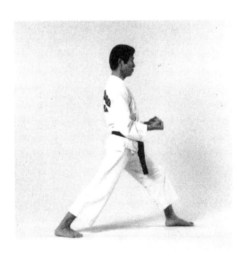

3. Execute an upset punch with twin fists.

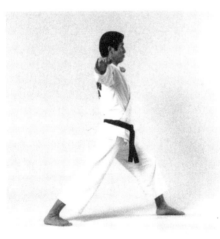

4. Execute a middle strike to sides with both knife-hands.

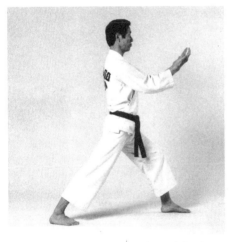

5. Execute middle inward strike with both knife-hands.

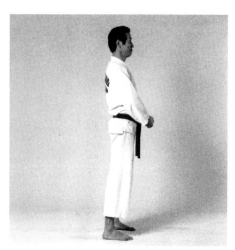

Parallel ready stance.

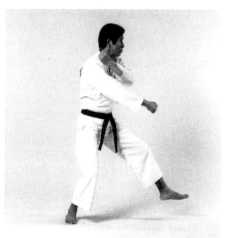

1. Prepare to execute an inner forearm circular block.

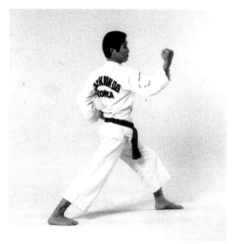

2. Move left foot to N, forming a left long walking stance while executing a high circular block to NE with the right inner forearm.

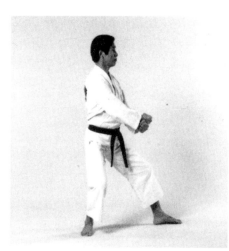

3. Execute a middle pressing block with X-fists while forming a left L-stance and pulling left foot.

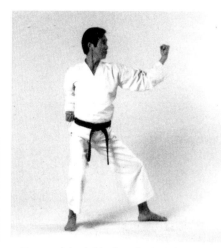

4. Execute a high block with the left inner forearm.

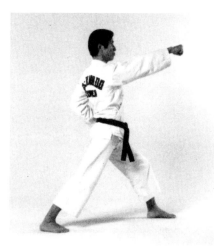

5. Execute a high punch with the right fist while slipping the left foot.

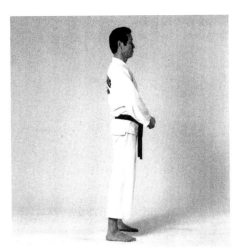

Parallel ready stance.

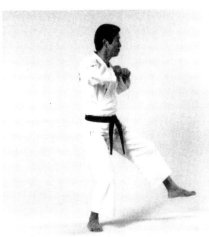

1. Prepare to execute the X-fist pressing block.

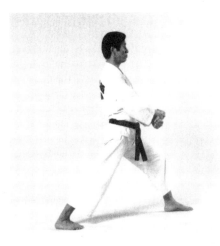

2. Move left foot to N, forming a left long walking stance while executing a pressing block with the X-fist.

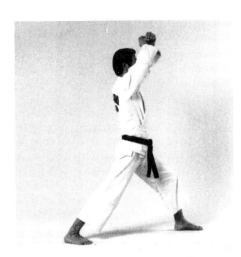

3. Execute a rising block with the X-fist.

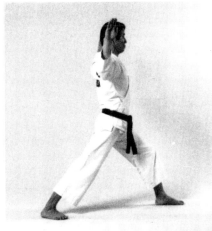

4. Execute a W-shape block with both knife-hands.

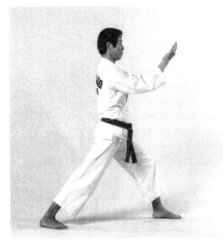

5. Execute a high inward strike with both knife-hands.

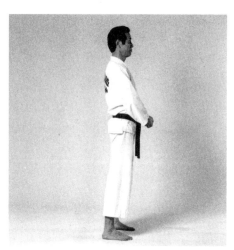

Parallel ready stance.

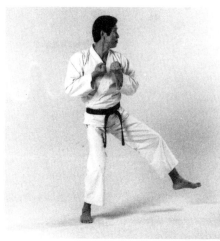

1. Prepare to execute a twin rising block.

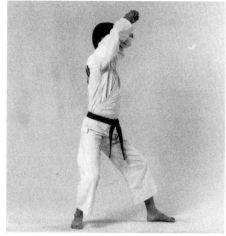

2. Move left foot to N, forming a left L-stance while executing a rising block with both outer forearms.

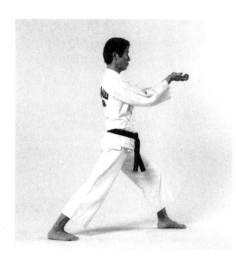

3. Execute a middle upward block with both palms while slipping the left foot.

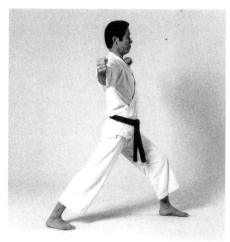

4. Execute a middle strike to sides with both back fists.

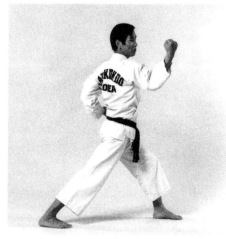

5. Execute a high circular block to NE with the right inner forearm.

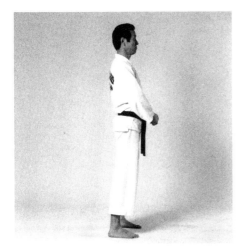

Parallel ready stance.

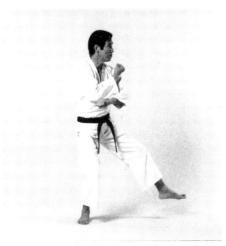

1. Prepare to right 9-shape block.

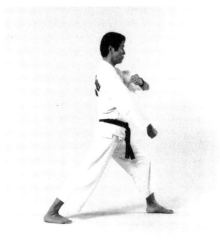

2. Move left foot to N, forming a left long walking stance while executing a right 9-shape block.

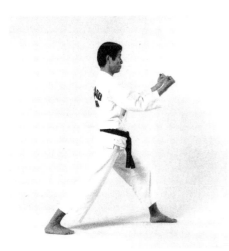

3. Execute a middle wedging block with the inner forearm.

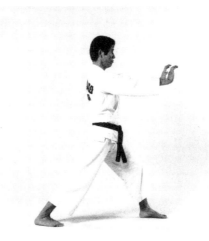

4. Execute a middle pushing block with both palms.

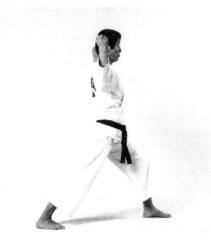

5. Execute a high W-shape block with the inner forearm.

Hand and Foot Techniques

This chapter is especially designed for highly advanced students and requires continuous kicking and jumping with accelerated hand movements. Proper mastering of hand and foot techniques help to improve hand and leg coordination for both attack and defense. Body balance and speed are also enhanced. When performed properly, the body movements flow smoothly and without interruption.

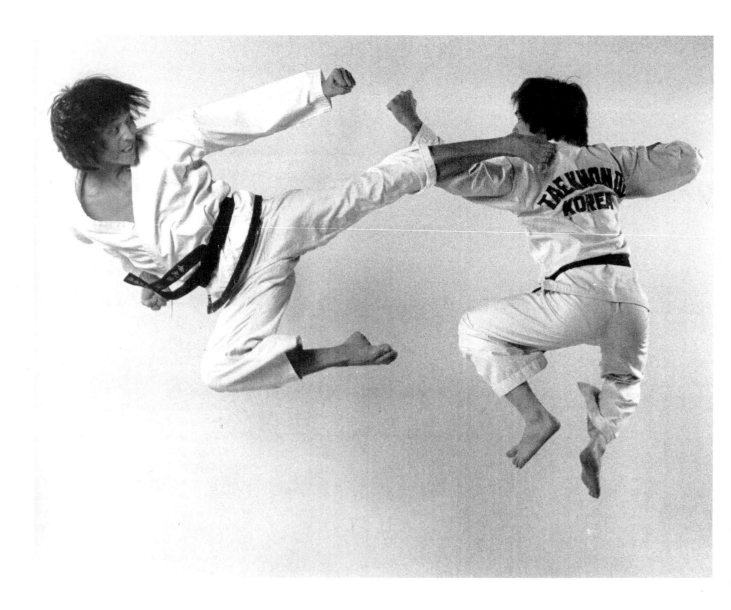

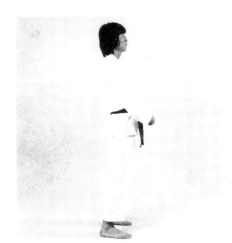

Parallel ready stance.

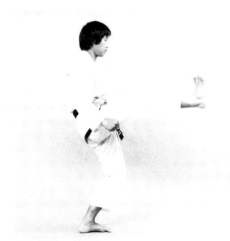

1. Execute a middle front snap kick to N with the right foot.

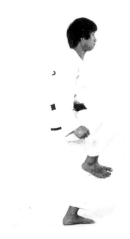

2. Prepare to execute jumping front snap kick.

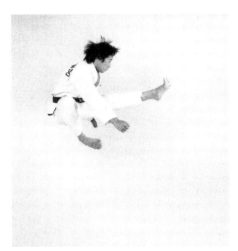

3. Execute jumping front snap kick to N with the left foot.

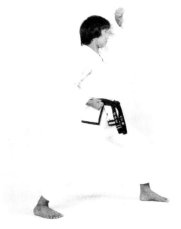

4. Land at N, forming a left long walking stance and execute a rising block with the left forearm.

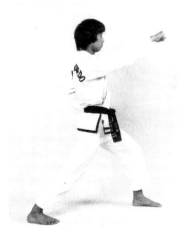

5. Execute a high punch to N with the right fist.

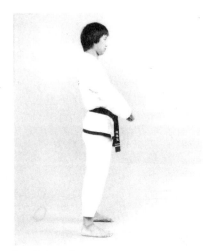

Parallel ready stance.

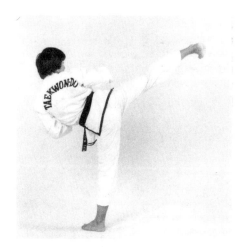

1. Execute a middle side-snapping kick to N with the right foot.

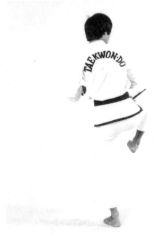

2. Prepare to execute jumping side kick.

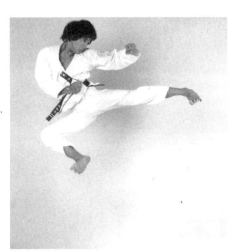

3. Execute jumping side-snapping kick to N with the left foot.

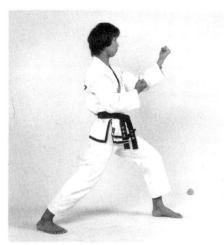

4. Land at N, forming a left long walking stance and execute a high block to N with the left double forearm block.

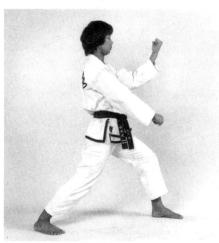

5. Execute low block to N with the right outer forearm.

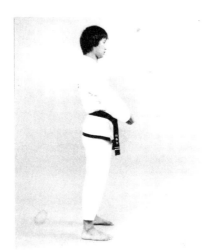

Parallel ready stance.

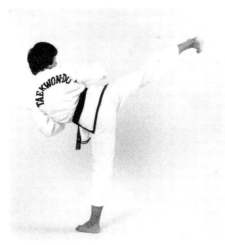

1. Execute middle turning kick to N with the right foot.

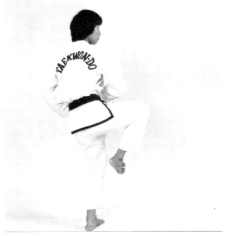

2. Prepare to execute jumping turning kick.

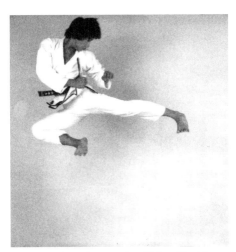

3. Execute jumping turning kick to N with the left foot.

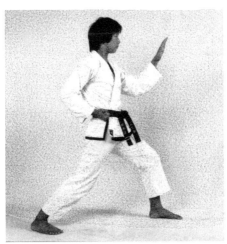

4. Land at N, forming a left long walking stance and execute a high side block to N with the left knife-hand.

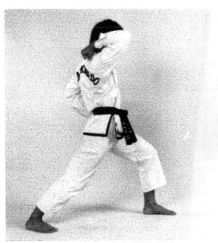

5. Execute upward strike to N with the right elbow.

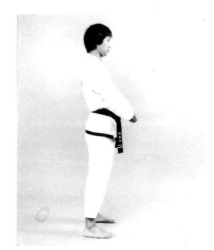

Parallel ready stance.

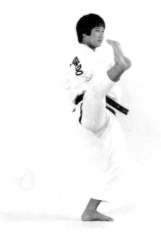

1. Execute a middle twisting kick to E with the right foot.

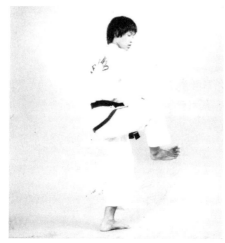

2. Prepare to execute jumping twisting kick.

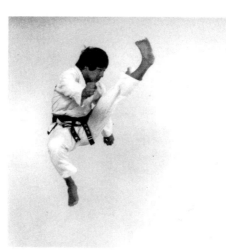

3. Execute jumping twisting kick to NW with the left foot.

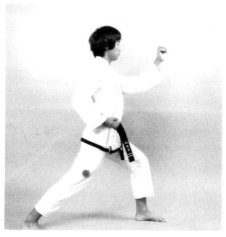

4. Land at N, forming a left long walking stance and execute a high side strike to N with the left back fist.

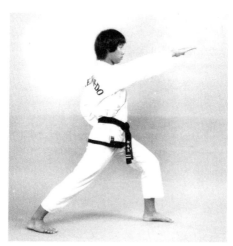

5. Execute high thrust to N with the right fingertips.

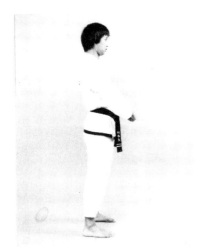

Parallel ready stance.

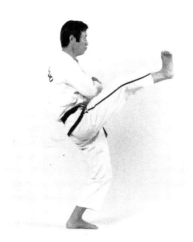

1. Execute middle crescent kick to N with the right foot.

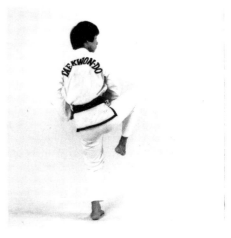

2. Prepare to execute jumping crescent kick.

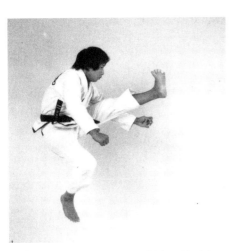

3. Execute jumping crescent kick to N with the left foot.

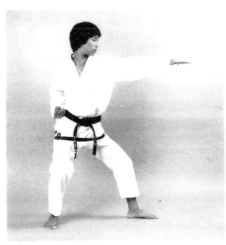

4. Land at N forming a left L-stance and exert middle strike to N with the left knife-hand.

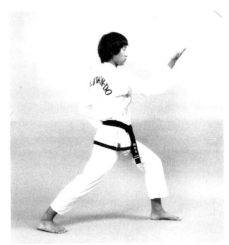

5. Execute high inward strike to N with the right knife-hand while slipping the left foot.

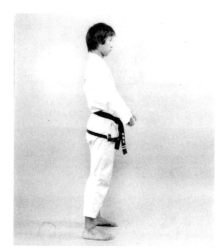

Parallel ready stance.

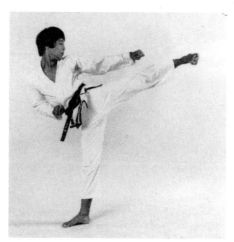

1. Execute middle side-snapping kick to N with the left foot.

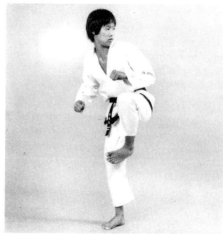

2. Prepare to execute jumping back side kick.

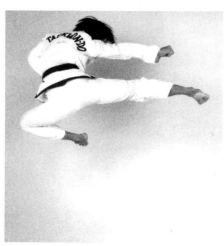

3. Execute jumping back snapping kick to N with the right foot while spinning to N clockwise.

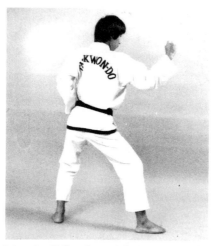

4. Land at N, forming a right L-stance and execute a high side strike with the right back fist.

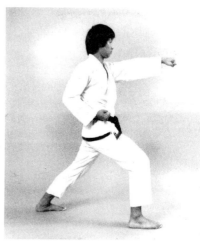

5. Execute middle punch to N with the left fist while slipping the right foot.

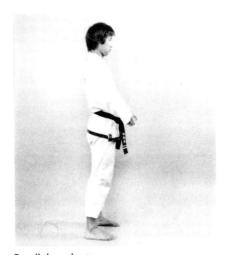

Parallel ready stance.

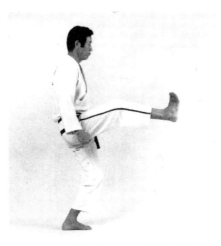

1. Execute middle front snap kick to N with the right foot.

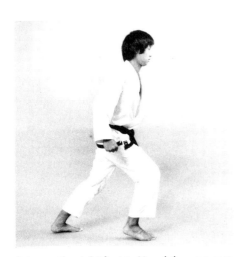

2. Lower the right foot to N and then prepare to execute jumping kick.

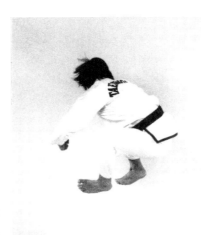

3. Spin clockwise at 180 degrees.

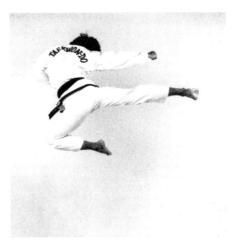

4. Execute flying side-snapping kick to N with the right foot while spinning clockwise at 360 degrees.

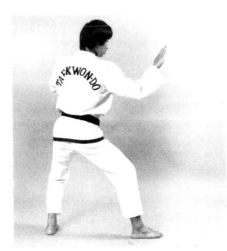

5. Land at N, forming a right L-stance and execute middle guarding block to N with the right knife-hand.

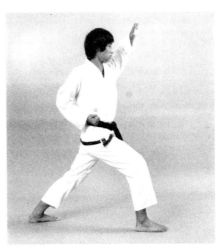

6. Execute rising block to N with the left knife-hand while slipping the right foot.

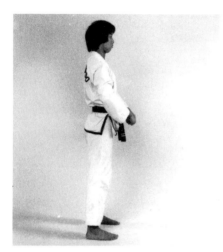

Parallel ready stance.

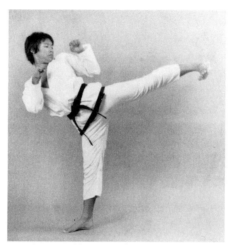

1. Execute middle turning kick to N with the left foot.

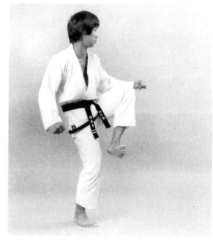

2. Prepare to execute jumping reverse turning kick

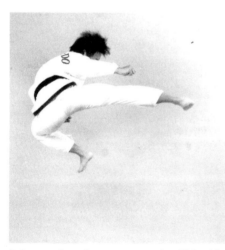

3. Execute jumping reverse turning kick with the right foot while spinning clockwise.

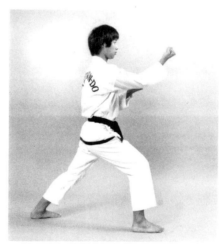

4. Land at N, forming a right long walking stance and exert high block to N with the right double forearm.

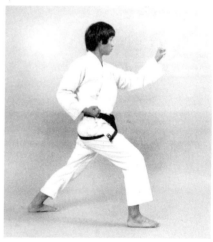

5. Execute high side block to N with the left outer forearm.

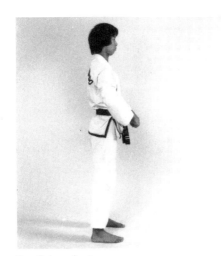

Parallel ready stance.

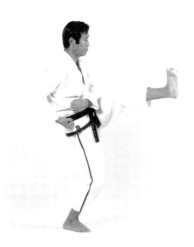

1. Execute middle crescent kick to N with the left foot.

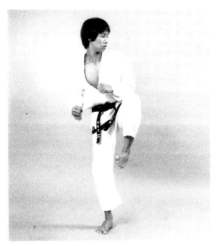

2. Prepare to execute jumping right reverse hooking kick

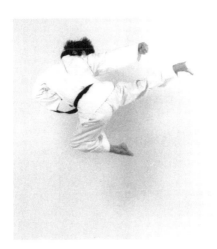

3. Execute jumping reverse hooking kick to N with right foot while spinning clockwise.

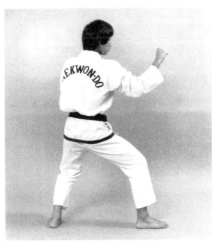

4. Land at N, forming a right L-stance and exert middle guarding block to N with the right forearm.

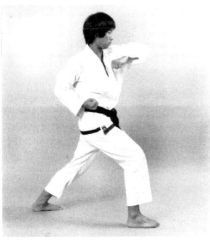

5. Execute middle side strike to N with the left elbow while slipping the right foot.

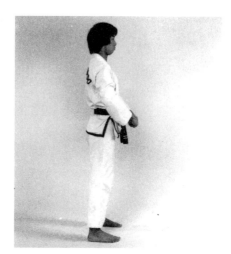

Parallel ready stance.

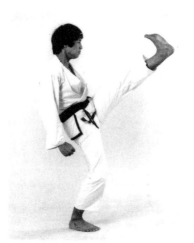

1. Execute middle downward kick to N with the left back heel.

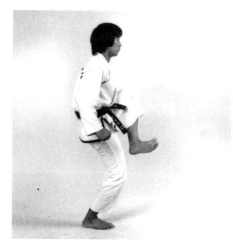

2. Prepare to execute jumping downward kick.

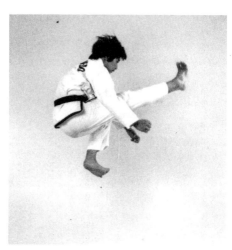

3. Execute jumping downward kick to N with the right back heel.

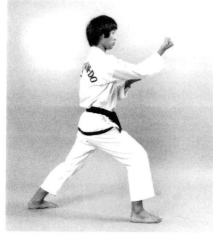

4. Land at N forming a right long walking stance and exert high block to N with the right inner forearm.

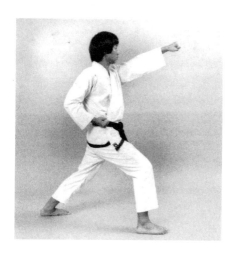

5. Execute high punch to N with the left fist.

Foot Techniques

Taekwondo is widely recognized for its superior foot techniques. The feet are used for blocking, deflecting, and attacking. The many foot variations offer the student a facility to improve balance and speed. Foot techniques in this chapter are for advanced students, for it requires fast and continuous foot movements in one action. Loss of leg control, power, and balance will result if the foot movement is not executed properly. With few exceptions, the foot should reach the target in a straight line in conjunction with a sharp twist of the hip and abdomen.

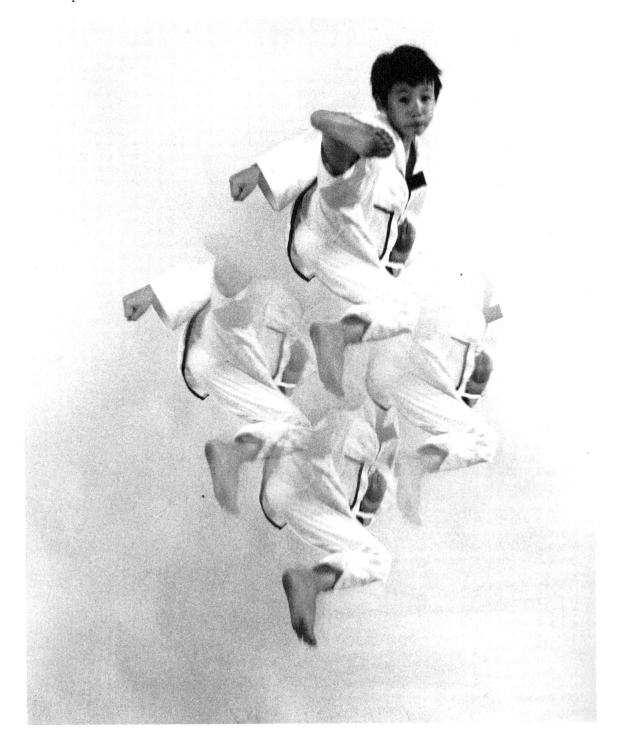

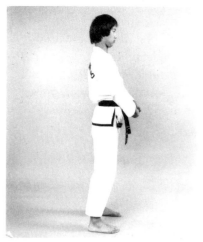

Parallel ready stance.

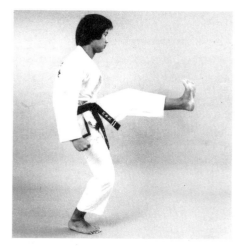

1. Execute middle front snap kick to N with the left foot.

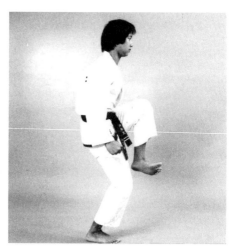

2. Prepare to side kick.

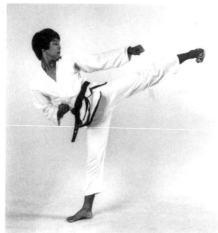

3. Execute middle side-snapping kick to N with the left foot.

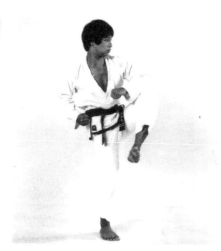

4. Prepare to execute side kick.

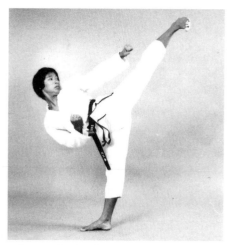

5. Execute high side-snapping kick to N with the left foot.

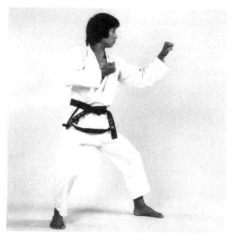

6. Lower the left foot to N forming a left L-stance with a forearm guarding block.

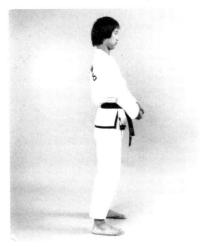

Parallel ready stance.

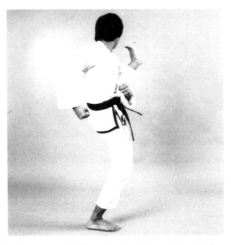

1. Execute middle twisting kick to W with the left foot.

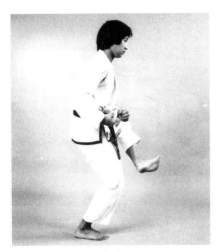

2. Prepare to turning kick.

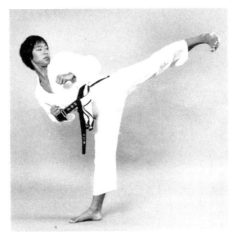

3. Execute middle turning kick to N with the left foot.

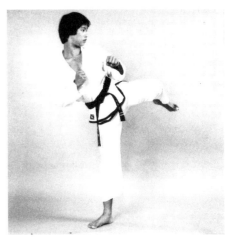

4. Prepare to turning kick.

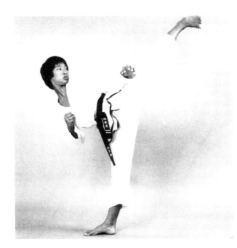

5. Execute high turning kick to N with the left foot.

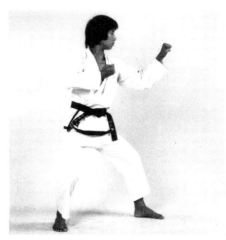

6. Lower the left foot to N forming a left L-stance with a forearm guarding block.

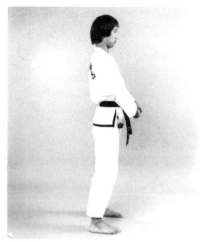

Parallel ready stance.

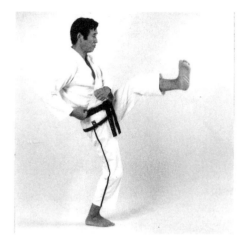

1. Execute middle crescent kick to N with the left foot.

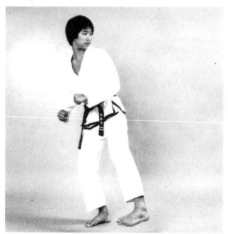

2. Prepare to reverse hooking kick.

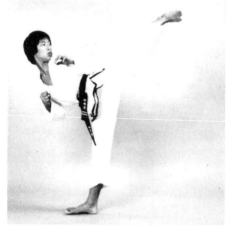

3. Execute high reverse hooking kick to N with the left foot.

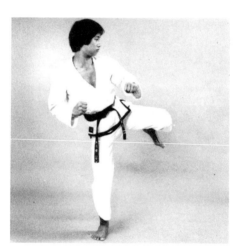

4. Prepare to side kick.

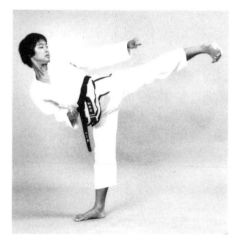

5. Execute middle side-snapping kick to N with the left foot.

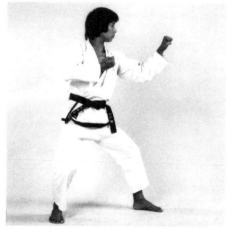

6. Lower the left foot to N forming a left L-stance with a forearm guarding block.

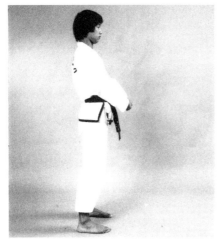

Parallel ready stance.

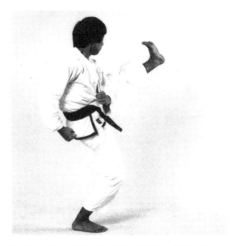

1. Execute middle twisting kick to NW with the left foot.

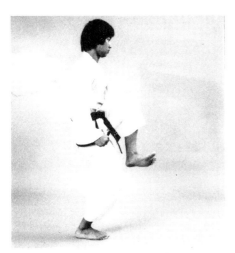

2. Prepare to execute turning kick.

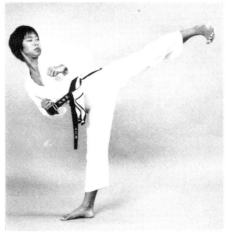

3. Execute middle turning kick to N with the left foot.

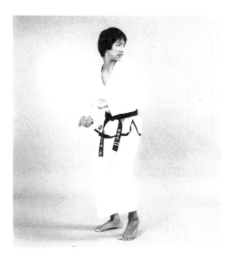

4. Prepare to execute reverse turning kick.

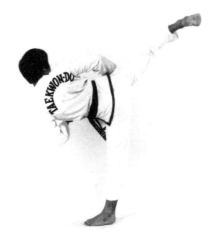

5. Execute high reverse turning kick to N with the right foot.

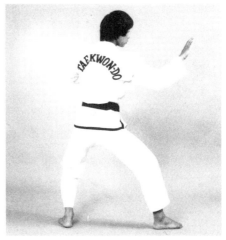

6. Lower the right foot to N forming a right L-stance with the knife-hand guarding block.

351 / Foot Techniques

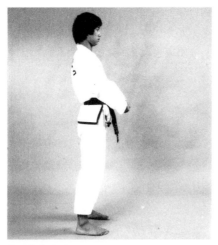

Parallel ready stance.

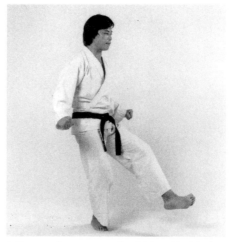

1. Execute lower sweeping kick to N with the left foot.

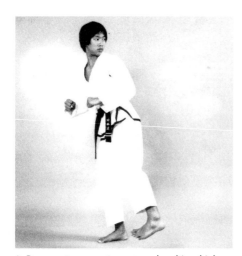

2. Prepare to execute reverse hooking kick.

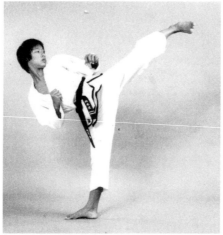

3. Execute high reverse hooking kick to N with the left foot.

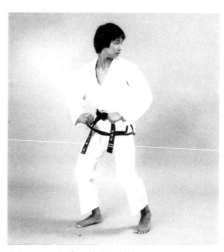

4. Prepare to back side kick.

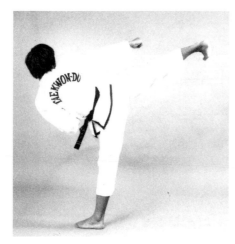

5. Execute middle back side-snapping kick to N with the right foot.

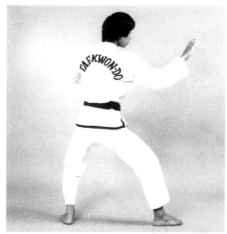

6. Lower the right foot to N forming a right L-stance with the knife-hand guarding block.

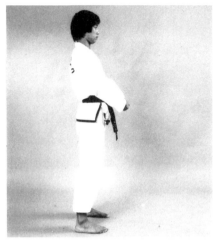

Parallel ready stance.

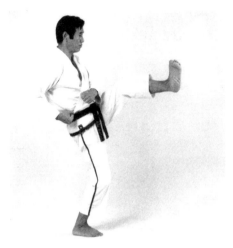

1. Execute middle crescent kick to N with the left foot.

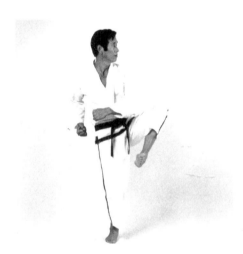

2. Prepare to side-snapping kick.

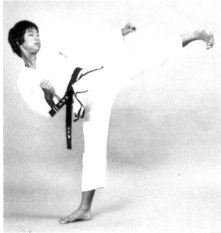

3. Execute middle side-snapping kick to N with the left foot.

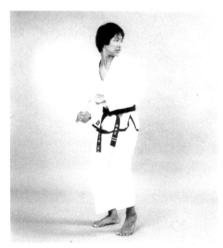

4. Prepare to execute reverse hooking kick.

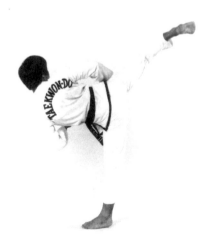

5. Execute high reverse hooking kick to N with the right foot.

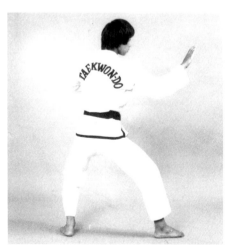

6. Lower the right foot to N forming a right L-stance with the knife-hand guarding block.

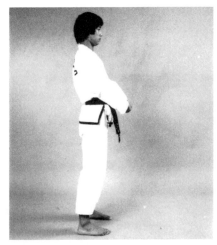

Parallel ready stance.

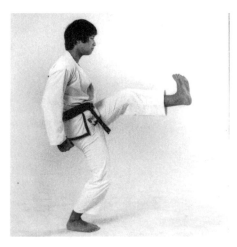

1. Execute middle front snap kick to N with the left foot.

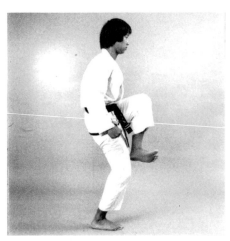

2. Prepare to execute jumping front snap kick.

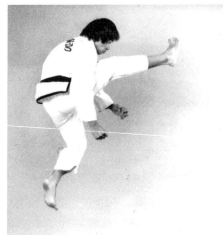

3. Execute jumping front snap kick to N with the right foot.

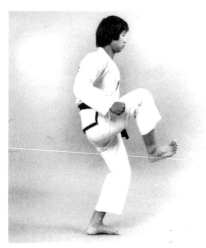

4. Land at N and then prepare to execute side kick.

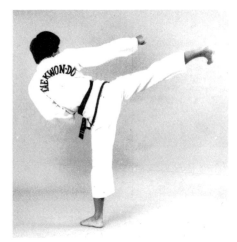

5. Execute middle side-snapping kick to N with the right foot.

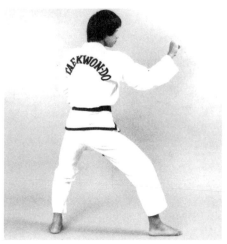

6. Lower the right foot to N, forming a right L-stance with the forearm guarding block.

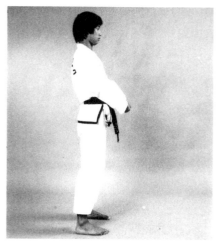

Parallel ready stance.

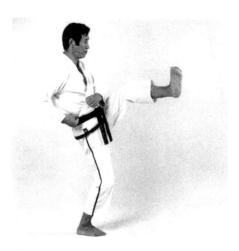

1. Execute middle crescent kick to N with the left foot.

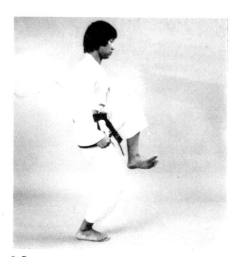

2. Prepare to execute jumping crescent kick.

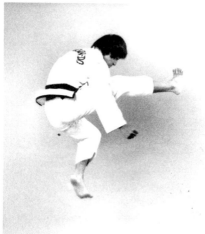

3. Execute jumping crescent kick to N with the right foot.

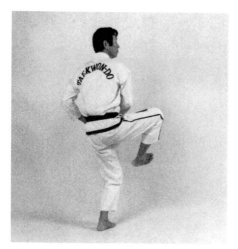

4. Land at N and then prepare to execute reverse hooking kick.

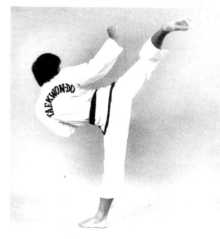

5. Execute high reverse hooking kick to N with the right foot.

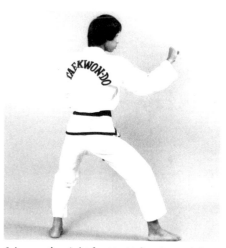

6. Lower the right foot to N, forming a right L-stance with the forearm guarding block.

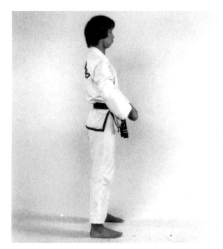

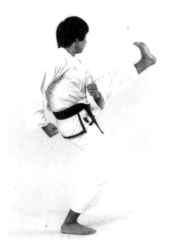

Parallel ready stance.

1. Execute middle twisting kick to NW with the left foot.

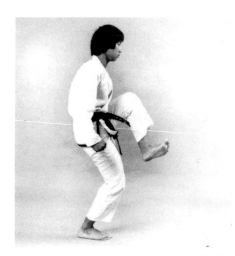

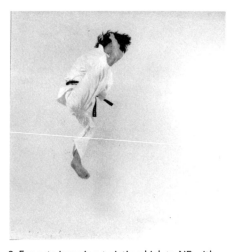

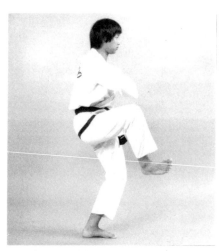

2. Prepare to execute jumping twisting kick.

3. Execute jumping twisting kick to NE with the right foot.

4. Land at N and then prepare to execute turning kick.

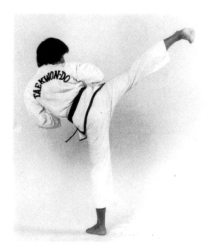

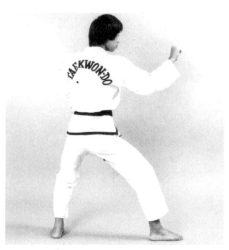

5. Execute high turning kick to N with the right foot.

6. Lower the right foot to N, forming a right L-stance with the forearm guarding block.

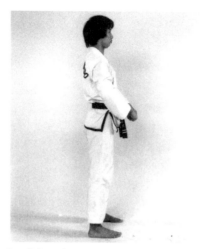

Parallel ready stance.

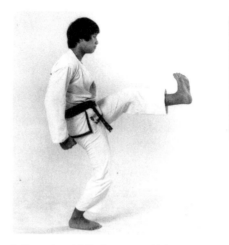

1. Execute middle front snap kick to N with the left foot.

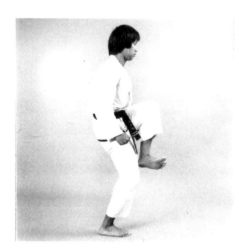

2. Prepare to execute twisting kick.

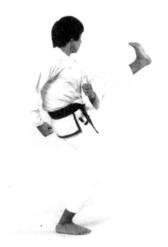

3. Execute middle twisting kick to NW with the left foot.

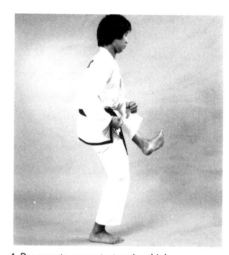

4. Prepare to execute turning kick.

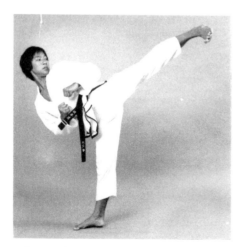

5. Execute high turning kick to N with the left foot.

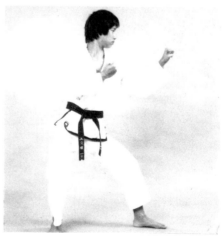

6. Lower the left foot to N forming a left L-stance with a forearm guarding block.

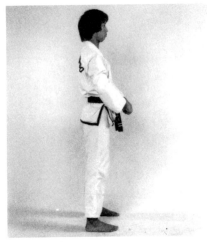

Parallel ready stance.

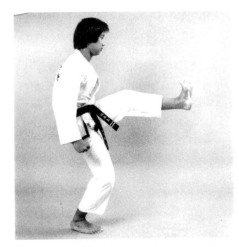

1. Execute middle front snap kick to N with the left foot.

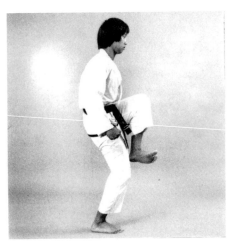

2. Prepare to execute jumping turning kick.

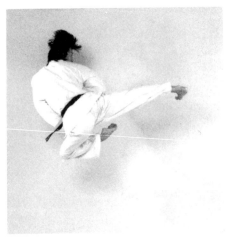

3. Execute jumping turning kick to N with the right foot.

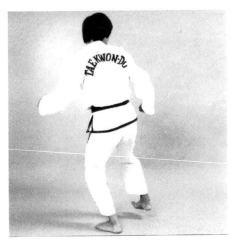

4. Land at N and then prepare to reverse turning kick.

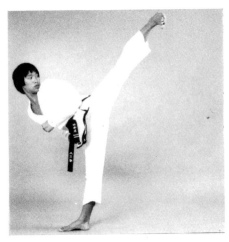

5. Execute high reverse turning kick to N with the left foot.

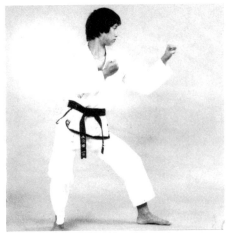

6. Lower the left foot to N forming a left L-stance with a forearm guarding block.

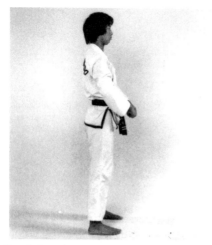

Parallel ready stance.

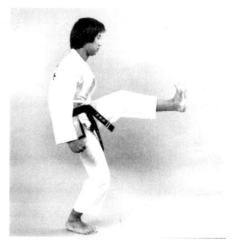

1. Execute middle front snap kick to N with the left foot.

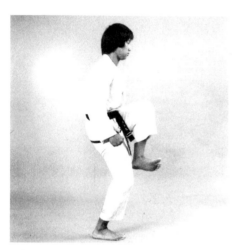

2. Prepare to execute jumping side kick.

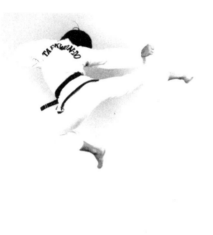

3. Execute jumping side-snapping kick to N with the right foot.

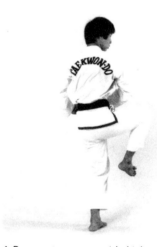

4. Prepare to execute side kick.

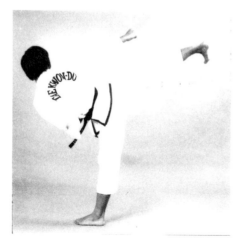

5. Execute middle side-snapping kick to N with the right foot.

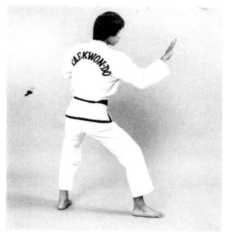

6. Lower the right foot to N forming a right L-stance with the knife-hand guarding block.

359 / Foot Techniques

Use of the Bag

The principle advantage derived from the use of the bag is that the student is free to bring into contact with his target his entire exertive strength, without the need to be wary of a human target. Practicing with the bag, therefore, improves the skill of hand and foot movements and actions, helping to perfect these movements. Above all, with intelligent use of the bag, overall power, balance, speed, and accuracy could be attained and successfully developed in a relatively short period.

During training, efficient jumps, kicks, and strikes with the legs and feet will determine how well you can control contact with your target. The front portions of the soles play a major role in almost all varieties of movements, whether in jumping or falling, blocking or striking. Turning on the ball (front sole) of the foot not only adds to an individual's soundness of balance for attack and defense movements, but also facilitates coordination of speed, power and timing.

The weight of the bag should also be taken cautiously into account prior to practicing. For adult beginners, use of a bag of 40 lbs, or less, would be ideal with careful calculation that the body will be able to withstand the new weight.

A 50-lb bag is considered suitable for a person who weighs 130 lbs or more and who has already worked up to a level of skill sufficient to be applied and developed with the use of the bag.

Wrong Positioned Kick

The bag can be a stationary target or swung to represent a moving target with varied weights. For example, if you kick a 40-lb swinging bag, the power will be doubled with its own power and your kicking power. The power will be stronger if the weight of the bag is heavier.

Whenever you practice swinging bag kicking, you should always remember to keep your foot in contact with the floor, and not to kick higher than halfway up the bag. If the time of contact is not correct, you will have bad results shown as follows.

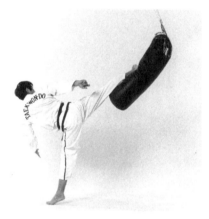

Losing balance.

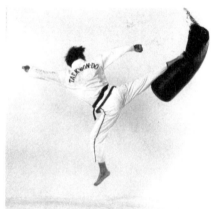

Hitting the leg.

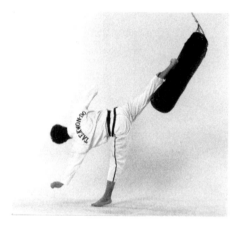

Hitting the leg.

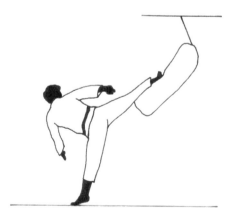

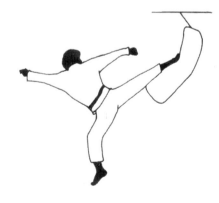

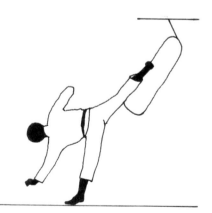

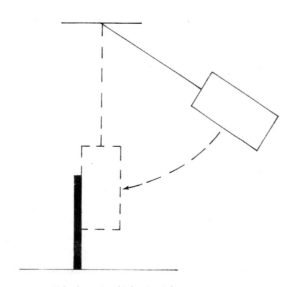

Side thrusting kick principle
1. Spring board fixed to ground.

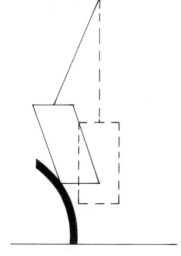

2. Yielding.

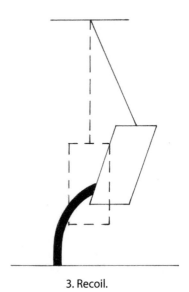

3. Recoil.

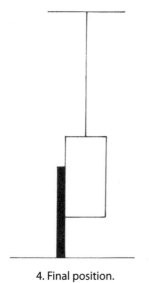

4. Final position.

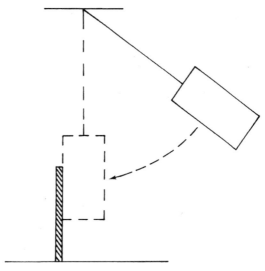

Side-snapping kick principle
1. Rigid wall.

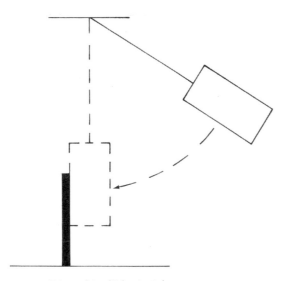

Side pushing kick principle
1. Spring board fixed to ground.

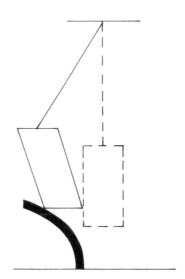

2. Yielding.

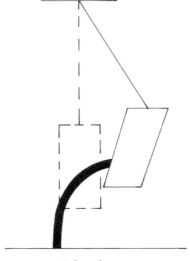

3. Recoil.

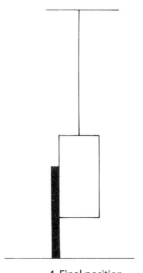

4. Final position.

Side-snapping Kick Principle

The side-snapping kick means to snap the bag to a stop when it reaches the focus of the vertical position. The kick should be directed to a focus point in the center of the bag. You should make use of the truncal power, for the power and speed of your body can be derived only from the trunk. The bag, if used correctly, can expedite the strengthening of leg and foot muscles.

The best way to turn the foot is to pivot on the ball of the foot pressed slightly to the floor. When you make a turn, your heel should not be too high because by doing so you will easily lose your balance.

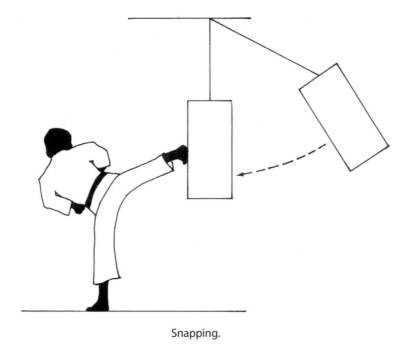

Snapping.

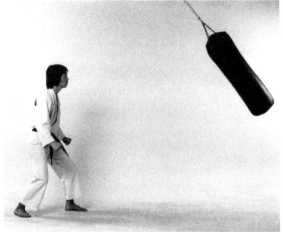

Ready.

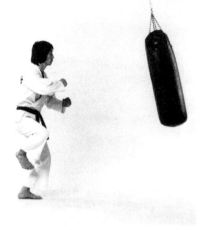

Ready to kick.

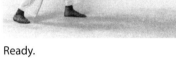

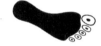

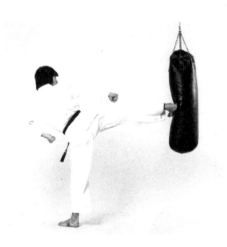

Snapping.

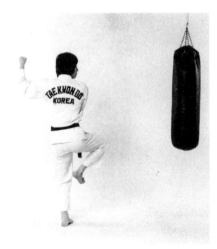

Withdraw.

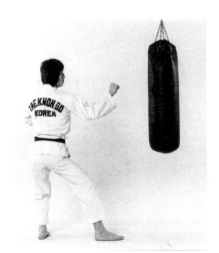

Ready stance.

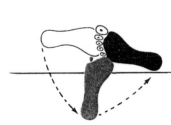

365 / Use of the Bag

Side Thrusting Kick Principle

The side thrusting kick is almost the same as explained in the side-snapping kick. The only difference is to snap and thrust onto the target (logically they are separate, but in practice, it is a continuous action). When you practice, it will be more effective to balance by slightly bending your upper body. The side thrusting kick is an ideal aid for perfecting timing and focus.

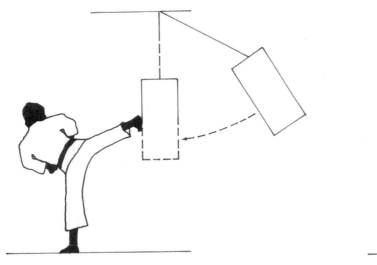

1. Snap.

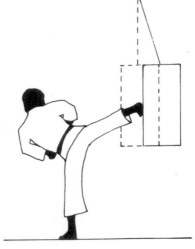

2. Thrust.

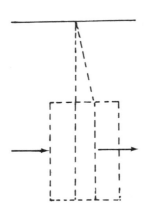

3. Snap thrust.

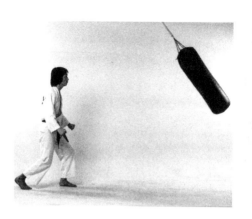

Ready.

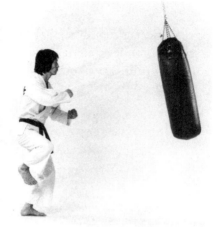

Ready to kick.

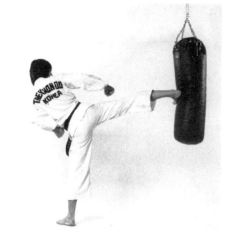

Snapping.

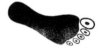

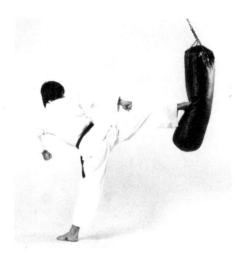

Thrusting.

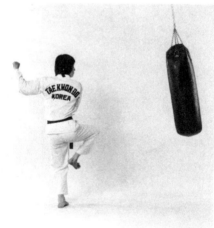

Withdraw.

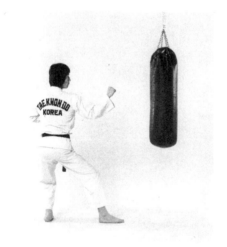

Ready stance.

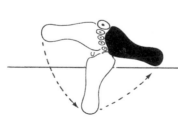

367 / Use of the Bag

Side Pushing Kick Principle

The side pushing kick means to contact and push the bag by bending the knee of the kicking leg when the bag reaches the vertical position. It is ordinarily used as a counterattack on an attacker, without giving great pain. The photographs below will give you an effective way of practicing.

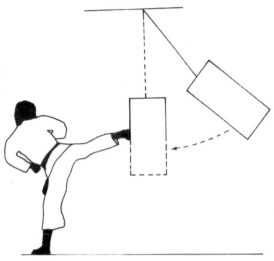

1. Contact.

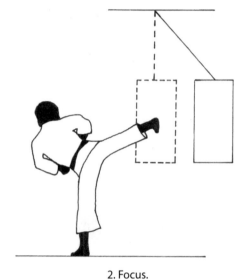

2. Focus.

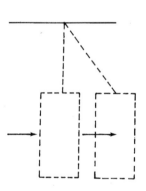

3. Contact focus.

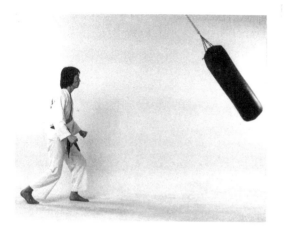

Ready.

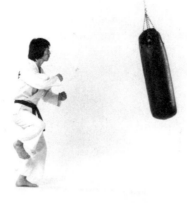

Ready to kick.

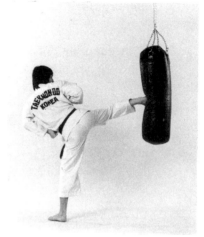

Contact.

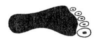

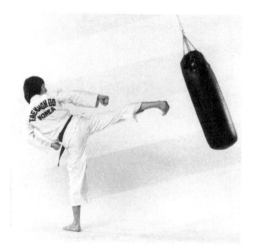

Pushing.

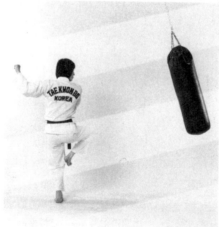

Withdraw.

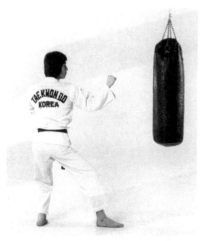

Ready stance.

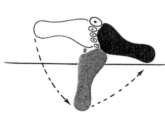

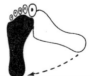

369 / Use of the Bag

Jumping Side Kick Principle

As explained before, snap, thrust, push, and kicks are all the same. The only difference for the jumping side kick is to kick with the jumping leg. After kicking, you have to land at the original position with a balanced body.

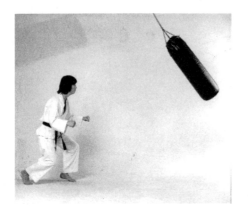

Ready to jump.

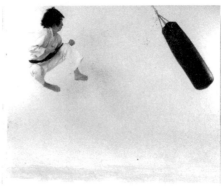

Jumping.

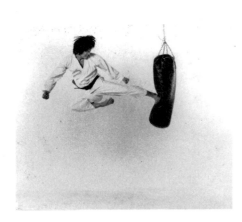

Snapping.

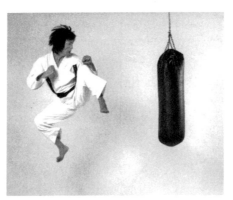

Landing.

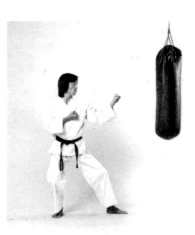

Landed.

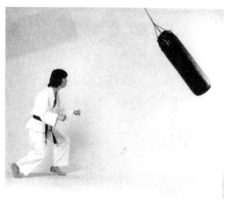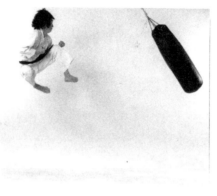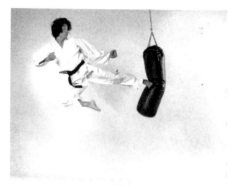

Ready to jump.

Jumping.

Snapping.

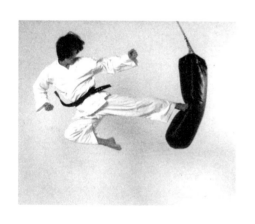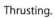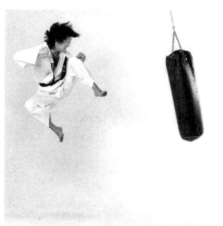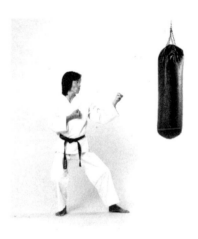

Thrusting.

Landing.

Landed.

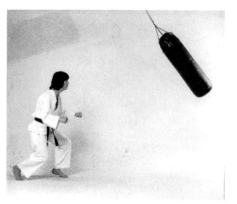

Ready to jump.

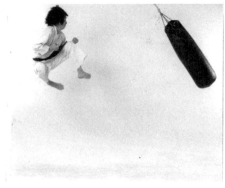

Jumping.

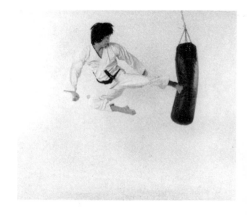

Contact.

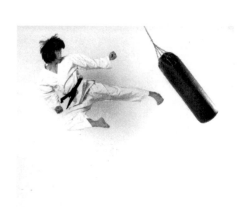

Pushing.

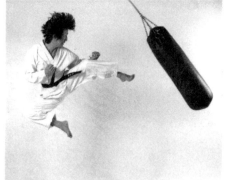

Landing.

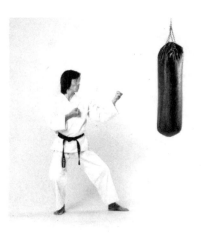

Landed.

Flying Side Kick Principle

Flying side kick means to kick with the left foot if you jump with the right foot, and vice versa. The advantages of the flying side kick are that you can kick from a far distance, and moreover the result will be more than double of your own power.

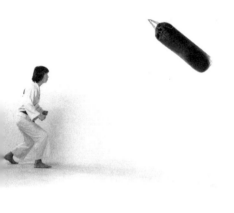

eady to jump.

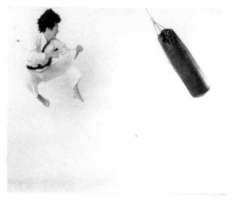

Jumping.

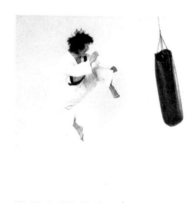

Flying.

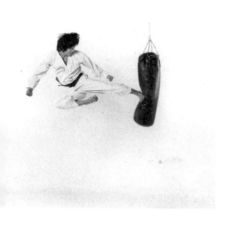

napping.

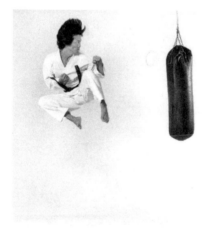

Landing.

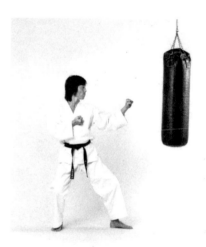

Landed.

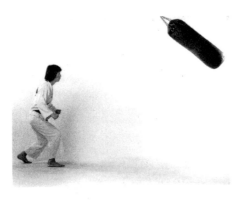

Ready to jump.

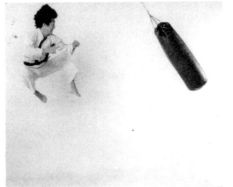

Jumping.

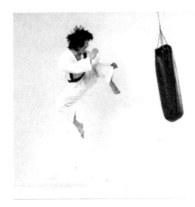

Flying.

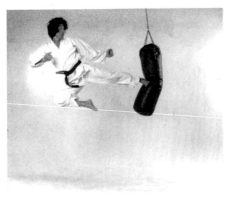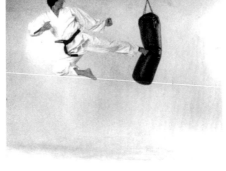

Snapping.

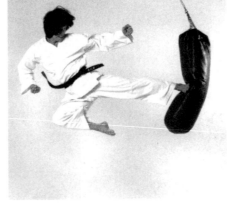

Thrusting.

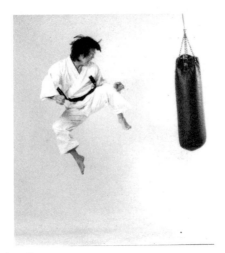

Landing.

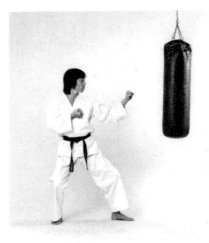

Landed.

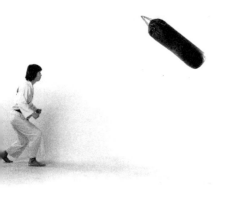 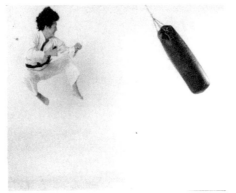 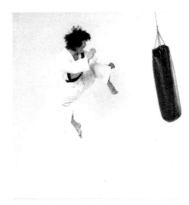

eady to jump.   Jumping.   Flying.

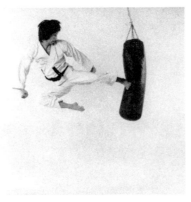 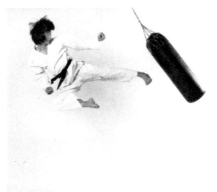

Contact.   Pushing.

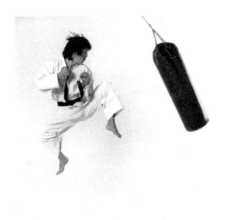 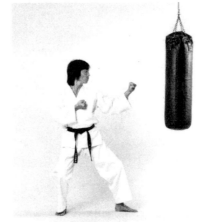

Landing.   Landed.

375 / Use of the Bag

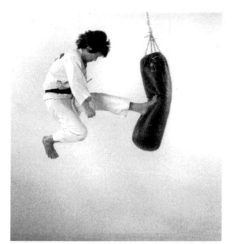

Jumping front kick.

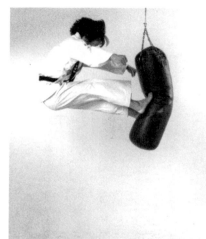

Jumping front twin foot kick.

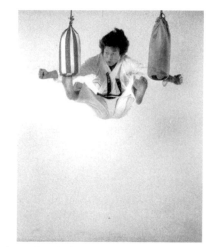

Flying double front kick.

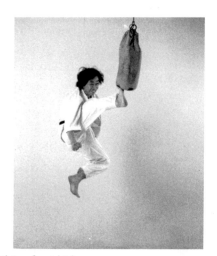

Flying front kick.

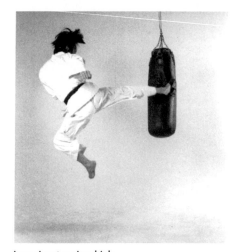

Jumping turning kick.

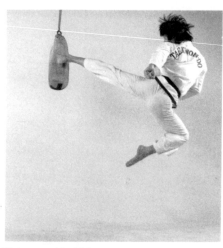

Flying turning kick.

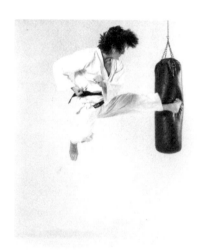

Jumping twisting kick.

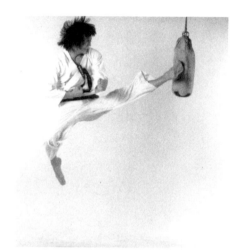

Flying twisting kick.

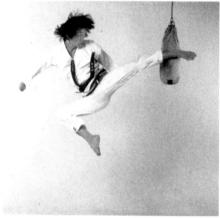

Flying reverse turning kick.

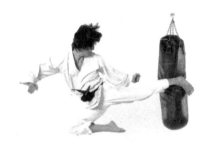

Jumping reverse turning kick.

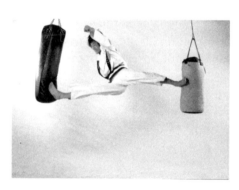

Flying double striding kick.

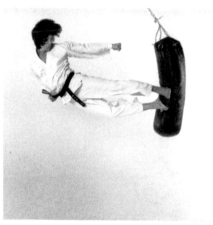

Jumping twin foot side kick.

Jumping Double Side Kick Principle

The outstanding feature of the jumping double side kick is the ability to attack both a lower and higher target in succession, while flying. Because double kicking is performed in one moment, it enables you to practice kicking at high speed.

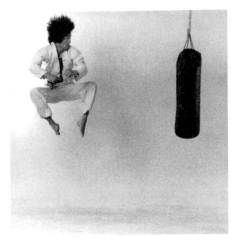

Jumping.

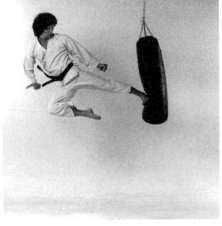

Lower kick.

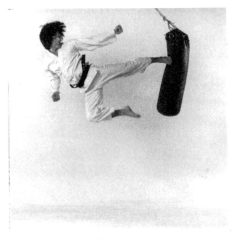

High kick.

Jumping 360 Spinning Mid-Air Kick Principle

This method of kicking is almost the same as the flying side kick; the only difference is that the kicking is executed while spinning in the air. This kick is useful after a fake movement, for the direction of the kick cannot be seen until the moment the kick is performed.

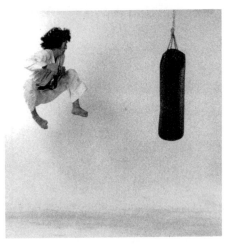

Jumping.

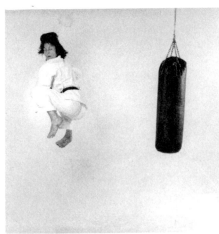

Turning 180.

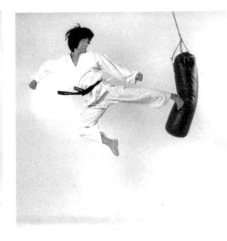

Kicking at 360.

APPENDIX

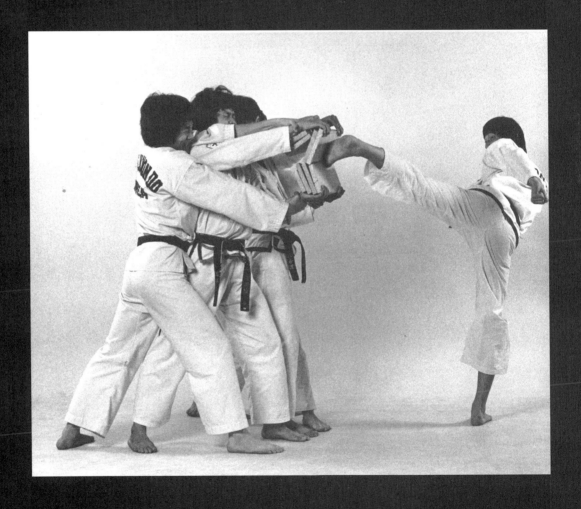

Use of Your Body Parts for Attack and Defense

The surface (or object) through which the force (power) is transmitted to an attacker's body is called the attacking tool. Any surface that intercepts or repulses an attack is called a blocking tool. Furthermore, every part where power can be easily concentrated is considered an attacking and a blocking tool. These tools are divided into parts of the hands and arms, parts of the feet and legs, and other parts of the body. Special care should be given to the selection of the appropriate tool for the distance, target, and desired results. This will require continual practice with firm dedication.

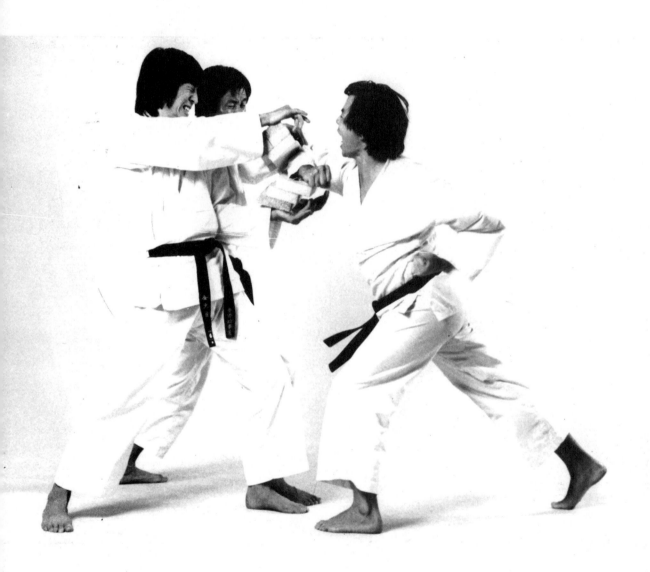

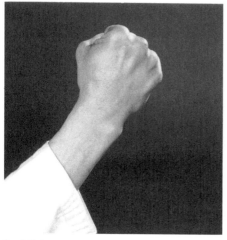

Back fist.

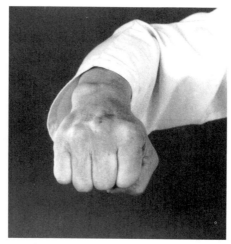

Fore fist.

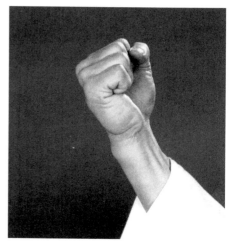

Side fist.

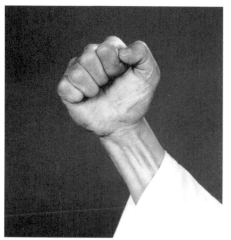

Under fist.

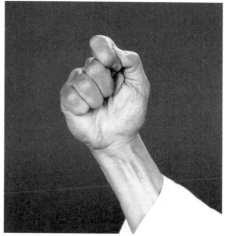

Fore-knuckle fist.

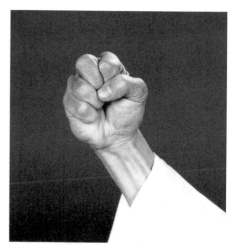

Middle knuckle fist.

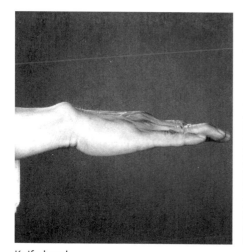

Knife-hand.

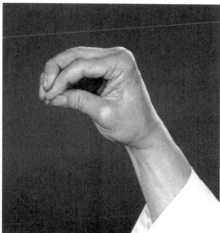

Close fingertip.

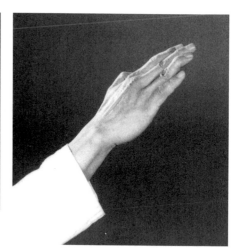

Flat fingertip.

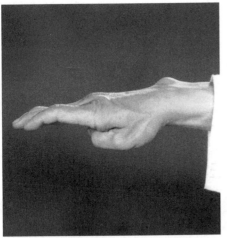

Reverse knife-hand.

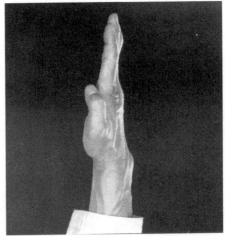

Straight fingertip.

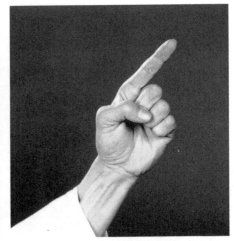

Forefinger.

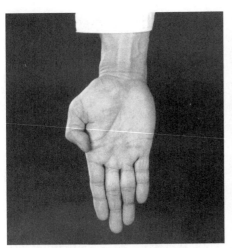

Upset fingertip.

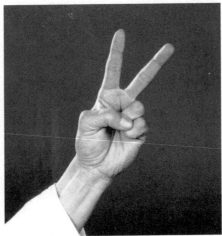

Double finger.

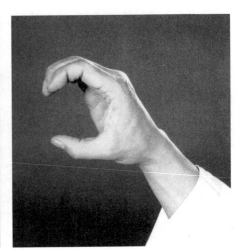

Press fingertip.

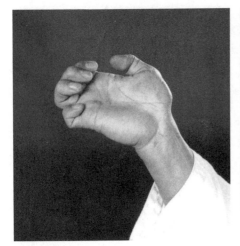

Base of knife-hand.

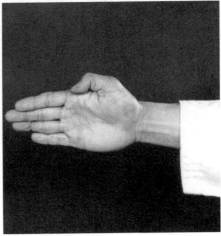

Finger belly.

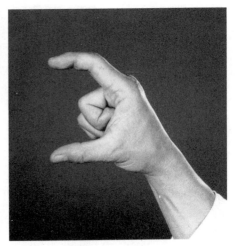

Finger pincers.

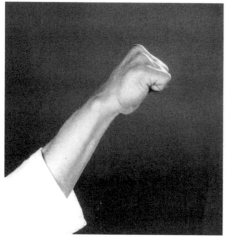

Outer forearm.

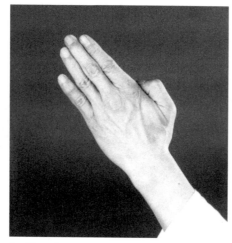

Backhand.

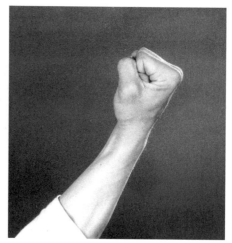

Inner forearm.

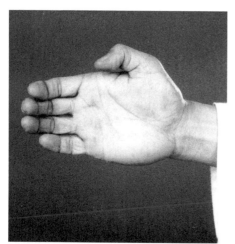

Palm.

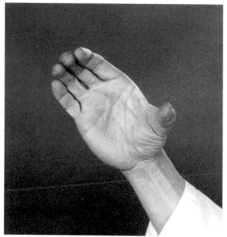

Arc-hand.

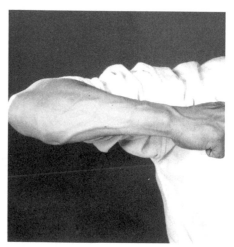

Elbow.

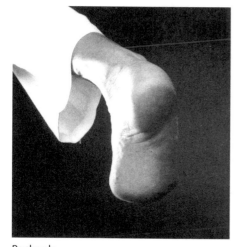

Back sole.

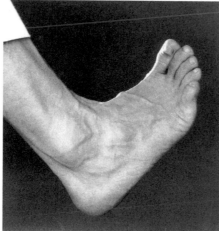

Toes.

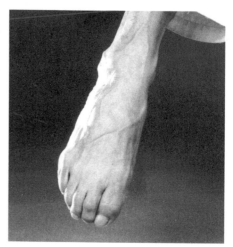

Instep.

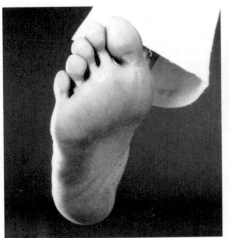

Ball of the foot.

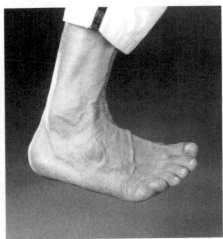

Footsword.

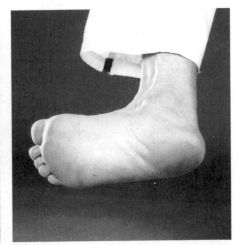

Side sole.

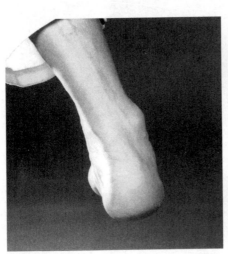

Back heel.

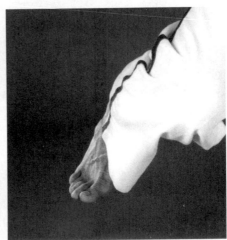

Knee.

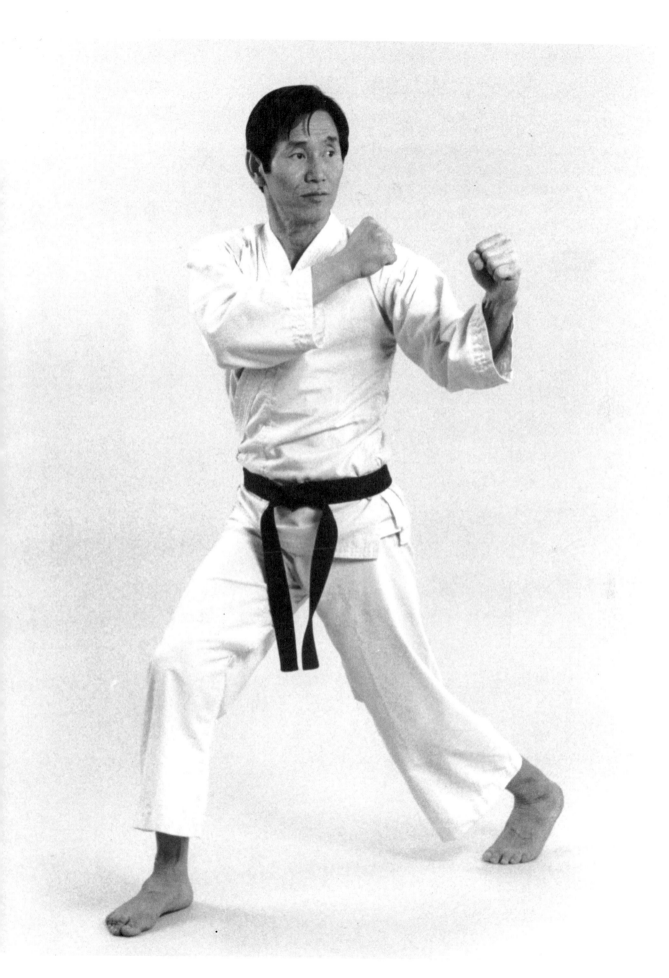

Stance

The movement of the entire body is largely dependent on posture, and a correct stance is most important in order to attack or defend properly and effectively. The controlling factors are stability, agility, balance, and flexibility. The basic principles to follow in forming a proper stance are to keep the back straight in almost all cases, relax the shoulders, and tense the abdomen muscles slightly. It is also important to face your body correctly and maintain correct equilibrium while keeping a little spring in your knees so that you can move quickly.

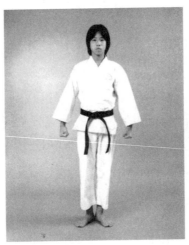

Attention stance.

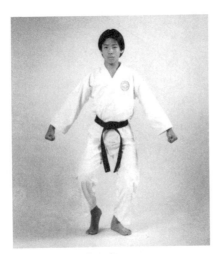

Right attention bending stance.

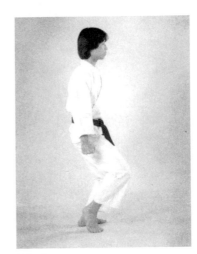

Side view.

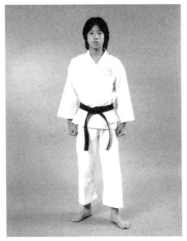 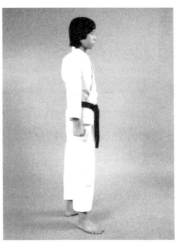

Left natural stance.

Side view.

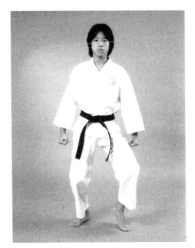 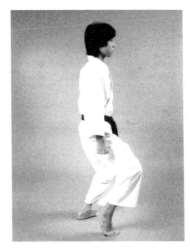

Left natural bending stance.

Side view.

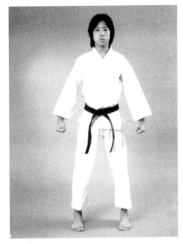

Parallel stance.

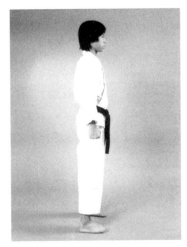

Side view.

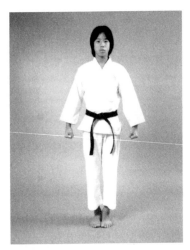

Close stance.

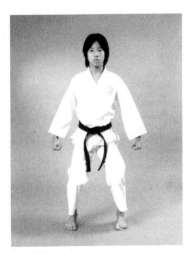

Parallel bending.

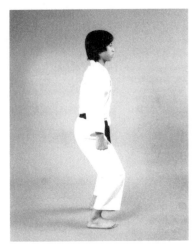

Side view.

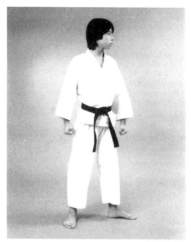

Left vertical stance.

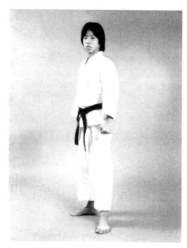

Front view.

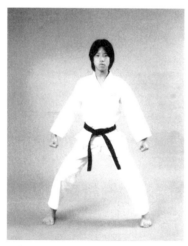

Riding stance.

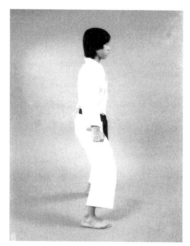

Side view.

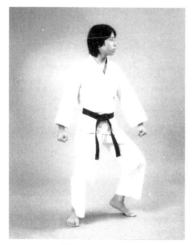

Left vertical bending stance.

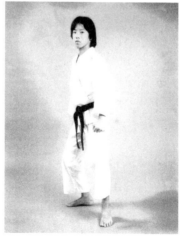

Front view.

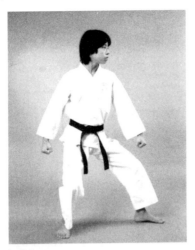

Left L-stance.

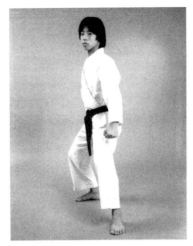

Front view.

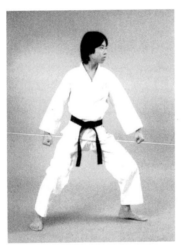

Left fixed stance.

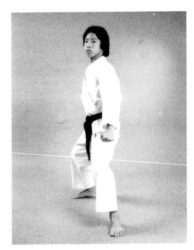

Front view.

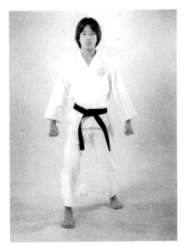

Right walking stance.

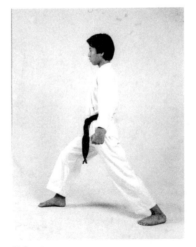

Side view.

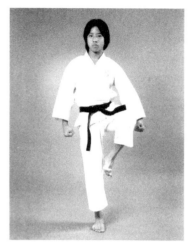

Right one-leg stance.

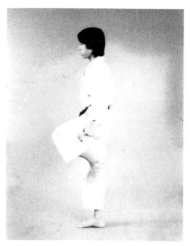

Side view.

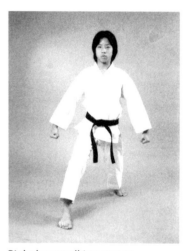

Right long walking stance.

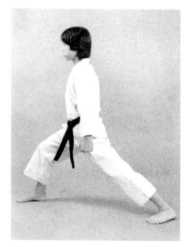

Side view.

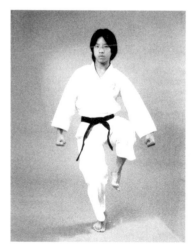

Right one-leg bending stance.

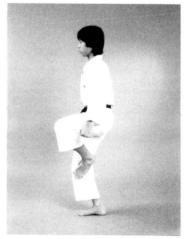

Side view.

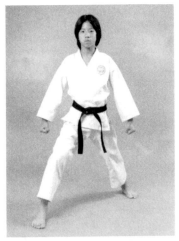

Right long walking lower stance.

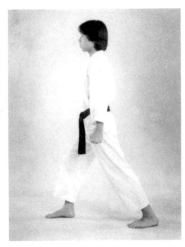

Side view.

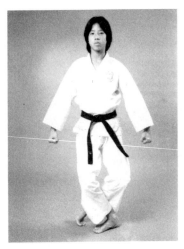

Right X-stance.

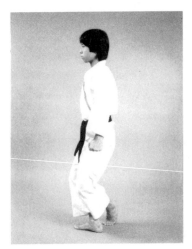

Side view.

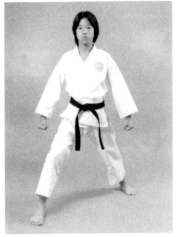

Right open walking stance.

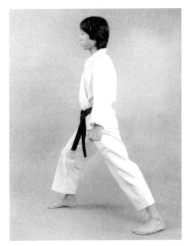

Side view.

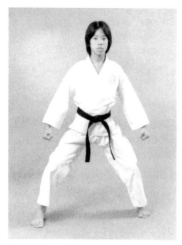

Right diagonal stance.

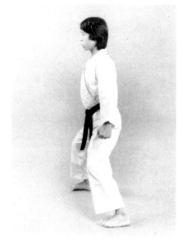

Side view.

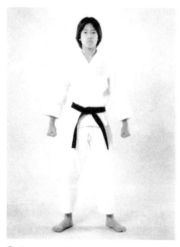

Outer open stance.

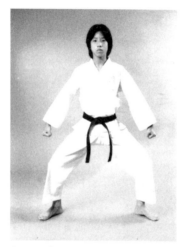

Open riding stance.

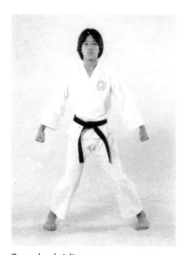

Crouched riding stance.

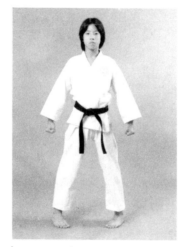

Inner open stance.

Vital Spots

Not everyone knows the names of the various parts of the human body; however, in taekwondo it is necessary for every student to have a basic knowledge of the structure of the human body and particularly its vital spots. The vital spots for taekwondo purposes are those sensitive or breakable points on the body that are most vulnerable to attack. It is essential for all students to familiarize themselves with the various degrees of vulnerability of each vital spot for effective offense, as well as defense. Regardless of how concentrated your power may be, if you miss the attacker's vital spots it will be difficult for you to get the better of him. The illustrations in the next pages show the vital spots used in taekwondo.

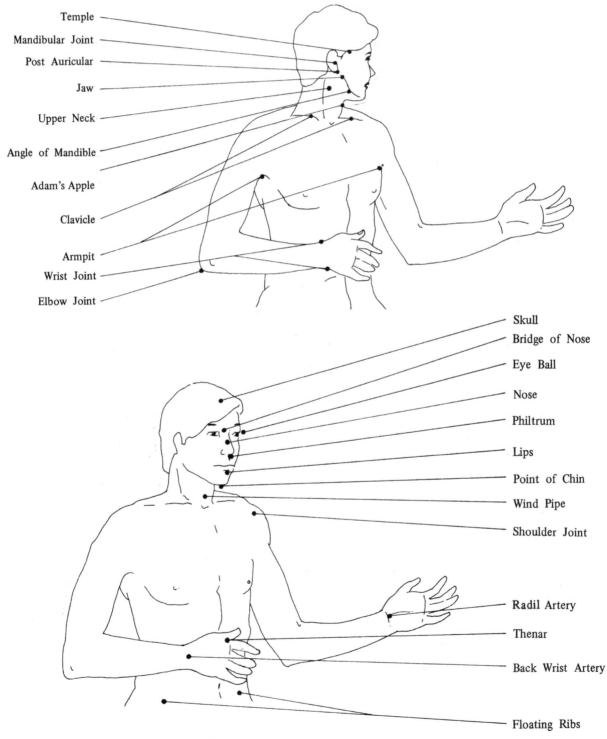

Temple
Mandibular Joint
Post Auricular
Jaw
Upper Neck
Angle of Mandible
Adam's Apple
Clavicle
Armpit
Wrist Joint
Elbow Joint

Skull
Bridge of Nose
Eye Ball
Nose
Philtrum
Lips
Point of Chin
Wind Pipe
Shoulder Joint
Radil Artery
Thenar
Back Wrist Artery
Floating Ribs

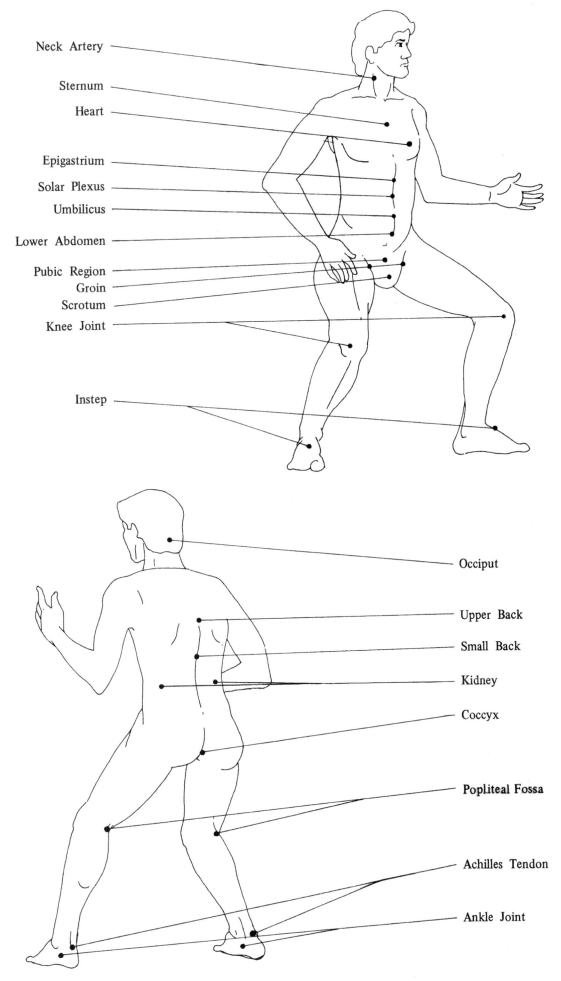

Neck Artery

Sternum

Heart

Epigastrium

Solar Plexus

Umbilicus

Lower Abdomen

Pubic Region

Groin

Scrotum

Knee Joint

Instep

Occiput

Upper Back

Small Back

Kidney

Coccyx

Popliteal Fossa

Achilles Tendon

Ankle Joint

395 / Vital Spots

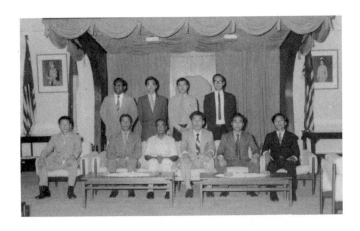

Instructor Kim, Bok Man was invited by the governor of Sarawak to his official residence in 1973.

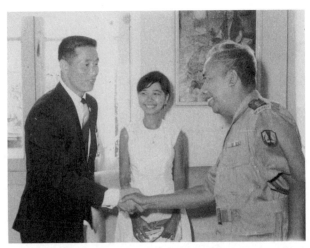

Mr. Kim, Bok Man visited the governor of Surabaya before the performance of a Taekwondo demonstration in 1968.

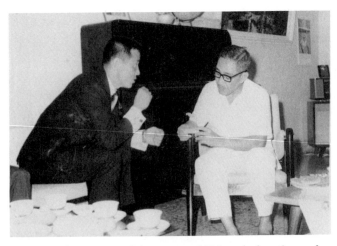

Mr. Kim, Bok Man visited the mayor of Malang before the performance of Taekwondo in Indonesia in February 1968.

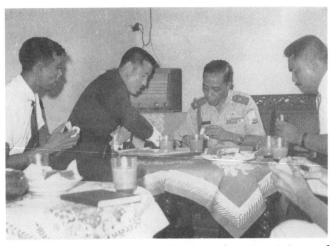

Mr. Kim, Bok Man was invited by the police commissioner of Surabaya before the performance of Taekwondo in Indonesia in February 1968.

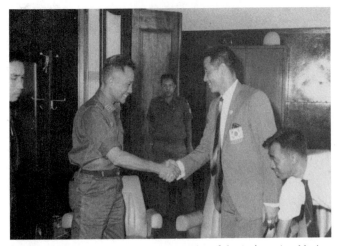

Mr. Kim, Bok Man visited the commander of the Indonesian Marine Corps before the performance of Taekwondo in Indonesia, 1968.

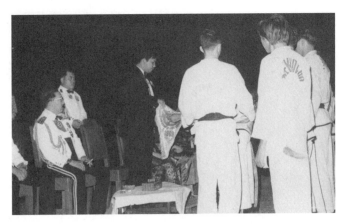

A pennant was presented to His Highness the Sultan of Brunei by the Brunei Taekwondo Association in 1969.

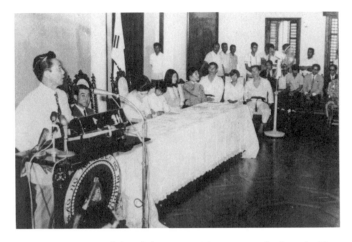

President Marcos of the Philippines giving a speech after the Taekwondo demonstration at Malacanang Palace in 1970.

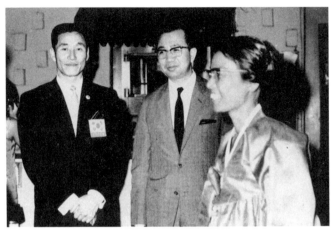

Mr. Kim, Bok Man with the Korean ambassador to Indonesia after demonstration in 1968.

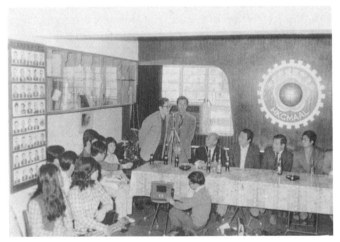

Mr. Kim, Bok Man, giving a speech at the Conference of the Hong Kong Chinese Martial Arts in 1973.

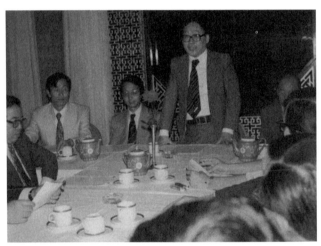

Mr. Peter H.C. Chiu, President of the Third Asian Taekwondo Championships, addressing the council after presenting a handsome donation to the Hong Kong Taekwondo Association.

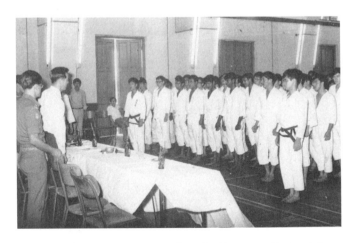

Mr. Kim, Bok Man, giving a speech to the Singapore National Army after the grading in 1969.

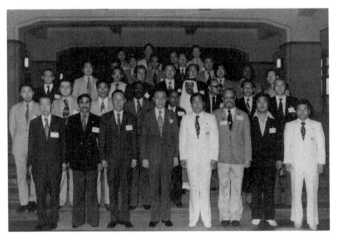

The prime minister of the R.O.C. posed with the team leaders of the World Invitational Taekwondo Tournament in Taipei, 1979.

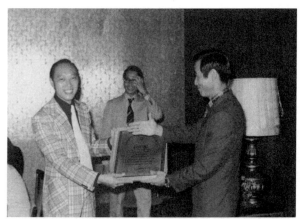

A commemoration plaque was presented to Mr. Kim, Bok Man by the President of the Hong Kong Taekwondo Association, Dr. Peter C.Y. Wong.

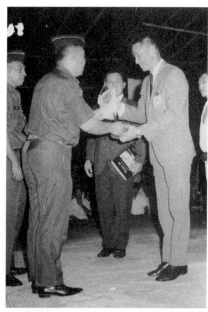

The Army commander of Semarang of Indonesia presented a pennant to Mr. Kim, Bok Man before a demonstration in 1968.

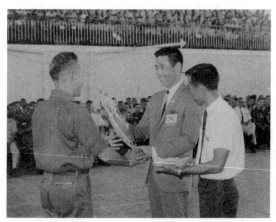

A pennant was presented by the Navy commander of Indonesia to Mr. Kim, Bok Man before a Taekwondo demonstration for Navy students, 1968.

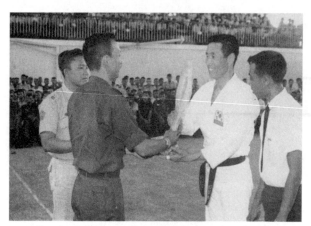

Presentation by Indonesian Marine commander to Mr. Kim, Bok Man before a demonstration, 1968.

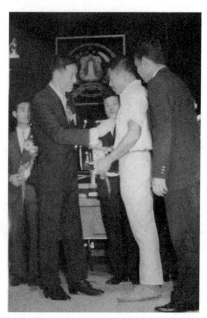

Mr. Kim, Bok Man presented a copy of his book to the commander of the Special Forces before the performance of Taekwondo in Indonesia, 1967.

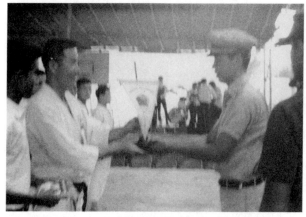

A pennant was presented by the chairman of the National Army Training School of Indonesia to Mr. Kim, Bok Man before a demonstration in 1968.

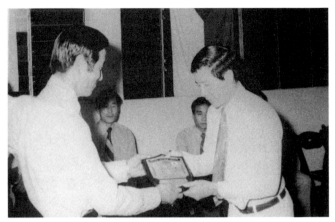

A commemorative plaque was presented to the secretary of the Sarawak Taekwondo Association by Mr. Kim, Bok Man in 1973.

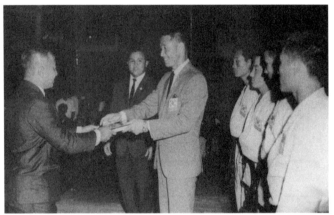

A commemorative plaque was presented to the chairman of the Malang Taekwondo Association by Mr. Kim, Bok Man before a demonstration of Taekwondo in 1968.

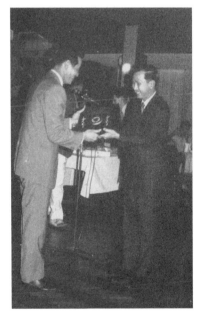

A commemorative plaque was presented to Mr. Kim, Bok Man by the chairman of the Singapore Chinese YMCA Taekwondo Association in 1968.

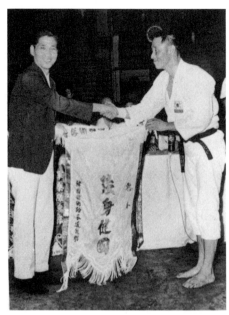

A pennant was presented by the chairman of the People's Association to Mr. Kim, Bok Man after the demonstration of Taekwondo in Singapore in 1968.

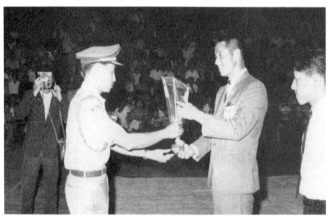

A plaque was presented by Commissioner of Police Bandung to Mr. Kim, Bok Man before a demonstration in 1968.

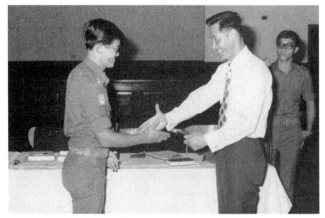

A plaque was presented by the chairman of the National Army Taekwondo Training School of Singapore to Mr. Kim, Bok Man in 1969.

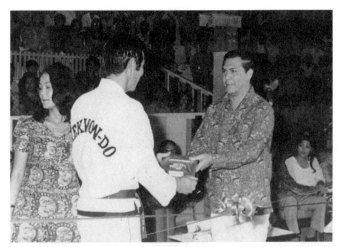

A commemoration plaque was presented to Mr. Kim, Bok Man by the president of the Sarawak Taekwondo Association, Mr. Wee, Boom Ping in 1973.

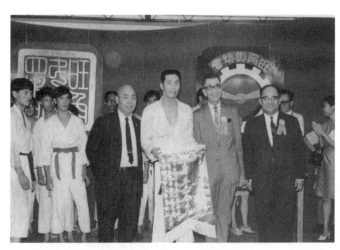

A pennant was presented by the president of the Hong Kong Chinese Martial Arts, Mr. Chan, Hon Chung, to Mr. Kim, Bok Man after a Taekwondo demonstration in 1968.

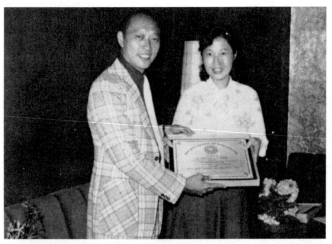

A plaque was presented by Mrs. Kim to the president of the Hong Kong Taekwondo Association, Dr. Peter C.Y. Wong.

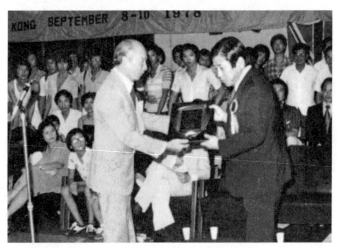

A commemorative plaque was presented to Dr. Kim, Un Young, president of the World Taekwondo Federation, by the secretary of the Hong Kong Amateur Sports Federation, Mr. Raymon Young, at the Third Asian Taekwondo Championships in 1978.

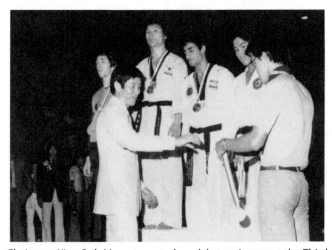

Chairman Kim, Bok Man presented medals to winners at the Third Asian Taekwondo Championships in Hong Kong, 1978.

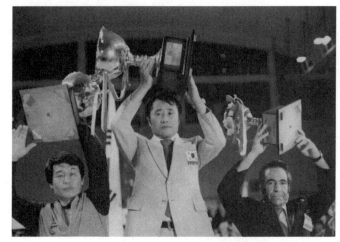

Winners at the Third Asian Taekwondo Championships in Hong Kong, 1978.

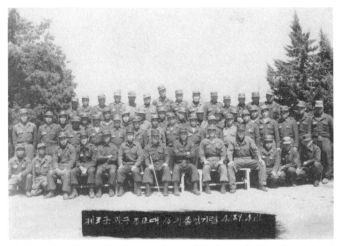

Mr. Kim, Bok Man with the members of Taekwondo Training School of the R.O.K. Armed Forces in Daejeon, 1956.

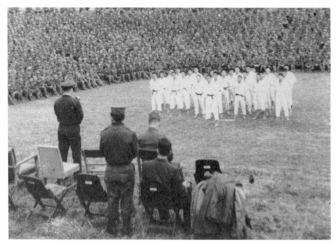

Mr. Kim, Bok Man gave a Taekwondo demonstration before the National Armed Forces in 1958.

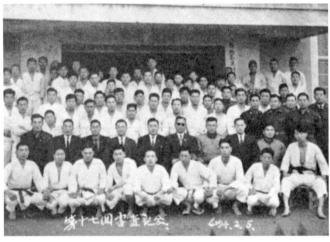

Mr. Kim, Bok Man at the Taekwondo Training School in the R.O.K. Armed Forces after grading in 1959.

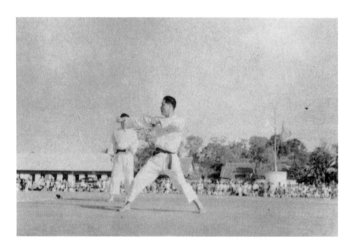

A Taekwondo demonstration by Mr. Kim, Bok Man in Saigon, 1959.

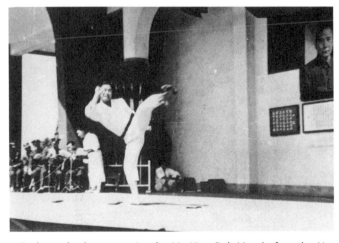

A Taekwondo demonstration by Mr. Kim, Bok Man before the National Army Training School of the R.O.C. in 1959.

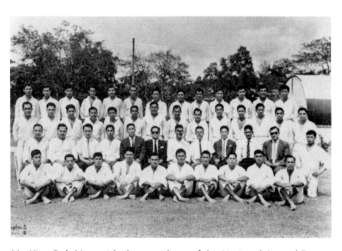

Mr. Kim, Bok Man with the members of the National Armed Forces of Malaysia after grading in 1963.

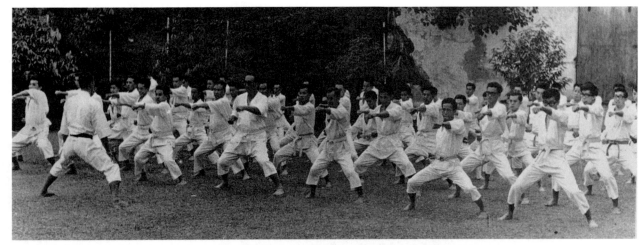

Mr. Kim, Bok Man, teaching the members of the Singapore Taekwondo Association in 1963.

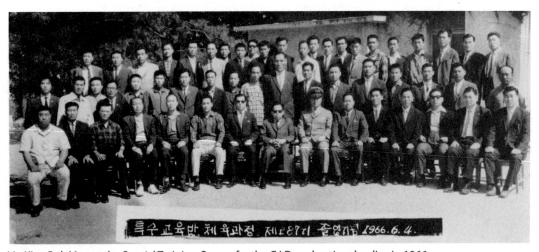

Mr. Kim, Bok Man at the Special Training Course for the C.I.D. and national police in 1966.

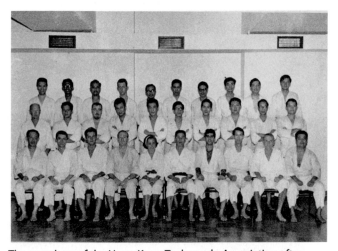

The members of the Hong Kong Taekwondo Association after grading in 1966.

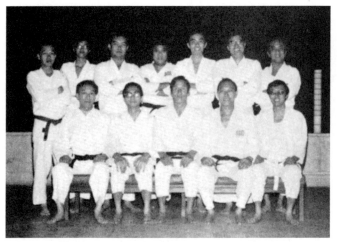

A group of doctors, members of the Hong Kong Taekwondo Association, posed with Instructor Kim, Bok Man, 1973.

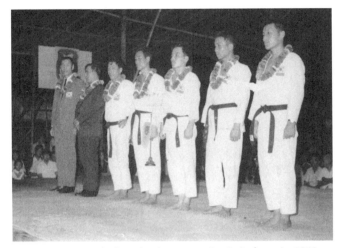

Korean instructors before the demonstration in Indonesia, 1968.

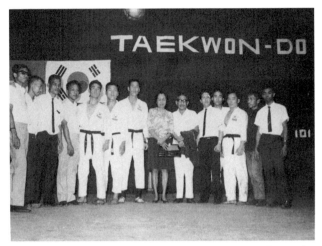

Mr. Kim, Bok Man had a commemorative photograph taken with the mayor at Malang before the demonstration in Indonesia, 1968.

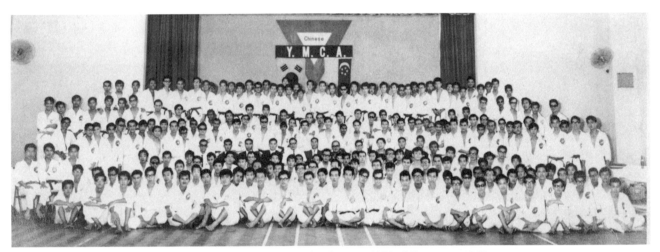

Mr. Kim, Bok Man with Taekwondo members after grading at the Chinese YMCA of Singapore, 1968.

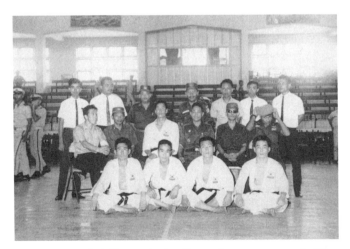

Instructor Kim, Bok Man and other Korean instructors posed with the commander of the Indonesian Marine Corps and the director of the Indonesian Naval Academy after a demonstration at the Naval Academy in Indonesia, 1968.

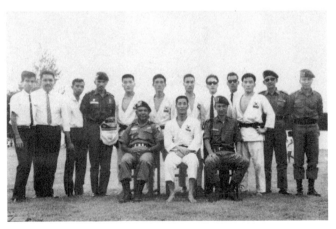

Mr. Kim, Bok Man posed with the members of the Academy of Police in Indonesia after a demonstration in 1968.

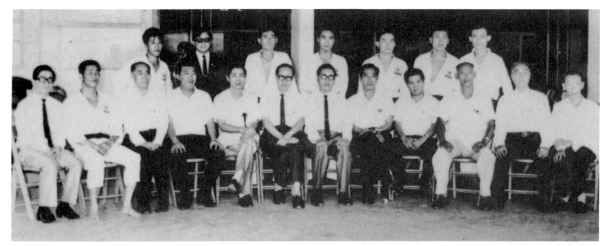

Mr. Kim, Bok Man with the chairman and members of Singapore's People's Association after a demonstration and press conference in Singapore, 1968.

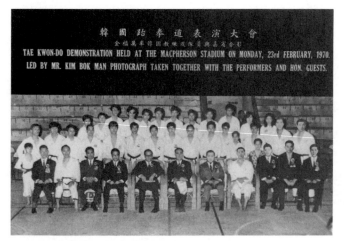

A Taekwondo demonstration at the Macpherson Stadium in Hong Kong 1970.

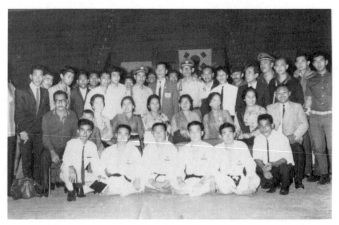

Mr. Kim, Bok Man with the members of the Commission of Police at Bandung after a demonstration in Indonesia, 1968.

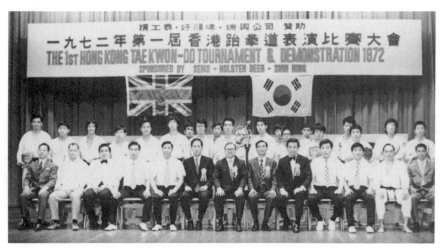

The First Hong Kong Taekwondo Tournament and Demonstration at City Hall, 1972.

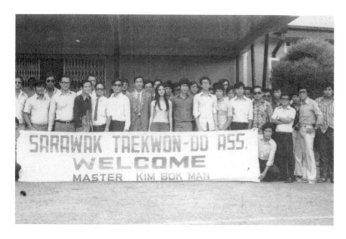

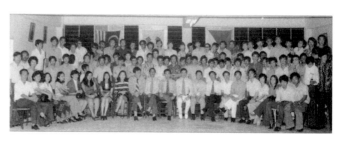

Mr. Kim, Bok Man was welcomed by the Sarawak Taekwondo Association in 1973.

Mr. Kim, Bok Man had a commemorative photograph taken with the members of the Sarawak Taekwondo Association in 1975.

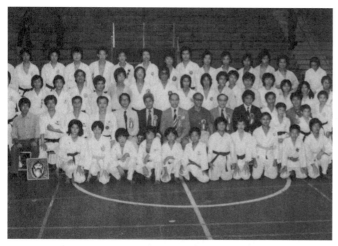

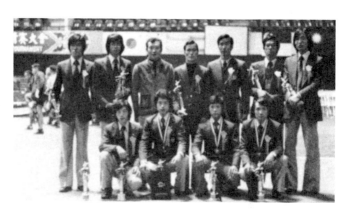

Mr. Kim, Bok Man with the members of the Hong Kong Taekwondo Association after a demonstration in 1977.

The Hong Kong team after the closing ceremony at the International Taekwondo Goodwill Tournament in Taiwan, 1977.

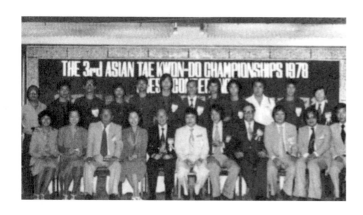

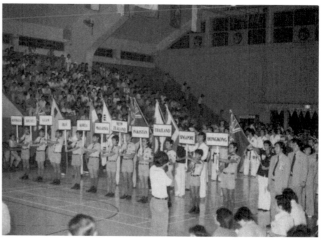

The Hong Kong team with the organizing committees of the Third Asian Taekwondo Championships in Hong Kong, 1978.

Opening ceremony at the Third Asian Taekwondo Championships in Hong Kong, 1978.

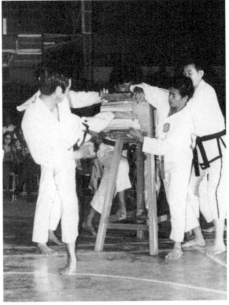

Indonesia, 1968.

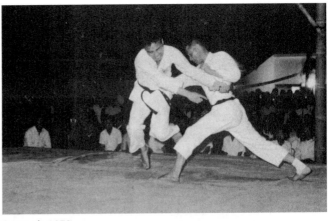

Sarawak, 1973.

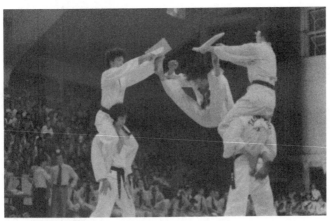

Hong Kong, 1978.

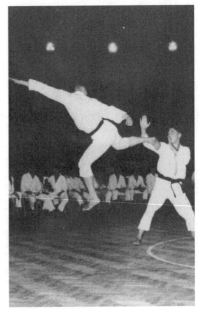

Malaysia, 1963.

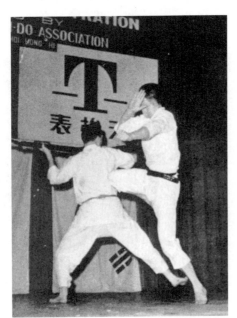

Hong Kong, 1966.

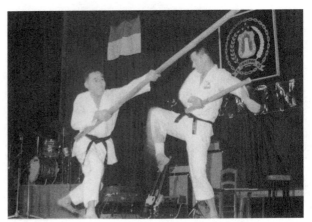

Indonesia, 1967.

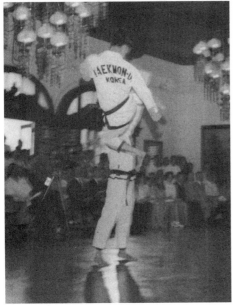

Philippines in 1970.

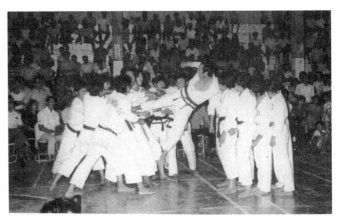

Sarawak, 1973.

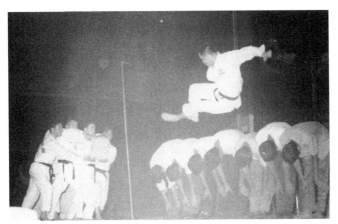

Indonesia, 1967.

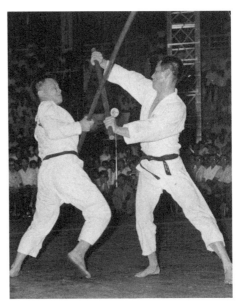

Singapore, 1968.

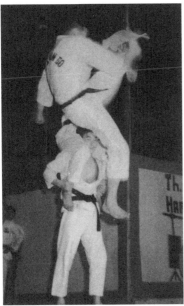

Indonesia, 1967.

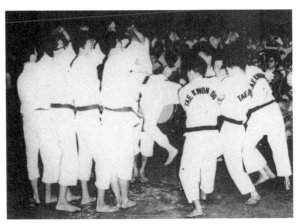

Indonesia, 1968.

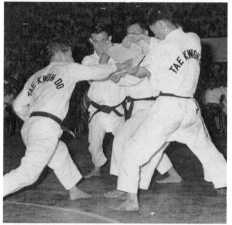

Singapore, 1968.

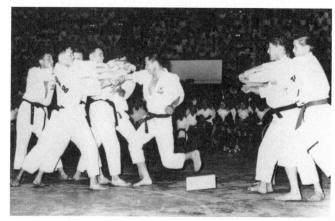

Singapore, 1968.

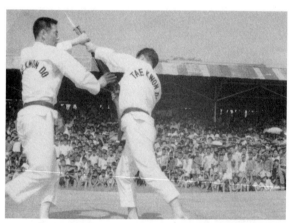

Singapore, 1968.

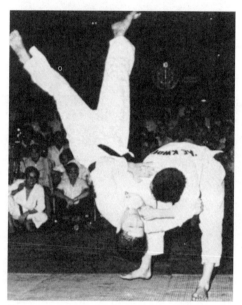

Singapore, 1968.

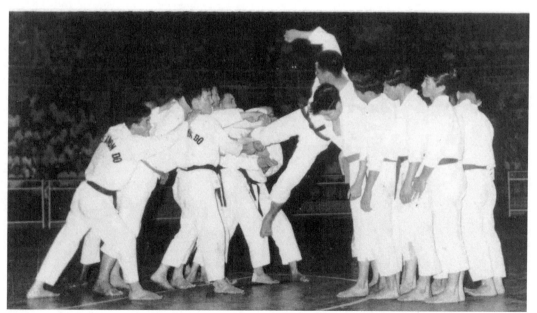

Malaysia, 1963.

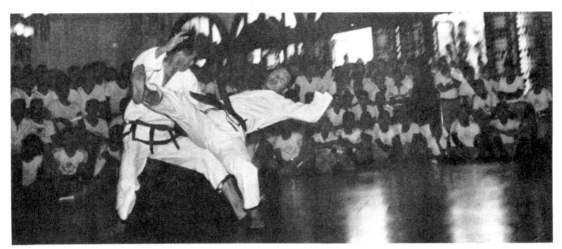

Philippines, 1970.

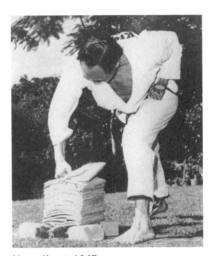

Hong Kong, 1967.

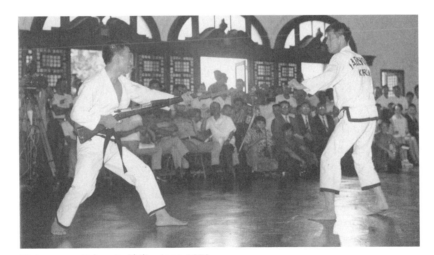

Malacanang Palace in Philippines, 1970.

About the Author

The man who inspires all interests in the martial arts is 78-year-old Kim, Bok Man, roving ambassador of taekwondo and pioneer of the art in Southeast Asia. Ironically, Kim once intended to devote his life to soccer, not taekwondo. As a teenager, he was one of Korea's top soccer stars. Equally at home on the cinder track, he also favored long-distance running. In 1948, at the age of 16, he was introduced to the ancient Korean foot-fighting art of Tae-Kyon, forerunner of taekwondo. This introduction changed not only Kim's athletic career but also the pattern of his life.

In 1950, Kim joined the army. It was during his army years that he honed his fighting skills and augmented his vast reservoir of knowledge about the Korean arts. Kim rose to the rank of sergeant major, and eventually he began teaching unarmed combat systems and techniques to other servicemen.

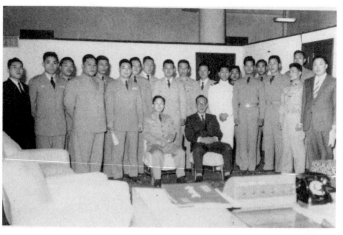

The First Asian Taekwondo Mission from the National Army leaders to South Vietnam and Taiwan in 1959.

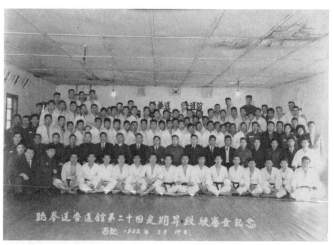

Directors and chief instructors from the National Armed Forces after having Taekwondo training courses in 1962.

In 1959, Kim visited Vietnam at the invitation of the South Vietnamese government to popularize and promote taekwondo to members of the police, military, and paramilitary establishments. Then, after giving countless demonstrations in and around Saigon, he moved on to Taiwan, also upon government invitation and performed before the Formosan police contingents and members of the National Armed Forces. Returning from abroad, he began to devote his time mainly to teaching. He traveled to other provinces to give lectures, demonstrations, and instructions.

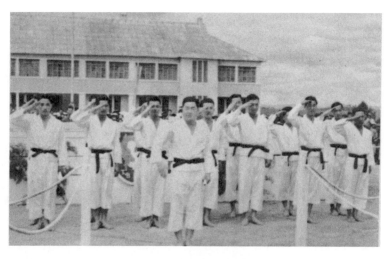

Taekwondo experts of the R.O.K. Armed Forces giving a salute before the 1959 demonstration in Vietnam.

Kim retired from the army in February, 1962, and in the year that followed geared himself up for a life devoted entirely to taekwondo. In 1963, he arrived in Malaysia accompanied by Woo, Jae Lim and another high-ranking Korean instructor. Demonstrations captivated audiences throughout the Malaysia Peninsula, including a command performance for the king of Malaysia and Tunku Abdul of Rahman, the prime minister. Before long, the work of the two Koreans resulted in the organization of the Malaysian Taekwondo Association. The Malaysian chief police officer pledged police support for the Association, and Khir, first chairman of the Association, relayed instructions from the king to impress upon Malaysian youth the necessity of learning this Korean art of self-defense. This was the first time Korean instructors traveled abroad under the name of taekwondo.

From Malaysia, Kim led a team of six Korean black-belts into Singapore in October 1963, starting with three public displays to packed audiences at the Gay World Stadium. Kim stayed on to foster the art, and quickly built up a strong following. He organized the Singapore Taekwondo Association.

In April 1965, Kim returned to Korea and revamped the entire structure of taekwondo. Definite teaching methods and training guidelines emerged, and the International Taekwondo Federation was formed in March 1966.

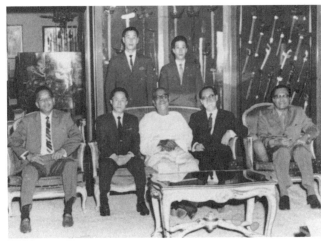

Mr. Kim, Bok Man and Mr. Woo, Jae Lim were invited by the Malaysian prime minister to visit his official residence during a visit to Malaysia in 1962.

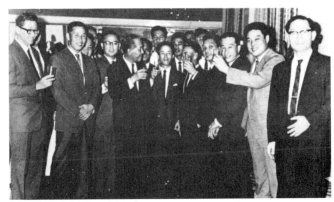

Mr. Kim, Bok Man with committee members celebrating the organization of the Singapore Taekwondo Association in 1963.

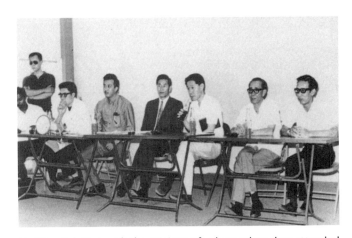

Mr. Kim, Bok Man with the minister of culture when they attended the Taekwondo grading in Singapore, 1968.

In 1966, Kim returned to the South East Asian circuit. Hong Kong is one of the few international crossroads of the world, so Kim selected this region as part of his master plan to spread and develop the Korean art in the Orient. He organized the Hong Kong Taekwondo Association in August 1967, and he brought in six assistants from Korea to carry on his initial work.

In 1968, Kim made several comprehensive teaching forays out of Hong Kong, starting with a group of six Korean instructors. They went to Indonesia at the invitation of the government. From Indonesia, Kim traveled back through Singapore and Malaysia at the invitation of the governments. Giving demonstrations and spending several months checking on the growth and development of his taekwondo schools in the region, he then went to Bangkok and provided the long-awaited impetus, which the infant Thai Taekwondo Association needed to properly get off the ground.

In 1969, Kim was invited to Brunei at the invitation of the Sultan of Brunei to participate in his birthday celebration. With his successful demonstration, he organized the Brunei Taekwondo Association. During his visit in Brunei, Kim also gave demonstrations to introduce taekwondo for the first time in the Malaysian states of Sabah and Sarawak.

Kim, the father of taekwondo, then returned to Hong Kong to prepare for the First Asian Taekwondo Tournament that was held in October 1969, in Hong Kong.

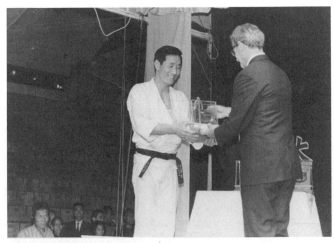

The Hong Kong Urban Consular, presenting a plaque to Mr. Kim, Bok Man in appreciation for a display of Taekwondo in 1969.

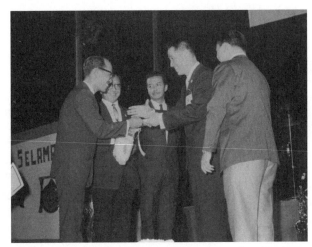

Presents were exchanged by Kim, Bok Man with police assistant commissioner of Indonesia before the performance of Taekwondo demonstration in 1968.

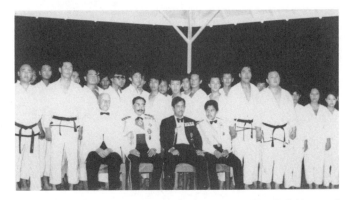

His Royal Highness the Sultan invited instructor Kim, Bok Man and the members of the Brunei Taekwondo Association to give a demonstration in honor of the Sultan's twenty-third birthday in 1969.

In 1970, Kim went to the Philippines at the invitation of President Marcos. Kim's reception by President Marcos was rewarding, and he left behind him a trail of followers under the auspices of the Philippines Taekwondo Association, which he founded.

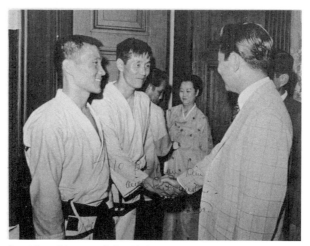

President Marcos of the Philippines greeted Instructor Kim, Bok Man after a performance of Taekwondo, which was introduced for the first time at the Malacanang Palace in 1970.

In 1971, Kim returned to his base in Hong Kong, and in 1972, the First Hong Kong Taekwondo Tournament and Demonstration was held at City Hall. Since then he has maintained a close watch over the regions in which he introduced taekwondo, making regular visits to the many different national associations.

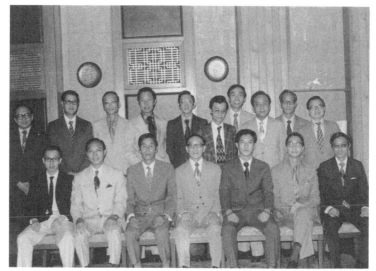

Mr. Kim, Bok Man posed with doctors, who were members of his association, after the Taekwondo Conference in Hong Kong, 1973.

In 1973, he went to Sarawak at the invitation of the Sarawak government to popularize and promote taekwondo to military members and the public. After successful demonstrations, he organized the Sarawak Taekwondo Association.

Then in 1975, he was again invited to Sarawak by His Excellency the Governor of Sarawak, Tun Datuk Patinggi Tuanku Haji Bujang, to attend the Sarawak Open Taekwondo Championships.

From Sarawak, he traveled back through Southeast Asia, checking on the growth and development of his Taekwondo Invitation Game. In 1977 he was invited to Chicago for the Third Taekwondo Championships.

In 1978, the Third Asian Taekwondo Championship was held in Hong Kong, organized by the Hong Kong Taekwondo Association.

In 1979, he was invited to the Fourth World Taekwondo Championships, which were held in Munich. From Munich, he traveled through several European countries to give lectures, demonstrations, and instructions.

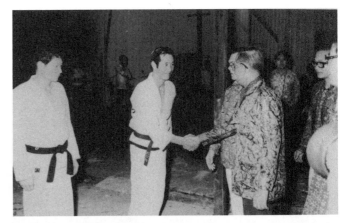

His Excellency the Governor of Sarawak, Tun Datuk Patinggi Tuanku Haji Bujang, greeted Instructor Kim, Bok Man before a performance of taekwondo, 1973.

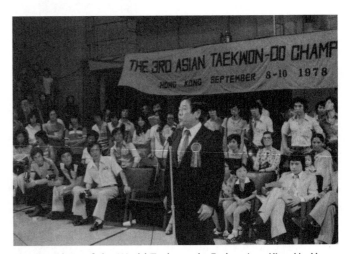

The President of the World Taekwondo Federation, Kim, Un Yong, gave the opening ceremony speech at the Third Asian Taekwondo Championship in Hong Kong, 1978.

Taekwondo under the eminent guidance of Mr. Kim, Bok Man has, in fact, passed the pioneer stage. This man has transformed the mystic and philosophic art of controlling physical and mental fitness into a complete series of well-developed and scientific forms of physical exercise, which definitely provides a splendid and worthwhile form of healthy and encouraging sport for people of all ages. It, therefore, gives me a great privilege to earnestly appeal to those who have already taken a keen interest in this refined modern art of graceful movements to help in further promoting and developing the technique of self-imposed moral discipline and paving the way for a classical appreciation of the beauty and value of human life.

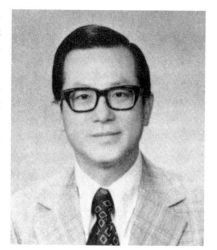

T.M. Ho

A.A.S.A., F.H.K.S.A., C.P.A.

Index

BOOKS FROM YMAA

6 HEALING MOVEMENTS
101 REFLECTIONS ON TAI CHI CHUAN
A WOMAN'S QIGONG GUIDE
ADVANCING IN TAE KWON DO
ANCIENT CHINESE WEAPONS
ANALYSIS OF SHAOLIN CHIN NA 2ND ED.
ARTHRITIS RELIEF — CHINESE QIGONG FOR HEALING & PREVENTION, 3RD ED.
BACK PAIN RELIEF — CHINESE QIGONG FOR HEALING & PREVENTION 2ND ED
BAGUAZHANG
CARDIO KICKBOXING ELITE
CHIN NA IN GROUND FIGHTING
CHINESE FAST WRESTLING — THE ART OF SAN SHOU KUAI JIAO
CHINESE FITNESS — A MIND / BODY APPROACH
CHINESE TUI NA MASSAGE
COMPLETE CARDIOKICKBOXING
COMPREHENSIVE APPLICATIONS OF SHAOLIN CHIN NA
DUKKHA — A SAM REEVES MARTIAL ARTS THRILLER
EIGHT SIMPLE QIGONG EXERCISES FOR HEALTH, 2ND ED.
ESSENCE OF SHAOLIN WHITE CRANE
ESSENCE OF TAIJI QIGONG, 2ND ED.
EXPLORING TAI CHI
FACING VIOLENCE
FIGHTING ARTS
INSIDE TAI CHI
KATA AND THE TRANSMISSION OF KNOWLEDGE
LITTLE BLACK BOOK OF VIOLENCE
LIUHEBAFA FIVE CHARACTER SECRETS
MARTIAL ARTS ATHLETE
MARTIAL ARTS INSTRUCTION
MARTIAL WAY AND ITS VIRTUES
MEDITATIONS ON VIOLENCE
MIND/BODY FITNESS — A MIND / BODY APPROACH
MUGAI RYU — THE CLASSICAL SAMURAI ART OF DRAWING THE SWORD
NATURAL HEALING WITH QIGONG — THERAPEUTIC QIGONG
NORTHERN SHAOLIN SWORD, 2ND ED.
OKINAWA'S COMPLETE KARATE SYSTEM — ISSHIN RYU
PRINCIPLES OF TRADITIONAL CHINESE MEDICINE
QIGONG FOR HEALTH & MARTIAL ARTS 2ND ED.
QIGONG FOR LIVING
QIGONG FOR TREATING COMMON AILMENTS

QIGONG MASSAGE —FUNDAMENTAL TECHNIQUES FOR HEALTH AND RELAXATION, 2ND ED.
QIGONG MEDITATION — EMBRYONIC BREATHING
QIGONG MEDITATION—SMALL CIRCULATION
QIGONG, THE SECRET OF YOUTH
QUIET TEACHER
ROOT OF CHINESE QIGONG, 2ND ED.
SHIN GI TAI—KARATE TRAINING FOR BODY, MIND, AND SPIRIT
SHIHAN TE — THE BUNKAI OF KATA
SUNRISE TAI CHI
SURVIVING ARMED ASSAULTS
TAEKWONDO — ANCIENT WISDOM FOR THE MODERN WARRIOR
TAEKWONDO — DEFENSE AGAINST WEAPONS
TAE KWON DO — THE KOREAN MARTIAL ART
TAEKWONDO — SPIRIT AND PRACTICE
TAI CHI BALL QIGONG—FOR HEALTH AND MARTIAL ARTS
TAI CHI BOOK
TAI CHI CHUAN — 24 & 48 POSTURES
TAI CHI CHUAN MARTIAL APPLICATIONS, 2ND ED.
TAI CHI CONNECTIONS
TAI CHI DYNAMICS
TAI CHI SECRETS OF THE ANCIENT MASTERS
TAI CHI SECRETS OF THE WU & LI STYLES
TAI CHI SECRETS OF THE YANG STYLE
TAI CHI THEORY & MARTIAL POWER, 2ND ED.
TAI CHI WALKING
TAIJI CHIN NA
TAIJI SWORD, CLASSICAL YANG STYLE
TAIJIQUAN, CLASSICAL YANG STYLE
TAIJIQUAN THEORY OF DR. YANG, JWING-MING
THE CROCODILE AND THE CRANE
THE CUTTING SEASON
THE WAY OF KATA—A COMPREHENSIVE GUIDE TO DECIPHERING MARTIAL APPS.
THE WAY OF KENDO AND KENJITSU
THE WAY OF SANCHIN KATA
THE WAY TO BLACK BELT
TRADITIONAL CHINESE HEALTH SECRETS
TRADITIONAL TAEKWONDO—CORE TECHNIQUES, HISTORY, AND PHILOSOPHY
WESTERN HERBS FOR MARTIAL ARTISTS
WILD GOOSE QIGONG
XINGYIQUAN, 2ND ED.

DVDS FROM YMAA

ANALYSIS OF SHAOLIN CHIN NA
ADVANCED PRACTICAL CHIN NA IN DEPTH
BAGUAZHANG 1,2, & 3 —EMEI BAGUAZHANG
CHEN STYLE TAIJIQUAN
CHIN NA IN DEPTH COURSES 1 — 4
CHIN NA IN DEPTH COURSES 5 — 8
CHIN NA IN DEPTH COURSES 9 — 12
EIGHT SIMPLE QIGONG EXERCISES FOR HEALTH
THE ESSENCE OF TAIJI QIGONG
FIVE ANIMAL SPORTS
KNIFE DEFENSE—TRADITIONAL TECHINIQUES AGAINST DAGGER
QIGONG FOR HEALING
QIGONG MASSAGE—FUNDAMENTAL TECHNIQUES FOR HEALTH AND RELAXATION
SHAOLIN KUNG FU FUNDAMENTAL TRAINING 1&2
SHAOLIN LONG FIST KUNG FU — BASIC SEQUENCES
SHAOLIN SABER — BASIC SEQUENCES
SHAOLIN STAFF — BASIC SEQUENCES
SHAOLIN WHITE CRANE GONG FU BASIC TRAINING 1&2
SIMPLE QIGONG EXERCISES FOR ARTHRITIS RELIEF
SIMPLE QIGONG EXERCISES FOR BACK PAIN RELIEF
SIMPLIFIED TAI CHI CHUAN
SUNRISE TAI CHI
SUNSET TAI CHI
SWORD—FUNDAMENTAL TRAINING

TAI CHI ENERGY PATTERNS
TAIJI BALL QIGONG COURSES 1&2—16 CIRCLING AND 16 ROTATING PATTERNS
TAIJI BALL QIGONG COURSES 3&4—16 PATTERNS OF WRAP-COILING & APPLICATIONS
TAIJI MARTIAL APPLICATIONS — 37 POSTURES
TAIJI PUSHING HANDS 1&2—YANG STYLE SINGLE AND DOUBLE PUSHING HANDS
TAIJI PUSHING HANDS 3&4—MOVING SINGLE AND DOUBLE PUSHING HANDS
TAIJI SABER — THE COMPLETE FORM, QIGONG & APPLICATIONS
TAIJI & SHAOLIN STAFF - FUNDAMENTAL TRAINING
TAIJI YIN YANG STICKING HANDS
TAIJIQUAN CLASSICAL YANG STYLE
TAIJI SWORD, CLASSICAL YANG STYLE
UNDERSTANDING QIGONG 1 — WHAT IS QI? • HUMAN QI CIRCULATORY SYSTEM
UNDERSTANDING QIGONG 2 — KEY POINTS • QIGONG BREATHING
UNDERSTANDING QIGONG 3 — EMBRYONIC BREATHING
UNDERSTANDING QIGONG 4 — FOUR SEASONS QIGONG
UNDERSTANDING QIGONG 5 — SMALL CIRCULATION
UNDERSTANDING QIGONG 6 — MARTIAL QIGONG BREATHING
WHITE CRANE HARD & SOFT QIGONG
YANG TAI CHI FOR BEGINNERS

more products available from...
YMAA Publication Center, Inc. 楊氏東方文化出版中心
1-800-669-8892 • info@ymaa.com • www.ymaa.com